Oxford Handbook of Public Health Practice

OXFORD
UNIVERSITY PRESS

Great Clarendon Street, Oxford OX2 6DP

Oxford University Press is a department of the University of Oxford.
It furthers the University's objective of excellence in research, scholarship,
and education by publishing worldwide in

Oxford New York

Athens Auckland Bangkok Bogotá Bombay Buenos Aires Calcutta
Cape Town Dar es Salaam Delhi Florence Hong Kong Istanbul
Karachi Kuala Lumpur Madrid Melbourne Mexico City Mumbai
Nairobi Paris São Paulo Shanghai Singapore Taipei Tokyo
Toronto Warsaw

and associated companies in Berlin Ibadan

Oxford is a registered trade mark of Oxford University Press
in the UK and in certain other countries

Published in the United States
by Oxford University Press Inc., New York

British Library Cataloguing in Publication Data

Data available

Library of Congress Cataloging in Publication Data

ISBN 0-19-263221-3

10 9 8 7 6 5 4 3 2 1

Typeset by Integra Software Services Pvt. Ltd., Pondicherry, India
www.integra-india.com
Printed in Great Britain
on acid-free paper by The Bath Press (Avon)

Oxford Handbook of Public Health Practice

Edited by

David Pencheon Public Health Observatory, Institute of Public Health, Cambridge, UK

Charles Guest National Centre for Disease Control, Commonwealth Department of Health and Aged Care; National Institute for Epidemiology and Population Health, The Australian National University, Canberra, Australia

David Melzer Department of Public Health and Primary Care, Institute of Public Health, Cambridge, UK

J.A. Muir Gray Institute for Health Sciences, University of Oxford, UK

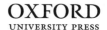

OXFORD
UNIVERSITY PRESS

Acknowledgements and thanks

The following helped in bringing this book to life:
Ibrahim Abubakur, Tim Albert, Peyman Altan, Heather Buchan, Val Busby, Melissa Canny, Hilary Charlesworth, Laura Diamond, Celia Duff, Derek Flannery, Alistair Grant, Rod Griffiths, Ulrike Harrower, Richard Himsworth, Nicola Howard, Chris Hyde, Rod Jackson, Tony Jewell, Kay Tee Khaw, Betty Kirkwood, Roz Lasker, Rosemary Lees, Geraldine Lockett, Chris Lord, Klim McPherson, Ruairidh Milne, Fiona Moss, John Newton, Richard Parish, Malcolm Perkin, Jem Rashbass, Dirk Ruwaard, Eileen Smith, Andrew Stevens, Pat Troop, Anna Wilkinson, Graham Winyard, Rosalie Woodruff, Jonathan Worters, Elizabeth Young, Ron Zimmern.

The following particularly helped with individual chapters: Tony Adams and Dorothy Broom (chapter 7.6) and Henry Foster and Emma Dexter (chapter 6.5)

Ruairidh Milne contributed extensively to the appendices.

Very special thanks to Helen Liepman and Kate Martin at Oxford University Press.

There is always one person who puts far more work into a book than is acknowledged through authorship or editorship. That person is Brenda McWilliams to whom all the editors and authors are heavily indebted.

Not every idea in this or any book can be traced to its source. We apologize for any omission here, and would be grateful to hear from readers with amendments, corrections or other suggestions, using the evaluation card.

DP, CSG, DM, JAMG

Editors' dedications

To the support and tolerance of my family and
colleagues, especially GL

DP

To all my family, especially Hilary, Stephanie and William

CSG

To Susan, Jonathan and Andrew

DM

To all those public health professionals who never get
thanked or sent a bottle of whisky at Christmas; in
gratitude for all we have learned from you and for your
commitment to health improvement

JAMG

Foreword

Originality, practical focus, and comprehensive coverage are not qualities normally found together in textbooks in the field of medicine and healthcare. In public health, the field, at least in Britain, is even thinner.

The Editors of this book have pulled off a remarkable feat—meeting these challenges and drawing together a team of diverse talents to do the thinking and writing. From values to decision making, from organizations to people, from strategy to team-working, the whole of public health practice is conceptualized in a fresh imaginative way.

Readers will find in this book the skills they use day-to-day but will seldom recognize themselves, they will identify needs and knowledge gaps which they had not previously acknowledged, and they will find inspiration in the examples of good practice.

The short chapter on using media advocacy to shape policy, the guide on writing to effect change, and the road map to find evidence are just a small number of examples of areas which would not be covered in other books yet are the very stuff of modern public health practice.

Osler, who graced Oxford with his inspirational presence nearly a century ago, once said 'No bubble is so iridescent or floats longer than that blown by the successful teacher'.

Oxford, with Muir Gray as its guiding light, is once again a metaphorical meeting place for ideas, inspiration, and great teaching.

Just as Laurent Blanc kissed the bald pate of Fabien Barthez before each game in France's glorious World Cup winning run, kiss the cover of the *Oxford Handbook of Public Health Practice* before you open it. You will have found a true soulmate.

Liam Donaldson
Chief Medical Officer
Department of Health

February 2001

Contents

List of contributors

Professor Gerard Anderson, Department of Health Policy and Management, The Johns Hopkins Schools of Medicine and Hygiene and Public Health, Baltimore, USA. ganderso@jhsph.edu

John Appleby, Director, Health Systems Programme, King's Fund, London, UK. j.appleby@kehf.org.uk

Dr Kate Ardern, Consultant in Public Health Medicine, Liverpool Health Authority, Liverpool, UK. kate.ardern@liverpool-ha.nhs.uk

Dr T-C Aw, Senior Lecturer in Occupational Medicine, Institute of Occupational Health, University of Birmingham, UK. t.c.aw@bham.ac.uk

Dr Gabriele Bammer, National Centre for Epidemiology and Population Health, The Australian National University, Canberra, Australia. gabriele.bammer@anu.edu.au

Dr Nick Banatvala, Consultant in Public Health Medicine, Suffolk Health Authority, Ipswich, UK. nick.banatvala@hq.suffolk-ha.anglox.nhs.uk

Dr Alex Barratt, Senior Lecturer in Epidemiology, Department of Public Health and Community Medicine, University of Sydney, Sydney, Australia. alexb@health.usyd.edu.au

Dr Martin Birley, International Health Impact Assessment Consortium, Liverpool School of Tropical Medicine, Liverpool, UK. m.birley@liverpool.ac.uk

Dr Paul Bolton, Center for International Emergency, Disaster and Refugee Studies, The Johns Hopkins University School of Hygiene and Public Health, Baltimore, USA. pbolton@jhsph.edu

Dr Cameron Bowie, Public Health Research and Consultancy, Chard, UK. cam.bowie@btinternet.com

Dr Peter Brambleby, Honorary Senior Lecturer in Public Health, University of East Anglia, Norwich, UK. peter.brambleby@norfolk.nhs.uk

Anne Brice, Director, Center for Library, Informatics and Knowledge, Institute of Health Sciences, University of Oxford, UK. anne.brice@hclu.ox.ac.uk

Dr Iain Buchan, Specialist Registrar in Public Health Medicine, Hertfordshire Health Authority, UK. iain@ukph.org

Dr Amanda Burls, Senior Clinical Lecturer in Public Health & Epidemiology, University of Birmingham, Birmingham, UK. a.j.burls@bham.ac.uk

Dr Martin Caraher, Centre for Food Policy, Thames Valley University, London, UK. martin.caraher@tvu.ac.uk

Dr Julia Carr, General Practitioner and Public Health Physician, Ministry of Health, Wellington, New Zealand. matheson.carr@xtra.co.nz

Professor Larry Chambers, Department of Clinical Epidemiology and Biostatistics, McMaster University, Ontario, Canada. chambers@fhs.csu.mcmaster.ca

Professor Simon Chapman, Department of Public Health and Community Medicine, University of Sydney, Sydney, Australia. simonc@health.usyd.edu.au

Associate Professor Robert Cumming, Department of Public Health and Community Medicine, University of Sydney, Sydney, Australia. bobc@health.usyd.edu.au

Dr Tom Davies, Director, East Anglian Cancer Registry, Cambridge, UK. twd10@medschl.cam.ac.uk

Dr Jennifer Dixon, Director, Health Care Policy Programme, King's Fund, London, UK. jdixon@kingsfund.org.uk

Dr Anna Donald, Honorary Fellow, Department of Public Health and Epidemiology, University College London, UK. a.donald@ucl.ac.uk

Professor Liam Donaldson, Chief Medical Officer, Department of Health, London, UK. liam.donaldson@doh.gsi.gov.uk

Professor Stuart Donnan, Public Health and Ethics, West Sussex Health Authority, UK. stuartdonnan@onetel.net.uk

Professor Martin Eccles, Centre for Health Services Research, University of Newcastle Upon Tyne, Newcastle Upon Tyne, UK. martin.eccles@ncl.ac.uk

Katie Enock, Public Health Specialist, Brent & Harrow Health Authority, London, UK. katie.enock@bah-ha.nthames.nhs.uk

Dr Vikki Entwistle, Health Services Research Unit, University of Aberdeen, Aberdeen, UK. vae@hsru.abdn.ac.uk

Professor Gene Feder, Department of General Practice and Primary Care, Barts and the London, Queen Mary's School of Medicine and Dentistry, London, UK. g.s.feder@mds.qmw.ac.uk

Professor Ray Fitzpatrick, Department of Public Health, Institute of Health Sciences, University of Oxford, UK. raymond.fitzpatrick@dphpc.ox.ac.uk

Dr Jeff French, Director of Communications and Planning, Health Development Agency, London, UK. jfrench@hda-online. org.uk

Dr Michael Frommer, Department of Public Health and Community Medicine, University of Sydney, Sydney, Australia. michaelf@health.usyd.edu.au

Dr Peter Gentle, Consultant in Public Health Medicine, North and East Devon Health Authority, Exeter, UK. peter.gentle@nedevon-ha.swest.nhs.uk

Professor Paul Glasziou, Department of Social and Preventive Medicine, University of Queensland Medical School, Australia. p.glasziou@spmed.uq.edu.au

Dr Caron Grainger, Medical Director, Warwickshire Health Authority, Warwick, UK. caron.grainger@wha-h.warwick-ha.wmids.nhs.uk

Dr Muir Gray, Director, Institute of Health Sciences, University of Oxford, UK. muir.gray@ihs.oxford.ac.uk

Professor Sian Griffiths, Director of Public Health, Oxfordshire Health Authority, Oxford, UK. sian.griffiths@oxon-ha.anglox.nhs.uk

Dr Chris Griffiths, Department of General Practice and Primary Care, Barts and the London, Queen Mary's School of Medicine and Dentistry, London, UK. c.j.griffiths@mds.qmw.ac.uk

Professor Jeremy Grimshaw, Programme Director and Professor of Public Health, University of Aberdeen, Aberdeen, UK. j.m. grimshaw@abdn.ac.uk

Dr Charles Guest, National Centre for Disease Control, Commonwealth Department of Health and Aged Care; National Centre for Epidemiology and Population Health, The Australian National University, Canberra, Australia. charles.guest@health.gov.au

Dr Jack Guralnik, Laboratory of Epidemiology, Demography and Biometry, National Institute on Aging, Bethesda, USA. jack_guralnik@nih.gov

Dr Margaret Guy, Consultant in Public Health Medicine, London Regional Office (NHS Executive), London, UK. margaret.guy@doh.gsi.gov.uk

Professor Gordon Guyatt, Department of Clinical Epidemiology and Biostatistics, McMaster University Faculty of Health Sciences, Ontario, Canada. guyatt@mcmaster.ca

Dr Fraser Hadden, Consultant in Communicable Disease Control, Suffolk Health Authority, Ipswich, UK. fraser.hadden@hq. suffolk-ha. anglox.nhs.uk

Philip Hadridge, Head of Planning and Development, NHS Executive (Eastern Region), Cambridge, UK. philip.hadridge@doh. gsi.gov.uk

Bec Hanley, Director, Consumers in NHS Research Support Unit, Help for Health Trust, Winchester, UK. bhanley@hfht.org

Professor Malcolm Harrington, Institute of Occupational Health, University of Birmingham, Birmingham, UK. jmharris@aol.com

Professor Ian Harvey, Professor of Epidemiology and Public Health, University of East Anglia, Norwich, UK. ian.harvey@uea.ac.uk

Dr Nicholas Hicks, Consultant in Public Health Medicine, Oxfordshire Health Authority, Oxford, UK. nicholas.hicks@public-health. oxford.ac.uk

Dr Alison Hill, Director, Public Health Resource Unit, Institute of Health Sciences, University of Oxford, UK. alison.hill@dphpc. ox.ac.uk

Professor Tony Hope, Director of Ethox, Institute of Health Sciences, University of Oxford, Oxford, UK. admin@ethox.ox.ac.uk

Peter Sotir Hussey, Department of Health Policy and Management, The Johns Hopkins Schools of Medicine and Hygiene and Public Health, Baltimore, USA. phussey@jhsph.edu

Professor Les Irwig, Department of Public Health and Community Medicine, University of Sydney, Sydney, Australia. lesi@health. usyd.edu.au

Professor Rachel Jenkins, Director of WHO Collaborating Centre, Institute of Psychiatry, Kings College, London, UK. r.jenkins@iop.kcl.ac.uk

Dr Edmund Jessop, Director of Public Health, West Surrey Health Authority, UK. edmund.jessop@wsurrey-ha.sthames.nhs.uk

Dr Yi Mien Koh, Director of Public Health, Kensington, Chelsea and Westminster Health Authority, London, UK. yimien.koh@ha. kcw-ha.nthames.nhs.uk

Professor Tim Lang, Professor of Food Policy, Centre for Food Policy, Thames Valley University, London, UK. tim.lang@tvu.ac.uk

Professor Stephen Leeder, Dean, Faculty of Medicine, University of Sydney, Sydney, Australia. steve@med.usyd.edu.au

Professor Annabelle Mark, Reader in Organisational Behaviour & Health Management, Middlesex University Business School, London, UK. a.mark@mdx.ac.uk

Dr Alan Maryon Davis, Consultant in Public Health Medicine, Lambeth, Southwark and Lewisham Health Authority, London, UK. alan.maryondavis@ob.lslha.sthames.nhs.uk

Dr Don Matheson, Deputy Director General, Public Health, Ministry of Health, Wellington, New Zealand.

Brenda McWilliams, Research Associate, Institute of Public Health, Cambridge, UK. bcm10@medschl.cam.ac.uk

Dr Jill Meara, Public Health Physician, National Radiological Protection Board, Didcot, UK. jill.meara@nrpb.org.uk

Dr David Melzer, Department of Public Health and Primary Care, Institute of Public Health, Cambridge, UK. dm214@aol.com

Dr Ruairidh Milne, Senior Lecturer in Public Health Medicine, National Co-ordinating Centre for Health Technology Assessment, University of Southampton, Southampton, UK. rm2@soton. ac.uk

Dr John Newton, Consultant Epidemiologist, Unit of Health Care Epidemiology, Institute of Health Sciences, University of Oxford, UK. john.newton@public-health.oxford.ac.uk

Professor Don Nutbeam, Head, Public Health Division, Department of Health, London, UK. don.nutbeam@doh.gsi.gov.uk

Dr Sarah O'Brien, Communicable Disease Surveillance Centre, London, UK. sobrien@phls.org.uk

Professor Joan Ozanne-Smith, Chair of Injury Prevention, Monash University Accident Research Centre, Melbourne, Victoria, Australia. joan.ozanne-smith@general.monash.edu.au

Dr Nick Payne, Consultant Senior Lecturer in Public Health Medicine, School of Health and Related Research, University of Sheffield, UK. n.payne@sheffield.ac.uk

Dr David Pencheon, Public Health Observatory, Institute of Public Health, Cambridge, UK. pencheond@rdd-phru.cam.ac.uk

Dr Angela Raffle, Consultant in Public Health Medicine, Avon Health Authority, Bristol, UK. angela.raffle@userm.avonhealth. swest.nhs.uk

Dr John Reynolds, Clinical Pharmacologist, John Radcliffe Hospital, Oxford, UK. djmr@doctors.org.uk

Dr George Rubin, Department of Public Health and Community Medicine, University of Sydney, Sydney, Australia. grubin@health. usyd.edu.au

Dr Gabriel Scally, Regional Director of Public Health, South West Regional Office (NHS Executive), Bristol, UK. gscally@doh.gsi.gov.uk

Dr Alex Scott-Samuel, Senior Lecturer in Public Health, University of Liverpool, Liverpool, UK. alexss@liverpool.ac.uk

Dr Fiona Sim, Associate Dean of Postgraduate Medicine, London Deanery and NHS Executive Regional Office, London, UK. fiona. sim@doh.gsi.gov.uk

Dr Chris Spencer-Jones, Consultant in Public Health and Primary Care, Dudley Health Authority, Dudley, UK. chris.spencer-jones@ dudley-ha.wmids.nhs.uk

Dr Nick Steel, Visiting Fellow and Specialist Registrar in Public Health Medicine, Institute of Public Health, Cambridge, UK. ns246@cam.ac.uk

Professor Andrew Stevens, Dept of Public Health & Epidemiology, University of Birmingham, Birmingham, UK. a.j.stevens@bham. ac.uk

Dr Roscoe Taylor, Public Health Physician, Central Public Health Unit, Rockhampton, Australia. roscoe_taylor@health.qld.gov.au

Dr Barry Tennison, Commission for Health Improvement, London, UK. barry@ukph.org

Dr Pamela Thomas, Consultant in Community Health, Research School of Social Sciences, Australian National University, Canberra, Australia. pamela.thomas@anu.edu.au

Dr David Tipene-Leach, Senior Lecturer in Maori Health, Auckland School of Medicine, Auckland, New Zealand. d.tipene-leach@ auckland.ac.nz

Michelle Tjhin, Department of Public Health and Community Medicine, University of Sydney, Sydney, Australia. mtjhin@health. usyd.edu.au

Dr Patrick Wall, Chief Executive, Food Safety Authority of Ireland, Dublin, Ireland. pwall@fsai.ie

Dr Jeanette Ward, Director and Associate Professor in Public Health, Central Sydney Area Health Service, Australia. jward@nah. rpa.cs.nsw.gov.au

Dr Nick Wareham, MRC Clinical Scientist, Institute of Public Health, Cambridge, UK. njw1004@medschl.cam.ac.uk

Dr Paul Watson, Director of Health Policy and Public Health, North Essex Health Authority, Witham, UK. paul.watson@ne-ha.nthames.nhs.uk

Dr Stuart Whitaker, Senior Research Fellow, Institute of Occupational Health, University of Birmingham, UK. s.c.whitaker@bham.ac.uk

Peter Wightman, Huntingdonshire Primary Care Group, St Ives, UK. peter.wightman@cambs-ha.nhs.uk

Dr John Wright, Consultant in Epidemiology and Public Health, Bradford Hospital NHS Trust, Bradford, UK. john.wright@bradfordhospitals.nhs.uk

Dr Ron Zimmern, Director, Public Health Genetics Unit, Cambridge, UK. ron.zimmern@srl.cam.ac.uk

Introduction

The last two decades of the twentieth century saw a renewal of interest in the eternal verities of public health, in disease prevention, communicable disease control, health protection, and health promotion. This was partly due to the realization that continued investment in clinical care brings diminishing returns, and partly because of the recognition that the problems tackled so successfully by public health actions in the last half of the nineteenth century and the first half of the twentieth century have not disappeared. In some cases, they are re-emerging as bacteria develop resistance to antibiotics and as new threats to health develop in the physical environment, both locally and globally.

Public health practice therefore continues to be a major force in the twenty-first century: there will be a need for guides such as this for those who make decisions. If clinicians spend their time discovering new ways of managing old diseases, public health practitioners are constantly relearning the old ways of managing newer patterns of disease.

The role of public health is to contribute 'to the health of the public through assessment of health and health needs, policy formulation, and assurance of the availability of services'.[1] As this handbook will show, many public health practitioners and teams make their biggest contribution through the development of health systems. A health system, in its broadest sense, is composed of 'personal health care, public health services and other inter-sectoral initiatives'.[2] It is rarely helpful to claim one part of such a system contributes more than another. A balanced view—and a balanced health system—should contribute to a fair and healthy society.

Many problems can be classified as public health problems, and public health problems and challenges can be classified in many ways (see table of contents). The challenge for public health practitioners is to cope with conflicting priorities for improving the health of populations.

As the scope of the public health challenge broadens, for example with the development of the new genetics and the renaissance of infectious diseases, it becomes impossible for any one individual to have a complete grasp of the knowledge needed to identify, analyse, and tackle the problems that influence their population's health. Public health practitioners therefore need a broad range of skills and selective depth in specialist knowledge areas. In particular, public health practitioners need to be skilled at finding and appraising sources of knowledge. The focus of public health practitioners on a population and its health needs should persist, even while other professional groups are specializing and sub-specializing to cope with the exponential growth of knowledge.

When public health is defined as the science and art of improving the population's health through the organized efforts of society,[3,4] using the techniques of disease prevention, health protection, and health promotion, these words are chosen carefully. This handbook outlines the important tasks and skills needed by today's public health practitioners to ensure these efforts are well directed and well made.

The handbook is structured around public health problems and the practical tasks needed to address them. It is designed to help new public health practitioners appreciate the scope, frameworks, and techniques in public health. In addition, it is a constant refresher, and reference guide for the more experienced practitioner.

We do not intend this handbook to be the last word in any area; rather, we have tried to present what might be considered the first words and the most important concepts in the essential activities of public health practice.

*

We assume that users of this handbook already have a basic understanding of epidemiology and statistics, in the same way as a textbook of medicine assumes the reader has a knowledge of anatomy and physiology. This handbook book covers the building blocks of public health practice. Those seeking the epidemiological and statistical foundations and detailed research methods will need to turn to other texts.[5,6,7,8]

Part 1 outlines the skills needed to assess and monitor the health of the population. We consider needs and health impacts. Part 2 outlines the technical skills needed to both identify the possible actions that can be taken and the methods of deciding between them. Rarely is this a neat sequential process of clarifying the problems, and finding the right knowledge to help address these problems. However, the chapters in this section lay out the skills needed at each stage of the process, whichever route might be most appropriate.

An underrated task of public health practitioners is that of turning complex and seemingly messy issues into soluble problems. Skills to find and assess the knowledge that underpins problem solving are carefully examined. Deciding on the most appropriate public health action almost always involves difficult, but important, choices. These choices are rarely simple, technical issues with quantitative answers. We therefore examine the approaches used in addressing the values and ethics in public health that cannot, and should not, be avoided in such decision making.

After applying these techniques, the issues may eventually become clearer, the options more obvious, and the decisions that need to be taken more apparent. Only then should the most appropriate methods of public health action be chosen and applied. The skills needed to take public health action across the spectrum are addressed in parts 3 and 4.

The influencing, making, and implementing of policy (whether by governments or by large multinational organizations), are addressed in part 3. This part of the handbook shows how science and rationality need to be combined with emotion and power (e.g. though the media) to achieve public health gains, not only through the *formulation* of policy but also in its *implementation*.

Part 4 presents the diversity and appropriateness of methods of taking direct action on the immediate determinants of public health. This section covers examples of the specific tasks facing public health: protecting and promoting health, and preventing disease through different techniques for different challenges, in different places and for different populations, around the globe.

The relative contributions of medical care and other public health measures to improvements in health have been hotly debated. However, the organization and delivery of health care is an area where many public health practitioners have the opportunity to play a significant role. Parts 5 and 6 present the tasks and skills needed to assess and assure the important dimensions of quality in health care organization and delivery. In addition, many of the principles outlined in this section are transferable to other services that influence the public's health.

The art of public health refers to the interpersonal and organizational skills needed to effect real change. Without these personal and organizational skills, the best evidence and the best intentions amount to nothing. Parts 7 and 8 cover the personal and organizational skills needed to create effective change in collaboration with other individuals and teams throughout the health system.

Part 9 completes the handbook with practical examples detailing the application of core principles from the rest of the book. The introduction to part 9 issues a challenge: the development of a casebook of public health achievements; a rigorous, but candid, analysis of failure as well as success. Please consider this as you complete the evaluation form, after you have had some experience of using the book.

*

The handbook is not intended to be read from start to finish. The order of the sections and chapters may imply that decisions and action do not take place until a complete assessment of the health of the population is performed. Life is rarely that simple. Most public health action around the world involves simultaneous firefighting of multiple real and perceived threats to public health. Many professionals therefore begin tasks with the scoping of apparent problems (part 2), rather than with the prior and more theoretical assessment of the real ones (part 1).

Throughout this handbook, we have tried to address, where possible, the ten core activities of public health as outlined by the US Health and Human Services Public Health Service:[9]

1. Preventing epidemics

2. Protecting the environment, workplaces, food, and water

3. Promoting healthy behaviour

4. Monitoring the health status of the population

5. Mobilizing community action

6. Responding to disasters

7. Assuring the quality, accessibility, and accountability of medical care

8. Reaching out to link high risk and hard to reach people to needed services

9. Researching to develop new insights and innovative solutions

10. Leading the development of sound health policy and planning.

Public health is centrally concerned with the pursuit of social justice and efficiency. Such achievements have sometimes only been possible because of opportunism, serendipity, and charisma. Nonetheless, learning and improvement are never complete for any of us. The processes outlined in this handbook should enable public health practitioners to improve old skills and learn new skills, all of which are needed to address the challenges, both local and global, in the twenty-first century.

DP, CSG, DM, JAMG

References

1. Institute of Medicine (1988), *The future of public health*, and Institute of Medicine / Stoto M, Abel C, and Dievler A (ed.) (1996), *Healthy communities—new partnerships for the future of public health*, both available from www.nap.edu (accessed 17 August 2000).

2. World health report 2000. *Health systems: improving performance*. World Health Organization, Geneva. www.who.int/whr (accessed 22 August 2000).

3. Acheson D (1988). *Public Health in England*. HMSO, London.

4. Last JM (ed.) (2001). *A dictionary of epidemiology*, (4th edn). Oxford University Press, Oxford.

5. Maxcy KF, Rosenau MJ, and Last JM (ed.) (1988). *Public health and preventive medicine*, (13th edn). Appleton and Lange, Norwalk Connecticut.

6. Detels R, Holland WW, McEwen J, and Omenn GS (ed.) (1997). *Oxford textbook of public health*, (3rd edn). Oxford University Press, New York.
7. Kerr C, Taylor R, and Heard G (ed.) (1998). *Handbook of public health methods*. McGraw-Hill, Sydney.
8. Donaldson LJ and Donaldson RJ (2000). *Essential public health*, (2nd edn). Petroc Press, Newbury.
9. US Health and Human Services Public Health Service (1995). *For a healthy nation: returns on investment in public health*. US Government Printing Office, Washington DC.

Part 1
Public health assessment

Introduction

If public health is the science and art of improving the health of populations, then measuring health status and assessing the health needs of populations are the universal starting points for most of its activities.

This part of the handbook assumes a basic knowledge of epidemiological principles, and aims to link these to the challenges faced in public health practice.

In chapter 1, we explore public health information, including both:

• qualitative information, conveying insights into the perception of risks, health problems, experiences, and outcomes

• quantitative information—essentially involving counts, either of people at risk, of health events, of people with a disease, or of outcomes.

Both forms of information are essential to most public health efforts, and in practice combining these approaches is almost always desirable.

Public health work would be much easier if the qualities and quantities it dealt with were clear cut, binary states. In practice, risks, diseases, and outcomes are complex and dimensional. Clinicians are used to categorizing people as either having or not having conditions, but in practice the boundaries of almost all diseases are unclear, and a full range of severity exists from the hardly perceptible to the catastrophic. Establishing what will be counted as a 'case' and what will be excluded is an essential step, yet the precise boundaries can have enormous impacts on the numbers included. The somewhat arbitrary nature of the definitions of the boundaries of health states results in much of the variability in routinely collected data: without meticulous definition and attention, classification errors and biases abound.

Many health issues are fairly stable over time and can be satisfactorily dealt with through special studies or routinely collected data. However, some health challenges require specific data collection systems linked to mechanisms for taking early public health action. Chapters 2 and 3 cover two examples of such systems, namely communicable disease surveillance (chapter 2) and cancer registries (chapter 3).

Assessing the health status of a population (chapter 4) and its health needs (chapter 5) are two linked and core activities. While health status assessments seek to identify the scale of health risks, morbidity, or mortality experienced by a population (usually relative to others), health needs assessment focuses also on available interventions for the problems faced. All too often, the health status of a population is threatened by new policies, projects, and programmes. Health impact assessment seeks to systematically chart these risks and opportunities, preferably before they become irreversible. The central aim is to identify ways of avoiding or mitigating the effects of such health threats.

Throughout the section, both the technical issues as well as the managerial or procedural issues are discussed. Sound information, and concern for data quality and accurate analysis, are part of the core scientific skills of public health practice. However, public health goes beyond analysis, and seeks to make a difference in the 'real world'. As a result, political, managerial, and procedural issues are central to the public health endeavour. Involving all stakeholders, especially patients and the public, helps to build an informed and active constituency to drive change. Nothing is more frustrating than completing a technically fine analysis of a public health problem only to find it ignored by those in a position to act. However logical the analysis, however technically correct the proposed action, nothing will happen without the support of the decision makers and their public—winning emotional involvement in public health analysis is vital. Throughout the section, advice and checklists are offered to maximize the chances of achieving change.

DM

1.1 Assessing information

Barry Tennison

Objectives

The aim of this chapter is to help the public health practitioner to:

- appreciate the subtleties of the varied forms of information about the health of a population and related matters
- develop a toolkit for thinking about the complexity of information and its uses.

The classification (taxonomy) of types of information given in this chapter should help the public health practitioner to:

- assess the completeness, accuracy, relevance and timeliness of available information
- decide which types of information are most appropriate for a particular public health task
- make optimal use of information which is not ideal, and assess the effects of its departure from perfection.

The use of the words 'data' and 'information'

Some people are purists. They will use the word 'data' (singular or plural) for raw numbers or other measures, reserving the word 'information' for what emerges when data are processed, analysed, interpreted, and presented. This has the virtue of making clear the sequence of steps that are involved in turning observations about the world into a form that is useful to those who wish to draw conclusions, and to act. This can be summarized in Figure 1.1.1.

In practice, many people use 'data' and 'information' more or less interchangeably, perhaps on the grounds of the greyness of some of these distinctions and steps (see chapter 2.5—'Managing public health information and knowledge'). However, in assessing the value of what emerges as information from these steps, the practitioner must bear in mind the fundamental issues which affect the quality of the data:

- *validity*—are the data capturing the concept or quantity the practitioner intends? Are the definitions and methods of data collection explicit and clear?
- *selection bias*—where the data mislead because they are not representative of the population or problem being considered, for example because of poor sampling

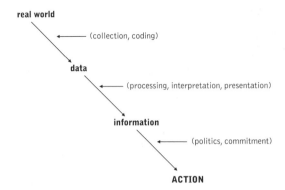

Figure 1.1.1 From reality to action.

- *classification bias*—where there is a non-random effect on putting data into groupings, for example in non-blind assessments of health outcome
- *statistical significance*—where, although differences seem apparent, analysis shows that they are reasonably likely to have occurred by chance (see for example Marshall and Spiegelhatter[1]).

What kinds of data sources are there?

In most countries, there are many different sources of information on the health of the population.[2] Different types of information vary in their 'C.A.R.T': (see chapter 1.2)

- Completeness
- Accuracy
- Relevance and/or Representativeness
- Timeliness.

Data sources also vary in the ease with which a 'base population' can be identified, for use in the denominator, for calculating rates. Typical data sources for local areas are summarized in Table 1.1.1.

A 'population health information' system can help in assembling data sources on a population. Such systems often involve a partnership between different agencies involved with a population, and the system can allow co-ordination of health information activities.

What does the information source describe?

Information about the health of a population can cover:

1. *Demography*: the basic characteristics of the population, such as age, sex, geographical distribution, and mobility

Table 1.1.1 Data sources.

Source	Strengths	Weaknesses
1. Routine data sources		
Population estimates Census or population registers	Usually reasonably good, especially if complemented by Local Authority (UK) or other government data	May be problems with small area estimates, especially between censuses
Birth/abortion notifications	Reasonably accurate; May contain other data	No complete data on spontaneous abortions; Non-standard coding
Mortality records	'Hardest' health data as death tends to be unequivocal; Total mortality reliable	Insensitive measure of health; Physician's cause of death specification often inaccurate/ incomplete; Non-fatal disease not reflected in mortality figures
Morbidity measures		
Infectious disease notifications (see chapter 1.2)	Certain diseases notifiable (mandatory); Generally adequate for monitoring trends	Often incomplete
Disease registers (see chapter 1.3)	Key group identified	Often doesn't cover whole country; May be missing people due to no contact or non identification
Impairment, disability and handicap	Functional status often more relevant than disease status	Usually available from surveys only
Health services data: access and supply, utilization, activity, costs	May be potentially relevant especially if condition almost always results in health care use—e.g. fractured femur	Likely to be incomplete; Data tend to identify health service activity and settings rather than receipt of (effective) interventions; Data quality may be poor
Data from other agencies—social care, housing, environmental risks, etc.	May be relevant	May be poor quality; May be incomplete; Categories and definitions may be incompatible

2. Surveys (see chapter 1.4)

National surveys, or surveys from other countries	Available; May be authoritative and highly relevant	Require 'modelling' to local population characteristics; May not be generalizable to local population; Quality variable
Previous local surveys	Relevant and usually appeal to a local audience	Quality variable
Local surveys to be commissioned	Can be tailor made	Often expensive

3. Qualitative data

Local descriptive accounts of environmental or social factors	May give a good understanding or stimulate research	The scale of health impact of identified problems may be difficult to assess
People's perceptions of how health problems affect them	May give a good understanding of what really affects people	Qualitative data can need careful handling, as details of context, background, and question wording can result in unstable responses

2. *Health-related characteristics or risk factors*, such as measures of deprivation, living conditions, employment, housing; or more medical factors or physiological measurements (e.g. blood glucose levels)

3. *Health need data*, such as the distribution of the indications for an intervention such as hip replacement[3] or the distribution of different thresholds for intervention

4. *Mortality*: the death experience of the population, including causes of death and variation according to the dimensions of person, place, and time

5. *Morbidity*: the health or illness experience of the population, including prevalence and incidence of diseases

6. *Health service use data*, such as diagnoses, interventions, and procedures, and health outcomes of interventions; it may be useful to distinguish patient interactions with *agents* (such as nurses or doctors) from their use of *settings* (such as hospital, day hospital, health centre, or home in using the health service)

7. *Health economic data*, often concerning the costs of interventions, and the distribution of activity and costs at marginal or average levels.

Clarity and judgement are needed about when one of these types of data is being used as a *proxy* for another. For example, where mortality data are firm and morbidity data poor in quality, with care mortality may be seen as a good proxy for morbidity: this might work well for certain kinds of heart disease or cancer, but very poorly for most mental health problems. Similarly, care is needed in moving from burden of disease (mortality, morbidity, or even more carefully, health service use) to health need.

In terms of how it is collected, assembled and made available, information can be routine or specially collected:

(a) **Routine**: collected, assembled, and made available regularly, according to well-defined and repeated protocols and standards; such data are usually part of a system of data collection by which information is:

• available at regular intervals

• intended to allow tracking over time

• codified according to national or international standards (for example, using the International Classification of Diseases* (ICD)).

(b) **Specially collected** for a particular purpose, without the intention of regular repetition or adherence to standards (other than those needed for the specific study or task); such data are usually:

• aimed at a specific, time-limited study or task

• codified according to the task in hand and the wishes of the investigators (sometimes in ignorance of the availability of suitable standard codes and methods).

Most of the data published in medical journals falls in the 'specially collected' category.

Table 1.1.2 gives important examples of information according to these dimensions.

Classification of intrinsic types of data

It is sometimes useful to categorize data as hard or soft. In fact, there is a spectrum from 'hard' to 'soft' data: data are never completely hard or soft.

(a) **Harder data** tend to be:

• precise (or intended to be precise)

• often numerical; if not, then coded according to a protocol

• reproducible, and likely to be similar even if the data collectors or individuals studied are varied.

(b) **Softer data** tend to be:

• qualitative, attempting to capture some of the subtlety of human experience

• often narrative or textual in form, at least as they are collected

• imbued with some subjectivity, due to the complexity of the personalities of the data collectors and the individuals studied.

Table 1.1.2 Dimensions of information.

	Mode of data collection	
	Routine	**Specially collected**
Demography	Census counts; Birth registration	Survey of homeless, roofless, and rough sleepers
Risk factors	Census details, such as housing conditions	Survey of ethnicity and CHD risk factors; Local survey of tobacco use
Mortality	Death registration; Coroner's records	Some cohort studies which capture deaths; Search for deaths probably due to suicide, using multiple sources
Morbidity	National health surveys (such as the Health Survey for England[4] or the National Health Interview Survey in the USA[5]); Disease notifications and registers	Case finding for an outbreak; Survey to establish prevalence of a specific disease; Most cohort studies
Health need	(Mainly proxies)	Survey of indications for hip replacement
Service use	Use of inpatient beds Attendances at outpatient department, emergency room, or physician's office	Observational study of use of a hospital department; Follow-up study of outcomes of hip replacement
Economic	Accounts of health service organizations; Comparative cost tables[6]	Costing of an existing or proposed service

(*Note*: some people will use the term 'soft' when they wish to imply that the data have inherent tendencies to imprecision, even if they are 'hard' in the sense of being numerical or strongly coded.)

Neither hard nor soft data are intrinsically better than the other (see Table 1.1.3 for examples). The utility of the information (in terms of better decision making) often comes from combining the two:

- harder data usually allow more precise analysis and comparisons, but may fail to capture subtleties
- softer data usually capture more of the 'truth' about the world, but often at the expense of emphasizing the uniqueness of circumstances, and are less likely to allow comparisons and conclusions.

The important thing to assess is *fitness for purpose*: are the existing or proposed data fit for the purpose for which they are intended, the conclusion to be drawn or the decision to be made? For example, for

Table 1.1.3 Examples of harder and softer data.

	Harder	Softer
Demography	Ethnic breakdown of a population according to a given ethnic classification; Proportion of houses with a bath	Narrative account of nature of a neighbourhood
Risk factors	Blood pressure; Proportion of smokers, non-smokers, and ex-smokers (according to precise definitions)	Patient experience of symptoms; Smoking 'careers' of teenagers
Mortality	Numbers dying of a specific disease; Survival data after specific interventions	Impact of deaths on the survivors
Morbidity	Prevalence of disease in a population at a moment in time; Numbers of admissions to a particular hospital	Reasons why a family doctor refers patients to hospital; Subjective quality of treatment given by a particular hospital

deciding the allocation of resources, one requires relatively hard data to obtain a degree of precision and transparency, so that the judgements involved are explicit. On the other hand, soft data may be useful in deciding on a change in the pattern of services provided. For example, when a client population (such as teenagers) seems to make poor use of current services: a well-designed qualitative survey may reveal some of the reasons, and a potential service configuration response. Softer data are also essential when capturing patient preference[7] or professional experiences.[8,9]

Absolute and comparative information

Often data about one location, one time, or one population are difficult to interpret in isolation; or worse, seem to beg obvious conclusions when in fact *comparison* with similar data elsewhere, previously or in another population, suggests a different conclusion or decision.

Comparative data are available on a local, regional, national,[10] or international level. WHO publishes comparative data between countries, for example on health spending as a percentage of GDP, and on comparative mortality and burden of disease.[11]

Experience shows the truth of the adage that the information you think you want is seldom the information you actually need; and the information you have seldom matches either need or want. The pragmatic public health practitioner must learn to cope with what is possible; not to set impossible standards; and to make the appropriate allowances, professionally, for shortcomings of the available information. Above all, the public health practitioner must not allow themselves or others to despair and to declare tasks impossible without the necessary information (which is in fact unavailable or impossible).

Here is a check-list of issues to consider when assessing data or a data source for fitness for purpose. None of these issues is absolute, and the balance of advantage and disadvantage must be assessed using judgement.

Check-list for assessing appropriateness and usefulness of data and data sources

1. Technical issues
   (a) Are the definitions clear and appropriate?
   (b) Are the target and study populations clear?
   (c) Are the data collection methods clear and sound?
   (d) How complete, accurate, relevant, and timely are the data? How much does this matter?
   (e) Do any differences that appear reach statistical significance, and what are the confidence limits or intervals? (Consider the use of a Bayesian approach[12]).

2. Issues relating to the conclusion or decision involved
   (a) Is the study population sufficiently representative of the target population for the purpose of the decision?
   (b) Do we need absolute or relative estimates, to make the best decision?
   (c) What precision is needed for the decision (taking into account confounding factors, random variation, and the influence of external factors such as resource availability, professional opinion, and politics)?
   (d) Would a simpler or existing data source suffice, for example by using comparative data; by extrapolating or interpolating, with care; or by transferring data from a similar or analogous situation?
   (e) Would qualitative information suffice, when habit automatically suggests quantitative data?

Conclusion

All too often, faced with a decision, there is a call for more information (or worse, a new information system). Frequently, either the available data are in fact, with care and interpretation, fit for the purpose of the decision needed; or the costs (including money, skills, burden of effort, and delay) of the new information or system are not commensurate with the problem faced. This check-list, and this chapter, should help the practitioner to balance what is needed with what is feasible and adequate.

Further resources

Abramson JH (1990). *Survey methods in community medicine*, (4th edn). Churchill Livingstone, London.

Abramson JH (1994). *Making sense of data*, (2nd edn). Oxford University Press, New York.

OECD Health care and policy data www.oecd.org/els/health/ (accessed 8 August 2000).

Your own national office of health statistics e.g. in the UK www.statistics.gov.uk (accessed 1 August 2000).

References

1. Marshall EC and Spiegelhalter DJ (1998). Reliability of league tables of in vitro fertilisation clinics: retrospective analysis of live birth rates. *BMJ*, **316**, 1701–5.

2. Detels R *et al.* (1997). *Oxford textbook of public health*. Oxford University Press, New York, Oxford.

3. Frankel S, Eachus J, Pearson N, Greenwood R, Chan P, Peters TJ, Donovan J, Smith GD, and Dieppe P (1999). Population requirement for primary hip-replacement surgery: a cross-sectional study. *Lancet*, **353(9161)**, 1304–9.

4. *Health survey for England* www.official-documents.co.uk (accessed 27 July 2000).

5. www.cdc.gov/nchs/nhis.htm (accessed 27 July 2000).

6. www.doh.gov.uk/nhsexec/refcosts.htm (accessed 27 July 2000).

7. Silvestri G, Pritchard R, and Welch HG (1998). Preferences for chemotherapy in patients with advanced non-small cell lung cancer: descriptive study based on scripted interviews. *BMJ*, **317**, 771–5.

8. Jain A and Ogden J (1999). General practitioners' experiences of patients' complaints: qualitative study. *BMJ*, **318**, 1596–9.

9. Dowie R (1983). *General practitioners and consultants: a study of outpatient referrals*. King Edward's Hospital Fund for London, London (distributed by Oxford University Press).

10. www.statistics.gov.uk (UK government statistics) (accessed 11 May 2001).

11. www.who.int/whosis/ (accessed 27 July 2000).

12. Spiegelhalter DJ, Myles JP, Jones DR, and Abrams KR (1999). Methods in health service research: an introduction to Bayesian methods in health technology assessment. *BMJ*, **319**, 508–12.

To understand God's thoughts, we must study statistics, for these are the measure of His purpose.

Florence Nightingale, 1860

1.2 Assessing acute health trends: surveillance

Fraser Hadden and Sarah O'Brien

What is surveillance?

Alexander Langmuir of the Centers for Disease Control in Atlanta, Last, and WHO all define surveillance in terms of the ongoing, systematic collection, collation, and analysis of data and the prompt dissemination of the resulting information to those who need to know so that an action can result.

Objectives

This chapter aims to describe:

- the *objectives* of surveillance
- the *types* of surveillance
- the *steps* involved in surveillance
- and the *limitations* of surveillance systems.

What are the objectives of surveillance?

The principal *objectives* are to:

- give *early warning* of changes of incidence—as with the recent increase in tuberculosis in many countries following a long period of decline
- detect *outbreaks* early
- *evaluate the effectiveness of interventions*—the introduction of new vaccines, for instance
- *identify at-risk groups*—surveillance might provide the impetus to establish, say, a neonatal BCG programme to prevent tuberculosis in children at higher than standard risk
- *help set priorities for resource allocation*—in general, surveillance systems alone do not contribute greatly to this as the importance of a condition is often a function of its health consequence and the treatments available for established cases, rather than simply its incidence.

The five characteristics that define surveillance are:

- *ease*—because surveillance data may be required speedily, the dataset and means of its collection must be simple
- *rapidity*—it is essential that surveillance data be available in real time if emergency action is required. Surveillance may, for instance,

indicate serious pathogens in the food chain and emergency action must follow to identify the locations and halt distribution of the contaminated food to the public. Given the importance of timeliness there is often a compromise between completeness of data and consistency. In general it is more important that a communicable disease surveillance system be consistent than completely accurate (see below)

- *standardized nature*—in order to identify trends over time, the data collected over time, and across geographical locations, must be consistent both in the means of collection and the definition of the data elements being collected. For instance, the definition of the notifiable disease category 'food poisoning' was expanded in 1992 to include diseases thought or known to be connected with the consumption of water. This expansion introduced a stepped increase in the number of food-poisoning cases notified in the following and subsequent years, and distorted the trends which had built up over past years

- *on-going nature*—as opposed to the time-limited nature of a survey

- *feedback*—this distinguishes a surveillance system from a database.

In practice, surveillance of communicable disease requires the integration, analysis, and interpretation of data from several different sources since no single system provides all the answers. The fact that data are derived from different sources and have often been collected in different ways increases the complexity of the surveillance process.

Types of surveillance

Surveillance can be classified into the following *types*:

- *passive*—where the data collator awaits its reporting, as with the British system of notifiable disease reporting

- *active*—where the data collator checks that the reporting agency is indeed collecting the source data, and doing so as completely as the collection mechanism allows

- *negative*—where the data collator presses the collector to report even the *absence* of cases. This is typically required for uncommon disorders so that the collator can be sure that a 'nil report' truly reflects zero incidence over the period and not simply a failure to report. Paediatric Surveillance Units around the world use negative reporting schemes.

Steps involved in surveillance

There are four *steps*:

(a) data collection

(b) data collation

(c) data analysis

(d) dissemination.

Action may or may not flow from the last.

(a) Data collection

There are many potential sources of communicable disease data. A few of the major ones used in the UK are:

- notifiable diseases—a selection of infective conditions are subject to compulsory notification by clinicians

- laboratory results—details of individual cases tend to be accurate, though demographic details of patients are often incomplete, and population denominators are usually lacking

- primary care 'spotter' practices—based on primary care units selected by their undertaking to report assiduously certain specified infectious diseases; a drawback is that the system is not necessarily representative of the whole population

- mortality data—numbers of deaths are reliable as the end-point is reliably defined—causes of death are much less reliably ascribed

- specific national administrative data systems, e.g. computerized systems supporting routine vaccination of children, and for assessing vaccination coverage.

The data collected must be defined precisely and understood by the collecting agency to avoid misclassification. Data must also be collected at regular intervals. Two examples of potential misclassification are given:

- the protozoal diseases giardiasis and cryptosporidiosis are often notified by GPs as cases of 'food poisoning'. Unless the GP has grounds for believing that the diseases arose from consumption of food or water, notification is incorrect. If the data collator accepts onto the record large numbers of cases, the true trend in food-poisoning incidence is distorted

- as diseases become rare, it may be that a case-definition becomes necessary or that it is accepted that the surveillance mechanism is no longer sufficiently refined to track its incidence. When measles was common, most cases notified as measles were genuinely so. Measles is now rare and only about 2% of notifications are genuine cases. Clearly, the notification system no longer provides useful trend data for measles.

Laboratory data might be considered intrinsically more reliable than notifiable disease data, but case-definitions are needed for this too. For example, the significance of an organism isolated from a site or specimen may mean little in itself. The clinical picture determines its importance.

Data collection intervals must be short for those conditions where rapid intervention may be needed.

The collection/collation process is only part of the overall delay between a case of disease arising and becoming known to the collator—other elements of the delay are:

- the incubation period of the disease
- the interval between the patient becoming ill and seeking medical help
- a potential interval between the patient seeking help and diagnostic specimens being taken
- the time for the laboratory result to be obtained.

These delays can sum to weeks. In addition, laboratory returns will not state the date of onset of illness. In this case, the date of specimen submission may have to be used as a proxy.

(b) Data collation

With the generalized availability of computers, it is tempting to think that a computerized database forms part of any worthwhile surveillance system, but this is far from universally so.

To track communicable diseases where emergency action may be required, data must be collated every day or two. Further, it must be apparent how each new element of data relates to data entered recently and more distantly. For this reason, paper-based systems have a role. If the collator simply marks on a sheet the cases of a disease as they arise, they can see immediately if the total number of cases over, say, a month is within expectations for the place and season or not. If not, the cases can be examined in more detail to see what is going on.

Computer databases have two drawbacks—the fixed overhead to starting them up and the skill and effort required to extract information from them. By contrast, anomalies that arise in a paper-based system almost force themselves upon the collator as they enter the data.

The computer does have a role in analysis of longer-term trends and in the management of data at regional and national levels. Although the term 'database' is used loosely for collections of data held on computer, true computer databases are not generally well-geared to mathematical manipulation of their data. It is better to use a spreadsheet, as these can readily accommodate the simple data that a surveillance system generates and are specifically designed for mathematical analysis and graphical representation. If data from each data source are put onto a different sheet, a modern spreadsheet can summate the data from these sources to generate the picture over a whole geographical area and to facilitate the production of reports.

(c) Data analysis

In general, analysis of surveillance data does not call for sophistic-ated data manipulation. The spreadsheet system described above can automatically generate summary data, including graphs of time-trends, for formal reports.

A major advantage of the spreadsheet approach is that, properly set up, it updates itself. Not only does this mean that a periodic report is simple to compile but that *ad-hoc* enquiries relating to disease incidence over a given period, which can obviously span more than one year, can be answered very rapidly.

(d) Dissemination

It is important that the original providers of data to the surveillance system are given feedback. Data providers may become disillusioned with servicing a system that yields nothing for them.

Beyond this, it is a courtesy to invite *ad-hoc* enquiries from data contributors. With a well-designed surveillance system, this involves the collator in minimal extra work and generates much goodwill.

Limitations of surveillance systems

As with all information sources, there are four potential shortcom-ings of surveillance systems, covered by the mnemonic 'C.A.R.T' (see chapters 1.1 and 1.4):

- completeness
- accuracy—is data classified correctly?
- relevance and/or representativeness
- timeliness—does data arrive in time for effective action to limit further cases to be instituted?

From a practical perspective, it is necessary to know what they are and their relative importance.

Completeness

The importance of completeness can be overstated. When used to trigger an acute intervention, surveillance systems are quite tolerant of incompleteness. When systems are used to compare data over successive years or from different geographical areas, it is important that the degree of incompleteness be consistent between all data contributors.

Some shortcomings of completeness are inevitable. If a data collator become aware of several cases of hepatitis A in a primary school, they can reasonably suspect that the data are incomplete, as most cases in this age-group will be asymptomatic. However, even the incomplete reporting will trigger action to prevent further spread of infection and may prompt investigation to ascertain the full number of cases in the school.

Accuracy

Accuracy is obviously most critical with diseases of low incidence where misdiagnosis or misclassification can generate a pseudo-outbreak and trigger inappropriate action.

Representativeness

The importance of representativeness is much more difficult to gauge. Such data as are routinely available from disparate sources suggest that geographical areas and surveillance systems vary widely in how well they represent the true picture of disease.

Timeliness

Timeliness is critical, as the prime purpose of nearly all surveillance is to trigger action. The definition of timeliness clearly depends on the nature of the disease under surveillance. For instance, measles, pertussis, and food-poisoning data must be received speedily, while malaria notifications are less time-critical.

Conclusion

It is important to remember the contribution surveillance can make when compared with the other tools available for assessing the health of populations:

- surveillance is an approximate science
- surveillance systems must be quick and easy to use
- surveillance systems are not data repositories—they must allow easy abstraction of information to be of any use.

Further resources

Carter A (1991). National Advisory Committee on Epidemiology Subcommittee. Establishing goals, techniques and priorities for national communicable disease surveillance. *Can J Infect Dis*, **2**, 37–40.

CDR Weekly. www.phls.co.uk (accessed 9 August 2000).

Chin J (ed.) (2000). *Control of communicable diseases manual*. American Public Health Association, Washington DC. *(Previously edited by Benenson.)*

Donaldson LJ and Donaldson RJ (2000). *Essential public health*, (2nd edn). Petroc Press, Newbury.

Eurosurveillance Weekly. www.eurosurv.org/ (accessed 9 August 2000).

Eylenbosch WJ and Noah ND (ed.) (1988). *Surveillance in health and disease*. Oxford University Press, Oxford.

MMWR. www2.cdc.gov/mmwr (accessed 9 August 2000).

Rushdy A and O'Mahony M (1998) on behalf of the PHLS Overview of Communicable Disease Committee. PHLS overview of communicable diseases 1997: result of a priority setting exercise. *CDR Report*, **8** (**suppl**).

WHO Weekly Epidemiological Record. www.who.int/wer/ (accessed 9 August 2000).

1.3 Assessing longer-term health trends: registers

David Melzer, John Newton, and Tom Davies

Objectives

The objectives of this chapter are to enable you to:

- understand disease registers in general
- understand cancer registries in particular
- use them efficiently
- be aware of the traps for the unwary.

Introduction

A disease register is a special form of clinical database. In compiling a population-based register, an attempt is made to identify and collect data on *all* cases of a disease or other health condition within a defined population. Many so-called registers do not in fact relate to a specified denominator population, being compiled from cases seen by a particular clinical unit or units. These are sometimes called 'clinically-rich' databases and are most useful for technology assessment and prognostic research rather than epidemiology or service planning. Considerable extra effort is required to compile a true population-based registry. However, this extra work is often justified and is rewarded by results that are independent of levels of supply of health care and inevitable clinical practice variations.

Registries are the organizations that support registers. They arrange systems to collect data on new cases having the condition of interest, and often also collect follow-up (longitudinal) data on identified cases. The resulting records are intended to be permanent, and the data are periodically analysed, tabulated, and reported.

Epidemiological registers can be based on cases defined according to:

- disease status: e.g. a diagnosis of cancer, psychiatric illness, coronary heart disease,[1] or diabetes
- risk factor status: e.g. exposure to radiation in an occupational cohort[2] or genetic factors, including twin status[3]
- interventions or treatments, for example, heart valve replacement or renal transplants.[4]

Disease registers are best suited to situations where disease or risk factor status do not tend to change over time. The disease in question also needs to be reliably diagnosed by different clinicians (i.e. there should be a robust diagnostic test) and there should generally be a continuing and specific health care need associated with the disease (e.g. for retinal screening in diabetics) or important epidemiological uncertainties (e.g. Creutzfeld Jacob disease).

Many registers are oriented toward service provision rather than epidemiology but these can be very useful for public health too. For example, 'at risk' registers might be used to plan adequate services for the protection of children. Registers of blind or otherwise disabled people are an important source of information on the needs of these groups (see chapter 1.2).

The data collected by registries vary widely, but often include personal identifiers, socio-demographic information, disease status (possibly including stage, severity, and co-morbidity), details of treatments and other interventions, and eventual outcomes. Registers that are used to investigate aetiology also collect information on risk factors.

There is a trend towards much more strict legislation on data protection in the UK and other countries. This will have considerable implications for disease registers, which have not always been set up in such a way that would satisfy the latest legislation. In future, explicit patient consent may be required for inclusion of cases on a register where the register is used for patient care purposes. Where the register is only for research, the arguments are less clear and opinions are divided. Epidemiologists argue that any requirement for consent can lead to selection bias and is anyway impractical for large-scale studies. In such cases, the public good may be deemed to override the need to respect the individual's autonomy provided the individual is not harmed in any way.

The suggestion that registers should only use anonymous data is not a helpful one. Patient names and addresses or equivalent unique personal identifiers are generally required to avoid double-counting of individuals and to enable follow-up data (for example from death certificates) to be correctly linked to previously registered cases. It is also very difficult to validate a register that does not allow cases to be identified so that disease status can be checked against some gold standard such as the clinical notes. Finally, a number of important studies have been done by linking data on individuals across more than one register.

A registry must establish systems to:

- maintain a reliable notification or identification of cases within the studied population

- ensure comparability of inclusion criteria onto the register: for a diagnosis, strict rules are needed to identify the studied condition, within an agreed classification

- minimize under-coverage—cases not being included when they should be

• ensure that duplication of cases within the register does not occur

• keep the register updated—removing those who have recovered, died, or moved out of the area.

Registries must usually also have resources for analysis and publication of reports, and be able to respond to requests for *ad hoc* analyses or data. Procedures for safeguarding confidentiality and maintaining ethical standards are needed, especially if identifiable data are held or shared with outside researchers. Research registries should be closely associated with appropriate research groups in the field to ensure that they remain relevant and accessible.

Maintaining a register is time and labour intensive and can be expensive. Maintaining motivation and interest is essential and often depends on the person organizing the register. Registers tend to get out of date quickly. It is essential that the objectives of any register are explicit and clearly justify the time and expense entailed. It is also crucial to evaluate quality continually as a poor register is of very little use and may be positively misleading.

How can registers help?

If case ascertainment is high, prevalence and incidence rates can be computed. Analysis of risks and aetiology can be explored, using individual as well as area characteristics. With follow-up data, outcomes can be measured, e.g. survival rates for cancer. If registers are maintained over time, they can produce evidence of change, e.g. in epidemics or in the effectiveness of interventions.

Registers can be used to assist in the management of chronic disease in clinical settings,[5] triggering follow-up care for people with, for example, diabetes or asthma within a primary care practice. Registers can also form the basis for clinical audit and quality improvement efforts. Psychiatric case registers have been used to evaluate community care services.[6]

An example of a disease register: a cancer registry

The cancer registration system is a unique world-wide resource, there being regional cancer registries covering between 1 and 15 million people in most countries in the world. Each registry is essentially a detailed list of all the cancers that have occurred since each registry was established (e.g. in the UK this was usually around 1970).

Cancer registries in Europe work together through the European Network of Cancer Registries.[7] World-wide, the International Association of Cancer Registries[8] co-ordinates registry activities. Population coverage is 100% throughout the UK and Republic of Ireland, Scandinavia, the Netherlands and Germany (from 1999), Canada, and nearly so in the USA. Registries in other countries have 100% coverage for sub-populations. Others are hospital based. International details can be found in *Cancer incidence in five continents.*[9]

Important features

Three important features of cancer registries should be remembered:

- cancer registries contain details of *diagnosed* cancers—they cannot tell you about cancers which we take to our grave without diagnosis
- the record starts at diagnosis and records features of the patient and the tumour at that time—there is often little further information until death is recorded (although more information should be available in the future)
- most are population based, providing a denominator for numbers of tumours in relation to the population of which the patients were members.

What is on the register?

Registries differ very slightly, but the minimum content is nationally defined. In the UK, for example, the registry includes details of:

- the patient—name, address, postcode, date of birth, sex, their doctors (in some registries now; in future, all)
- the tumour—site, histological type, and possibly grade and stage at diagnosis (how advanced the tumour is)
- date of diagnosis
- treatment during the first six months after diagnosis date, and cause of death.

Many registries will keep extra data on each patient and tumour, and there will be links between multiple tumours in the same patient.

Cancer registries *do not* compile mortality statistics in the UK. These come from the Office for National Statistics[10] and refer to date of death and residence at death. This type of arrangement also applies to other countries. On receipt, the place and date of death is added to the patient's record, to enable registries to calculate survival from diagnosis. Note that cancer mortality data are classified by year and place of death no matter when or where the diagnosis was made. Survival data refer to place and date of diagnoses.

What can the data be used for?

For each type of tumour and type of patient, it is possible to calculate:

- *incidence* of cancer, and trends in incidence
  These can be used to make projections in demand and to help judge the effectiveness of preventive strategies. Given knowledge of the population size, migration, and all-cause mortality, projections of incidence are fairly reliable for up to ten years. Projections of prevalence, the proportion of the population with cancer at any one time, are much less reliable. The definition of prevalence has

to be the number of people diagnosed as having cancer and who will still be alive, but this does not distinguish those cured from those still being treated. It is very difficult to forecast the future degree of success of treatment. Projections can be improved by only counting people as prevalent cases for a period after diagnosis when that group's mortality is higher than the population average for that age and sex group, based on past experience

• *survival* of people with cancer, and trends in survival
   Trends in survival can be used to make projections and to help judge the effectiveness of treatment.

Examples of uses of registry data:

• a recent study in England measured survival in patients treated in different types of hospital, those with oncology departments and those without. The comparison was made after adjusting for cancer stage, age, and sex. For patients aged under 75 with some cancers (ovary, breast, and rectum) survival was better in hospitals with oncology departments

• one can sometimes compare survival between modes of treatment. This is not true of all cancer registries at present, but it will be in future. The problem is that for specific cancers, numbers are too small for reliable analysis, so you have to amalgamate data from different years. An example of using the cancer registry to monitor treatment outcomes comes from Ontario. The question posed was whether breast implants were a risk factor for cancer. Plastic surgeons gave permission for data to be collected on their patients, cases with breast implants, and controls with other operations. The cancer registry data were used to measure the incidence in both groups; breast cancer was rarer in women with implants.[11]

Patients can be selected for research studies into the cause and treatment of disease, but this usually means gathering more information from the patients' notes or the patients themselves.

Using registry data

All registries produce routine reports, usually on incidence and survival. Thus, if your enquiry is simple, just take the report off the shelf. If the enquiry is more complex, or if you are not quite sure what you need, the registry will advise you. However, there are some questions you will always be asked, so you must know:

• which cancers you are interested in—cancers are classified by site (lung, brain, rectum, etc.) and type (adenocarcinoma, teratoma, etc.)

• which people you are interested in—by age, or date of birth, year or age band (e.g. 35–40, or born between 1920 and 1930); sex; area of residence (in the UK usually health district; any combination of postcodes can be used, but must be in the region covered by the registry)

• which year of diagnosis.

Most registries are willing to provide data from which individuals cannot be identified. If individuals are to be identified, release will depend on other factors, mainly related to ethical and confidentiality issues. These are spelt out in the UK Association of Cancer Registries Policy Document but procedures are similar to those established by the International Association of Cancer Registries. To summarize, you can have named data, if you are the patient or the patient's doctor, or if you want the data for the benefit of the patient, or the direct benefit of others, or for audit. For genetic counselling you need the consent of living relations, and for research you need research ethics committee permission.

Analysing the data

Before you obtain the data, you must have a reasonably detailed idea of what you intend to do with them. Essentially, the analytical skills you need are epidemiological and statistical, as with any investigation of this kind, but you must be quite clear what problems you are trying to solve, and whether any questions you ask will do it. All registries employ statisticians or epidemiologists, part of whose job is to advise on the use and the limitations of the data.

The limitations of the data

Cancer registries are the main source of epidemiological information on cancer. They are developing very quickly, but at the moment they:

• will not tell you about cancer more than 30 years ago (at least for the whole of the UK)—before that, you have to rely on mortality information—other countries are similar though many have been started more recently

• will not tell you about hospital activity; they will tell you about patients resident in that region, but patients from outside the registry region will be entered on their home registry, and patients from outside the UK probably will fall through the net

• will not tell you about patients diagnosed within the last year— registries cannot provide survival data for a period longer than the time since diagnosis, e.g. five-year survival in patients diagnosed last year—actually, approximations and projections can be made but they are not particularly accurate

• will not tell you what has happened between six months after diagnosis and death. Unless there is active follow-up, some deaths may be missed—this also applies to local recurrence and prolonged treatment.

Myths and shortcomings

As with any large systems, there are both shortcomings and myths, e.g. malignant hypertension being registered as a cancer. All humans make mistakes, but not as gross as that one, and even if they did, validation checks would stop the registration. Nevertheless, mistakes do occur, but they are rare and not normally major. Cases are missed, and sometimes duplicated, but the limiting factor is the quality of clinical notes.

Registries are often said to be years out of date. Nationally this is true, because national statistics offices (e.g. ONS) have to wait for the slowest contributor, but nowadays contracts specify publication of data after 18 months. The data are never 100% complete because occasional data may appear years after diagnosis.

Conclusion

Cancer Registries and Intelligence Units are very powerful epidemiological tools, and are developing quickly in terms of data gathered and processed. They have data going back 30 years for the whole population for most diagnosed cancers, and intelligent use is extremely rewarding.

Further resources

Andersson E, Nilsson T, Persson B, Wingren G, and Toren K (1998). Mortality from asthma and cancer among sulfite mill workers. *Scand J Work Environ Health*, **24**(1), 12–7.

Davies T (ed.) (1995). *A guide to the use of cancer registries.* UK Association of Cancer Registries, Cambridge.

Donaldson L (1992). Registering a need. *BMJ*, **305**(6854), 597–8.

EUCAN (1995). European Network of Cancer Registries. IARC* (International Agency for Research on Cancer, Lyon) www-dep.iarc.fr/encr.htm (accessed 2 August 2000)

Ferlay J, Bray F, Sankila R, and Parkin DM. EUCAN: Cancer Incidence, Mortality and Prevalence in the European Union 1996, version 3.0. IARC CancerBase No. 4. Lyon, IARC Press, 1999. Available on CD-ROM. Limited version available from www-dep.iarc.fr/eucan/eucan.htm (accessed 2 August 2000)

Goldberg J, Gelfand HM, and Levy PS (1980). Registry evaluation methods: a review and case study. *Epidemiologic Reviews*, **2**, 210–20.

Klaucke D, Buehler J, Thacker S, Parrish R, Trowbridge F, and Berkelman R (1988). Guidelines for evaluating surveillance systems. *MMMR*, **37**(S5), 1–18.

UK Cancer Research Campaign (CRC). *Vital statistics on cancer.* www.crc.org.uk (accessed: 9 August 2000)

Weddell JM (1973). Registers and registries: a review. *Int J Epidemiol*, **2**(3), 221–8.

References

1. Moher M, Yudkin P, Turner R, Schofield T, and Mant D (2000). An assessment of morbidity registers for coronary heart disease in primary care. *British Journal of General Practice*, **50**, 706–9.

2. Davies T and Williams L (ed.) (1994). *Cancer registry handbook*. UK Association of Cancer Registries, Cambridge.

3. Ljungquist B, Berg S, Lanke J, McClearn GE, and Pedersen NL (1998). The effect of genetic factors for longevity: a comparison of identical and fraternal twins in the Swedish Twin Registry. *J Gerontol A Biol Sci Med Sci*, **53**(6), M441–6.

4. Berthoux F, Jones E, Gellert R, Mendel S, Saker L, and Briggs D. *Epidemiological data of treated end-stage renal failure in the European Union (EU) during the year 1995: report of the European Renal Association Registry and the National Registries.*

5. Dawson A and Ferrero M (ed.)(1996). *Chronic disease management registers: proceedings of a workshop*. The Stationery Office, London. www.the-stationery-office.co.uk/index.htm (accessed 11 May 2001).

6. Tansella M (2000). Do we still need psychiatric case registers? *Acta Psychiatr Scand*, **101**(4), 253–5.

7. www-dep.iarc.fr/encr.htm (accessed 27 July 2000).

8. www-dep.iarc.fr/iacr.htm (accessed 27 July 2000).

9. Parkin DM, Ferlay J, Whelan, SL, Raymond L, and Young J (1998). *Cancer incidence in five continents*, Vol. VII. IARC, Lyon.

10. www.statistics.gov.uk/ (accessed 9 August 2000).

11. Holowaty EJ and Lee G (1999). *Do breast implants prevent breast cancer?* 21st Annual Conference International Cancer Registries, Lisbon.

1.4 Assessing health status

Peter Gentle

Objectives

Assessing the health of a population is a fundamental part of many public health activities. Doing assessments well is challenging, as there are usually problems in obtaining the necessary data and in balancing alternative approaches. Assessments of health status can support policy reviews, goal setting, a needs assessment programme, or efforts to improve resource allocation.

The objectives of this chapter are to identify the principles of assessing the health of a defined population and to provide some practical advice.

Assessing population health status

There are many types of population health assessment, but the usual steps in performing an assessment are:

* define the purpose of the assessment
* define the population concerned and any comparator populations
* define the aspects of health to be considered
* identify and review existing data sources
  * are good local data available?
  * are routine local or national statistics available?
  * are relevant published surveys available?
* select the most appropriate existing data
* make good use of the data, analyse appropriately (e.g. adjusting for population composition, deriving suitable measures, and perhaps modelling future trends)
* consider if specific issues require specially collected data: should a special survey be undertaken?
* communicate the results of the assessment
* evaluate the health assessment.

Be clear about the purpose

The starting point, defining the purpose, is especially important. A tendency to have an extensive unfocused list of objectives must be resisted, as well as the temptation to examine interesting but irrelevant issues.

The most important reasons to assess the health status of a defined population are to:

- support *needs assessment*, establishing whether particular health problems exist in a given population, characterizing the problems, and identifying the potential for avoidable mortality and morbidity
- support *policy making* through informing the public, professional groups, and decision-makers about the nature and distribution of health challenges, and the definition of the problem. This includes Health Impact Assessment (see chapter 1.6)
- support *planning and implementation*, improving resource allocation, target setting, and helping targeting of health and other services
- support *evaluation* of interventions, programmes, or policies (see part 5)
- identify important areas where *research* is needed.

Define the aspects of health to be considered

Health can have a variety of meanings, and the World Health Organization takes a very broad view. Health is seen as having physical, emotional, and social dimensions. In practice, you may want to use a more restrictive definition, but you should always be aware of broad aspects of health.

Box 1.4.1 **The World Health Organization's view of health**

Health is the extent to which an individual or group is able:

- to satisfy needs
- to realise aspirations
- to change or cope with their environment.

Health is a resource for everyday life, not the objective for living: it is a positive concept emphasising social and personal resources as well as physical capabilities.[1]

Profiles of the health status of populations can present data on both

- the determinants of health status (see list below)
- the measures of the status itself (see list below).

Assessments may relate to health overall or just cover one or more aspects.

Scope of health status measures for populations

1. *Determinants of health* (endogenous and exogenous) (adapted from Ruwaard *et al.*[2])

1.1 susceptibilities: markers, genetic factors (e.g. prevalence of sickle cell trait, Apo e4 gene), or endogenous susceptibilities

1.2 physical, emotional, social, economic, and environmental influences

1.3 health attitudes and health-related behaviours

1.4 health protection, collective prevention, health promotion

1.5 health and social care, both physical and mental.

2. *Health status*

2.1 self-assessed health status (including the experience of having the health problem)

2.2 symptom incidence and prevalence

2.3 disease incidence and prevalence

2.4 disability, impairment, or handicap

2.5 mortality.

Who defines health for a particular study may be crucial. It may be the individual with a health problem, or a professional expert, or society as represented by e.g. government policy.

Define the population

Defining the population of interest is critical. Population size, structure, and the period of observation covered can have powerful effects on the numbers of cases of disease or disability: data are therefore usually expressed as proportions (e.g. the number of people with diabetes per thousand population at a particular point in time) or rates (the number of new cases per thousand population per year). For certain purposes such rates may need adjustment for potential confounding variables (e.g. age, sex, socioeconomic status or ethnicity) to allow valid comparison with other populations.

Often geographical identifiers are used to frame the population studied, using for example, postcodes. Problems can arise with population estimates for small areas, especially those projected from a census that is relatively distant in time. If small areas are being studied, errors in estimates of population numbers and composition can result in dramatic but erroneous findings.

Review the available data

Comprehensive population health assessments are based on a wide range of data of different types. In order to maintain some framework to all the data items being used, consider the simple dimensions of data as used by Stevens and Gillam:[3]

• local vs. national data

• routine vs. *ad hoc* data

• quantitative vs. qualitative data

The interrelationship of these dimensions can be represented as a cube (Figure 1.4.1).

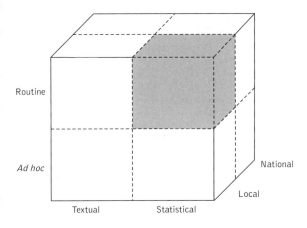

Figure 1.4.1 The data cube, showing a small cube representing routine local statistical information. (Adapted from Stevens and Gillam.[3])

While local data are required for assessing the health of the local population, it may not be available, and so national (or indeed international) data may be used, if the local population is felt to be typical of these bigger populations as a whole. Data from similar localities (e.g. in terms of levels of deprivation) or national data may of course be used for comparative purposes.

Quantitative data are usually necessary to answer questions such as 'How many people have a particular condition?' *Qualitative approaches* are well suited for exploring such issues as what it is like to be disabled, or perceptions about the effects and tolerability of risks from industrial pollutants. Qualitative data can be very valuable and tends to be insufficiently used.

Much data are collected *routinely* by census offices, health service providers, local and central government, and others. In addition, some of the many *ad hoc* studies that have been carried out locally or elsewhere may be relevant to a particular issue. Weaknesses of routine data collection systems include non-standard or inconsistent approaches to coding and data collection, and limited availability due to cost and privacy policies.

Much useful data are recorded as part of clinical care or collected by health care providers. However, very great care is needed in using such data: not all people with a health condition receive treatment (or they may be treated by other providers). Clinicians usually record information just for clinical purposes rather than for analytical purposes. The absence of a positive record (e.g. of smoking) may mean a true negative or that the information was not sought. The definition of a condition (and whether to treat it) may vary substantially from clinician to clinician, causing large differences between areas. Confidentiality issues must be addressed.

Select data carefully

At first sight there seems to be so much data available that assessing health should not be much of a challenge. However, Finagle's Law is usually proved correct in public health work: the data we have are not what we want; the data we want are not what we need; the data we need are not what we can get.

There are detailed descriptions of sources and approaches to using health-related data elsewhere in this handbook. Relevant, detailed, and accurate data are seldom available directly, and so data collected for other purposes have to be used appropriately to give an indirect assessment.

In considering the use of any data, think about how they have been obtained. People often assume that the quality and relevance of the data are satisfactory for the intended purpose. But those recording the data may well not use consistent terms or criteria and this can have a major impact. It is usually better to use good data from elsewhere than poor local data.

Remember that organizations that collect data often publish only some of it and may make other data available. They will often advise on data quality and relevance for particular purposes.

The use of international data needs great care, as different countries may use different definitions and data collection processes.

When the source has been identified, the questions in Table 1.4.1 should be asked.

Make good use of the data

Those assessing the health of populations should always be suspicious of any data, but they should not be paralysed by the above list of potential problems with data sources. If the purpose remains clear, direct or indirect measures of the studied risks or health problems can usually be derived, sometimes by assembling fragments of evidence from different sources.

In progressing from data to information, the five forms of health information identified by Ruwaard[4] form a useful framework:

- recording the situation at one moment in time for individual variables
- recording trends over time for individual variables
- simultaneously recording a series of different variables
- describing relationships between different indicators
- making forecasts with the help of modelling.

Table 1.4.1 Questions to be asked of data.

Validity of data for your purpose	
Relevance	Are the data relevant to the issue?
Definition	Have the data items been defined usefully for your purpose?
Conceptual bias	Are there conceptual biases in the data source (e.g. has data collection been structured to benefit the organization that has produced it?)
Timeliness	Are the data still sufficiently up to date?
Generalizability	Are the data relevant to your population?
Technical quality of data	
Recording	Have the data been entered properly according to the definitions?
Completeness	Have all been included—or a random sample used?
Bias	Are there classification or selection biases? (see chapter 1.1)
Appropriate aggregation	If the data are already aggregated, has this been done properly?
Quality of the analytical methods	
Appropriate adjustment or modelling	Can adjustment be made for your population structure (e.g. age/sex standardization, weighting for social group or ethnic composition?) Is modelling necessary?
Summary measures used	Are the summary measures useful? (e.g. do you require a measure of absolute risk while only relative risk is reported?)
Statistical significance	Are the numbers big enough to allow an adequately precise estimate?
Practical questions	
	Will confidentiality policies allow the relevant use of the data?
	What is the cost likely to be?
	Are the data available in machine-analysable form?

The purpose of the assessment will determine the nature of the analyses chosen. Common purposes include:

- comparing findings for the population with other similar populations or larger populations, or comparing health status observed with that expected for the type of population
- describing the relative health of parts of the population (areas or social groups), identifying inequalities (see chapter 6.7)

- comparing health trends over time
- estimating the extent of potentially preventable health problems
- describing the likely health impact of environmental and social factors (see chapter 1.6)
- describing the impact of health problems in terms of people's experience of health problems.

Some general approaches that may help include:

- using data from larger populations or special studies, if thought to be comparable
- adjusting data statistically for confounders, e.g. allowing for population age, sex, and social differences
- using evidence-based proxy measures (e.g. estimating all deaths due to smoking from those due to lung cancer[5])
- combining data from several years, to reduce statistical uncertainty
- giving broad estimates or ranges, if uncertainties exist (observed differences may be very large)
- making logical deductions from patterns of data
- seeing whether different analyses give similar results.

A number of technical analyses on the available data might be helpful, for example:

- elementary measures such as prevalence (point or period), incidence, etc.
- calculating relative rates or ratios of standardized mortality or morbidity e.g. standardised mortality ratio (SMR)
- calculating years of life lost before a given age (e.g. before age 70) in the studied population, perhaps by risk factor or condition
- calculating and comparing life tables and life expectancy

One challenge is analysing data on both mortality and morbidity patterns together. Chronic conditions such as arthritis and depression cause a great deal of disability, but relatively few deaths. A number of methods of measuring and comparing the burden of disease by suitably combining disability and death data have been developed, including:

- disability free life expectancy[6]
- disability-adjusted life years (DALYs*)[7,8] (see Figure 1.4.2)

On occasions, data from different systems can be linked if a unique or probabilistic identifier is available (see chapter 5.2).

Geographical information systems[9] can be used to map differences in any of the risk or health status measures.

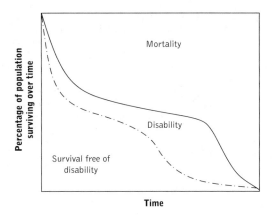

Figure 1.4.2 Disability-adjusted life years over time. (Adapted from Murray, Salomon, and Mathers.[9])

Carry out a local study, if necessary

Health issues can be sufficiently pressing and the available data so limited that a case exists for conducting a specific study, with fresh data collection. At national or state level, this situation arises relatively frequently. At local level, a survey or longitudinal study should only be carried out if time is available and the value of the data to be provided justifies the cost. Again, it is essential to be clear about the purpose. There is always a tendency to ask too many interesting questions or record too many findings. As well as being unnecessarily expensive, this may reduce the response rate, for example if a questionnaire appears too complex. Key features of a successful survey are:

- clear aim
- well designed, with enough statistical power to address the studied issue
- good instrument selection, ensuring measures are valid and reliable
- good planning and management of the study logistics and resources, including interviewer training and data recording
- adequate arrangements for timely data entry, analysis, and reporting.

Communicate results effectively

Occasionally a large set of data is produced for reference purposes, for subsequent expert analysis. But usually the information is used to inform the process of identifying opportunities to improve health, and while experts may be involved, the information usually needs to be communicated to a general audience. The communication methods required need careful consideration and co-ordination. This becomes most apparent when communicating with the press (see chapters 3.5 and 7.4).

When communicating results, a full description of the analytical methods used together with their limitations and assumptions may well be inappropriate. If so, the assessor must take great care to provide a fair assessment and ensure that the typical audience will gain the right impression (for example by resisting the temptation to use a false origin for a bar chart, even if it spoils the impact). The assessor must however be prepared and able to justify the methods in detail if requested.

Key points about health status analyses to consider in a written or oral communication are:

+ think through its purpose

+ don't leave it to the reader to deduce relevant points from a mass of data—quote specific data to make a point

+ ensure confidentiality for participants in surveys, and ensure this is made clear to everyone

+ don't be too sophisticated—many people in the target audience will not have much background knowledge of the issue.

Evaluate your health status assessment

Those of us engaged in public health emphasize the importance of assessment to others. This should begin at home. It is important that our work is assessed using tools such as audit—perhaps using the headings of this section.

Further resources

Last JM (1998). *Public health and human ecology.* Appleton and Lange, Stamford, Connecticut.

McDowell I and Newell C (1996). *Measuring health. A guide to rating scales and questionnaires.* Oxford University Press, New York.

Murray SA and Graham LJC (1995). Practice based health needs assessment. *BMJ*, **310**, 1443–8.

Stevens A and Raftery J (ed.) (1997). *Health care needs assessment*, (2nd series). Radcliffe Medical Press, Oxford.

Streiner DL and Norman GR (1995). *Health measurement scales: a practical guide to their development and use*, (2nd edn). Oxford University Press, Oxford.

Wright J (ed.) (1998). *Health needs assessment in practice.* BMJ Books, London.

References

1. WHO (1998). *Health promotion glossary*. World Health Organization, Geneva. WHO/HPR/HEP/98.1 www.who.int/hpr/docs/glossary.pdf (accessed 9 August 2000).

2. Ruwaard D, Kramers PGN, Berg Jeths A van den, and Achterberg PW (1994). *Public health status and forecasts: the health status of the Dutch population over the period 1950–2010*. National Institute of Public Health and Environmental Protection, Bilthoven, the Netherlands. The Hague: Sdu Uitgeverij, pp. 30–3.

3. Stevens A and Gillam S (1998). Needs assessment: from theory to practice. *BMJ*, **316**, 1448–52.

4. Ruwaard D, Kramers PGN, Berg Jeths A van den, and Achterberg PW (1994). *Public health status and forecasts: the health status of the Dutch population over the period 1950–2010*. National Institute of Public Health and Environmental Protection, Bilthoven, the Netherlands. The Hague: Sdu Uitgeverij, pp. 159–61.

5. Peto R, Lopez AD, Boreham J, Thun M, and Heath C Jr (1992). Mortality from tobacco in developed countries: indirect estimation from national vital statistics. *Lancet*, **339(8804)**, 1268–78.

6. Robine JM, Romieu I, and Cambois E (1999). Health expectancy indicators. *Bull World Health Org.*, **77(2)**, 181–5.

7. Morrow RH, Hyder AA, Murray CJ, and Lopez AD (1998). Measuring the burden of disease. *Lancet*, **352(9143)**, 1859–61.

8. Murray CJ and Lopez AD (1997). Global mortality, disability, and the contribution of risk factors: Global Burden of Disease Study. *Lancet*, **349(9063)**, 1436–42.

9. Murray CJL, Salomon JA, and Mathers C (2000) A critical examination of summary measures of population health. *Bull World Health Org*, **78(8)**, 981–94.

10. de Lepper MJC, Scholetn HJ, and Stern RM (ed.) (1995). *The added value of geographical information systems in public and environmental health*. Kluwer, Dordrecht. *(On behalf of the World Health Organization for Europe.)*

1.5 Assessing health needs

John Wright

Objectives of this chapter

Health needs assessment is a systematic method of identifying unmet health and health care needs of a population and making changes to meet these unmet needs. Health needs assessment is used to improve health and other service planning, priority setting, and policy development.

This chapter will describe why health needs assessment is important and what it means in practice. Most clinical health professionals are familiar with assessing the health needs of individual patients. Professional training and clinical experience teaches a systematic approach to this assessment, before starting treatment that the health professional believes to be effective. Such a systematic approach has often been missing in assessing the health needs of local or practice populations.

The following example (Box 1.5.1) shows what happens when you do a health needs assessment systematically. In this case, it revealed an inequitable matching of need and health care services.

Box 1.5.1 **Example 1: Epidemiological health needs assessment: coronary heart disease**[1]

Objective: To assess whether the use of health services by people with coronary heart disease reflected need.

Setting: Health district with a population of 530,000.

Methods: The prevalence of angina was determined by a validated postal questionnaire. Routine health data were collected on Standardised Mortality Ratios; admission rates for coronary heart disease and operation rates for angiography, angioplasty, and coronary heart disease. Census data were used to calculate Townsend scores to describe deprivation for electoral wards. Prevalence of angina and use of services were then compared with deprivation scores for each ward.

Results: Angina and mortality from heart disease were more common in wards with high deprivation scores. However, treatment by revascularization procedures was more common in more affluent wards.

Conclusion: The use of revascularization services was not commensurate with need. Steps should be taken to ensure health care is targeted to those who most need it.

Defining need

An understanding of health needs assessment requires a clear definition of need. Need, in the sense used in this chapter, implies the capacity to benefit from an intervention. 'To speak of a need is to imply a goal, a measurable deficiency from the goal and a means of achieving the goal'.[2]

Health needs assessment is not the same as population health status assessment (see chapter 1.4). Health needs assessment incorporates the concept of a capacity to benefit from an intervention. It therefore introduces an assessment of the effectiveness of relevant interventions to supplement the identification of health problems. Health needs assessment should also make explicit what benefits are being pursued by identifying needs for intervention.

Economists argue that the capacity to benefit is always greater than available resources and that health needs assessment should also incorporate questions of priority setting through considering the cost-effectiveness of the available interventions (see chapter 2.6).[3]

Approaches to needs assessment

A number of approaches to needs assessment have been suggested,[4] including:

- 'epidemiologically based' needs assessment—combining epidemiological approaches (specific health status assessments) with assessment of the effectiveness and possibly the cost-effectiveness of the potential interventions
- comparative—comparing levels of service receipt between different populations
- corporate—canvassing the demands and wishes of professionals, patients, politicians, and other interested parties.

In this chapter, an epidemiological and qualitative approach to determining priorities is explored. This incorporates clinical effectiveness, cost-effectiveness, and patients' perspectives.[5] While comparisons of health service usage are commonly used as indicators of needs, population-based usage rates typically vary markedly between areas, often for unexplained reasons. In addition, the links between usage rates and improved health outcomes is often hard to demonstrate.

The distinction between individual needs and the wider needs of the community is important to consider when assessing needs. If individual needs are ignored then there is a danger of a top down approach to providing health and other services, reflecting what a few people perceive to be the needs of the population, rather than what they actually are.

Health needs assessment involves the active identification of need rather than a passive response to demand. Health needs can be differentiated into needs, demands, and supply and are not restricted to health care needs. Health needs include wider social and environmental determinants of health such as deprivation, housing, diet, education, and employment. Health needs should ideally be 'met', but also may be unmet (e.g. waiting lists, undiagnosed hypertension, ignored moderate depression) or 'overmet' (e.g. prescribing antibiotics for sore throats).

Box 1.5.2 **Different aspects of health needs**

Felt needs: what people consider and/or say they need
Expressed needs: needs expressed by action e.g. visiting a doctor
Normative needs: what health professionals define as need

Assessing health needs provides the opportunity for:

• assessing the population's health status (see chapter 1.4), describing the patterns of disease in the local population and the differences from district, regional, or national disease patterns

• learning more about the needs and priorities of patients and the local population

• highlighting areas of unmet need and providing a clear set of objectives to work towards to meet these needs

• deciding rationally how to use resources to improve the local population's health in the most effective and efficient way

• influencing policy, interagency collaboration, or research and development priorities.

Importantly, it also provides a method of monitoring and promoting equity in the provision and use of health services and addressing inequalities in health (see chapter 6.7).[6]

A framework for assessing the health needs of a population

Box 1.5.3 summarizes the questions or steps involved in a formal health needs assessment project. The process seldom follows a simple linear progress through the steps—often needs assessments develop from several steps concurrently. Health needs assessment can be approached in much the same way as doing a jigsaw, so that different pieces are put together to give a complete picture of local health.

Box 1.5.3 **Questions to be answered in a formal health needs assessment project**

1. *What is the problem?* Identify the health problem to be addressed in the defined population.

2. *What is the size and nature of the problem?* Carry out a health status assessment for the population, covering the relevant areas of ill-health and/or potential health gain.

3. *What are the current services?* Identify the existing services and interventions being delivered, including, where relevant, the service targeting, quality, effectiveness, and efficiency.

4. *Identify interventions by asking what patients want.* Consult.

5. *Identify interventions by reviewing the scientific knowledge.* Find and appraise.

6. *Consult professionals and other stakeholders.*

7. *What are the most cost-effective solutions?*

8. *What are the resource implications?* Choose between competing ways of meeting needs (competing interventions) and decide on competing priorities—resources are always limited.

9. *What are the recommendations and the plan for implementation?*

10. *What are the outcomes to evaluate change?* Identify the expected health gains.

Needs assessment needs careful preparation

Undertaking needs assessment involves identifying the right issue, using the right technical methods, and managing the process effectively. Start with attention to defining the task. Objectives should be clarified and should be as simple and focused as possible. Care should be taken not to raise over-ambitious expectations. The right project team should be convened, with all relevant stakeholders, including (as relevant to the issue) the service funders, the clinicians, and the users (public involvement) (see chapter 8.2). Good leadership is important (see chapter 7.1), as is clear and effective communication during the project, especially if there is multi-agency involvement. Access to relevant information and informants should be sought at an early stage.

What is the health issue?

The health problem on which to focus the needs assessment exercise should be clearly identified. A health problem may come to attention from many sources, including the results of a population health status assessment, input from patients or stakeholders, government priority setting, or the scientific and professional literature.

An initial clarification of the issues can be valuable. A first step in clarifying the definition of the needs problem is a search of the health and social science databases for the topic. A review of the published health literature will provide a national and international perspective about the health topic and provide methods and results (for example case definitions, disease incidence and prevalence, current provision of health services) that may be applicable to the local population.[7] A search of grey literature sources (for example public health professional bodies and government health department databases) can also provide useful models and information.

After initial clarification, it should become apparent whether the problem justifies a full and systematic needs assessment.

What is the size and nature of the problem?

With a working definition of the health problems in mind, relevant health status data can then be collected. This should aim to establish:

- how many people in the studied population are likely to be suffering from the target condition or conditions
- what their characteristics are
- to what extent they are already receiving appropriate interventions.

Accurately estimating how many people would benefit from each of the potential interventions is desirable but often difficult. Previous chapters provide a guide to sources of information.

What are the current services?

There are several sources of data on health care in the locality. Hospital activity data can provide information on hospital admissions, diagnoses, length of stay, operations performed, and patient characteristics. Clinical indicators can provide information on the comparative performance of hospitals and health authorities.

Health care provision (e.g. numbers of family doctors per capita; number of operations per capita) is often compared to national or international norms, although there is rarely evidence of a link between provision and health outcome.

What do professionals, patients, and other stakeholders want?

Consult a wide range of stakeholders to describe local health needs. Local health professionals in primary and secondary care will have valuable contributions to make about the health needs of their local community. Other stakeholders such as health authorities, local government agencies, and voluntary groups are also important contributors, not only for their knowledge and beliefs, but also to engage them in the assessment and encourage ownership and eventual implementation of the results.

Consult users, carers, and the public (see chapter 8.2). Health services have been historically weak at involving users and the public in decision making about local health care. With increasing recognition of the importance of obtaining greater public involvement, various methods have been used, including:[8]

- *citizens' juries*: Local people who are representative of the population are selected to sit on a jury for a specified period of time. Members are presented with information from different experts on health topics and debate the issues surrounding them

- *health panels*: Standing panels of local people representative of population. These can be large (>1000 people) panels which are surveyed at regular intervals about key health issues, or smaller panels where the members meet and discuss different topics. Members are replaced at regular intervals

- *focus groups*: Groups of 6–12 participants with a facilitator who encourages discussion about health topics, which is recorded on tape or by an observer

- *interviews*: Interviews with randomly or purposefully selected individuals to canvass their views and opinions. Users, carers, or other stakeholders (e.g. community leaders) can all be valuable contributors

- *questionnaires*: These allow structured information to be collected from a large sample of local people on one or more health topics. Such surveys can provide information on user satisfaction, perceived needs, and use of health services. Other generic health measures such as quality of life scores,[9] or disease specific measures can also be included.

What are the most appropriate and cost-effective interventions?

An essential part of a health needs assessment is the review of the clinical effectiveness and cost effectiveness of interventions that can address the identified health needs. Evidence about the effectiveness of health interventions or services can be found in databases of good quality systematic reviews such as the Cochrane Library,[10] or publications such as the *Effective Health Care Bulletins*.[11] The United States Agency for Healthcare Research and Quality[12] and its National Guidelines Clearinghouse[13] can also be good source of effectiveness information, and information on professional consensus on treatment. Where there is limited evidence of effectiveness of interventions then professional consensus about best practice may have to be relied on.

What are the resource implications?

If needs are to be matched to limited available resources so that as much need as possible is met, then economic appraisal, including cost effectiveness information, must be considered. At a practical level this involves:[14]

- determining how resources are currently spent (programme budgeting—see chapter 2.6)
- defining options for change (marginal analysis) by specifying alternatives:
  (a) identify potential services for more resources
  (b) identify services which could be provided at the same level of effectiveness but at reduced cost, releasing resources for (a)
  (c) identify services which are less cost effective than those identified in (a)
- assessing the costs and benefits of the principal options
- decide on the best option, aiming to increase investment in (a) and reduce investment in services identified in (b) and (c).

The second example in this chapter (see Box 1.5.4) shows how the needs assessment process can help plan services, using generalizable research and local surveys involving users.

Implementation

In drawing a needs assessment together, the collected information should be collated, analysed, and presented, usually in report form. A summary of key findings is very useful in communicating the results to the decision makers and those who will be affected by the decisions.

Reporting results however is not an end in itself. This is where too many health needs assessments end, when they should only just be beginning. Building agreement to a practical implementation plan for meeting the unmet needs is an essential part of needs assessment.

Does assessing need create change?

Factors that will increase the likelihood of needs assessment leading to change are:

- consideration of the potential resource implications of the assessment from the beginning (discussion between commissioners and assessors)
- methodological rigour to ensure the results are valid and believed
- ownership of the project by relevant stakeholders from the start and effective involvement during the work
- effective dissemination of the results (see chapter 6.9)

* the existence of a practical plan for implementing the necessary actions to partly or fully meet the identified unmet needs.

Box 1.5.4 **Example 2: Needs-based services for people with multiple sclerosis[15]**

Background: With rising health care costs, limited resources, and the move to a needs-led health care system it has become increasingly important to purchase and plan health services that match resources to patient needs. The aim of this study was to assess the health needs of a community-based cohort of people with multiple sclerosis (MS) in the metropolitan city of Leeds and to define the current service provision.

Methods: Work undertaken included a systematic review of the literature; focus groups with people with MS and their carers; in-depth interviews with representatives of service providers, purchasers, and voluntary organizations; and in-depth interviews with 30 people with MS randomly selected from the Leeds population-based register and stratified according to age, gender, household, duration of MS, and disease course.

Results: Five major themes emerged: information needs, emotional support for people with MS and their families, access to services (particularly respite care and rehabilitation services), increasing public awareness of MS, and maintaining independence.

Outcome: This health needs assessment provided a framework for reorganization of the services provided for people with MS in Leeds. A Patient Information Group was established for new diagnoses. An Information Resource Centre was set up for patients and carers. Patient-held records are being piloted. A dedicated MS clinic with multi-disciplinary input is now operational.

Conclusion

Health needs are not static, and any assessment will only provide a snapshot of the needs of the local population. These needs and the health and social care services that try to address them are always changing and it is important to return to the assessment work, to review it and update it, and to evaluate the impact it has had.

Further resources

Murray SA (1999). Experiences with 'rapid appraisal' in primary care: involving the public in assessing health needs, orientating staff, and educating medical students. *BMJ*, 3(**18**), 440–4.

National Health Service Management Executive (1991). Assessing health care need. Department of Health, London.

Wright J (1998). *Health needs assessment in practice*. BMJ Books, London.

References

1. Payne N and Saul C (1997). Variations in use of cardiology services in a health authority: comparison of coronary artery revascularisation rates with prevalence of angina and coronary mortality. *BMJ*, **314**, 256–61.
2. Wilkin D, Hallam L, and Dogget M (1992). *Measures of need and outcomes in primary health care*. Oxford Medical Publications, Oxford.
3. Donaldson C and Mooney G (1991). Needs assessment, priority setting, and contracts for healthcare: an economic view. *BMJ*, **303**, 1529–30.
4. Stevens A and Raftery J (ed.) (1997). *Health care needs assessment*, (2nd series). Radcliffe Medical Press, Oxford.
5. Wright J, Williams DRR, and Wilkinson J (1998). The development of health needs assessment. In *Health needs assessment in practice*, (ed. J Wright), pp. 1–11. BMJ Books, London.
6. Rawaf S and Bahl V (1998). *Assessing health needs of people from minority ethnic groups*. Royal College of Physicians, London. www.rcplondon.ac.uk (accessed 10 August 2000).
7. Stevens and Raftery 1997, Rawaf and Bahi 1998, 4 and 6 above.
8. Jordan J, Dowswell T, Harrison S, Lilford R, and Mort M (1998). Whose priorities? Listening to users and the public. *BMJ*, **316(7145)**, 1668–70.
9. Bowling A (1997). *Measuring health: a review of quality of life measurement scales*, (2nd edn). Open University Press, Buckingham.
10. Cochrane Library. www.update-software.com/ (accessed 27 July 2000).
11. Royal Society of Medicine Press. *Effective Health Care Bulletins*. www.york.ac.uk/inst/crd/ehcb.htm (accessed 26 July 2000).†
12. The United States Agency for Healthcare Research and Quality. www.ahrq.gov/ (accessed 25 January 2001).
13. National Guidelines Clearinghouse. www.guideline.gov/index.asp (accessed 27 July 2000).
14. Scott A and Donaldson C (1998). Clinical and cost effectiveness issues in health needs assessment. In *Health needs assessment in practice*, (ed. J Wright), pp. 84–94. BMJ Books, London.
15. Ford HL and Gerry EM (1999). Needs based services for people with MS. *Multiple Sclerosis*, **5**, S48.

....

† EHCBs are bi-monthly publications for decision makers which examine the effectiveness of a variety of health care interventions. They are based on a systematic review and synthesis of research on the clinical effectiveness, cost-effectiveness, and acceptability of health service interventions. This is carried out by a research team using established methodological guidelines, with advice from expert consultants for each topic. The bulletins are subject to extensive and rigorous peer review (accessed 26 July 2000).

1.6 Assessing health impacts on a population

Alex Scott Samuel, Kate Ardern, and
Martin Birley

Objectives

By reading this chapter you will become familiar with:

- emerging concepts of health impact assessment (HIA)*
- emerging methods of HIA
- an approach to conducting comprehensive prospective HIAs on major public policies, programmes, and projects.

Definition

Health impact assessment is 'the estimation of the overall effects, of a specified action on the health of a defined population'.[1] The actions concerned may range from projects (e.g. a housing development) to programmes (e.g. urban regeneration) to policies (e.g. integrated transport strategy).

HIA builds on the generally accepted understanding that a wide range of economic, social, psychological, environmental, and organizational influences determine a community's health. It is important to try to estimate the effects of these influences on health. Ideally, such work should be *prospective* and so should precede the start of the project, programme, or policy concerned.

The aims of prospective HIA are:

- to assess the potential health impacts, both positive and negative, of projects, programmes, and policies
- to improve the quality of public policy decisions by making recommendations that are likely to enhance predicted positive health impacts and minimize negative ones.

The importance of health impact assessment

Health impact assessment is an important public health method as it:

- focuses on social and environmental justice (it is usually the already disadvantaged who suffer most from negative health impacts)
- involves a multi-disciplinary, participatory approach
- involves positive encouragement of public participation in the debate about public health issues and public policy or planning issues

- gives equal status to qualitative and quantitative assessment methods
- makes values and politics explicit and opens the issues to public scrutiny
- demonstrates that health is far broader than health care issues
- improves the quality of decision making in health and partner organizations by incorporating the need to address health issues positively into planning and policy making.

Health impact assessment is increasingly being adopted internationally:

Europe

There is considerable interest in HIA in the European Community, with pressure from the European Parliament to incorporate it into the development of all EU policy. In Sweden, HIA has been used at a local government level to assist in achieving local public health targets and in pointing the way to 'healthier' decision making.[2] The WHO European Centre for Health Policy, together with other European partners, has initiated a project to bring together available experience and try to reach a degree of consensus on how HIA can best be used to improve health policy development. More specifically, the project is designed to:

- clarify the basic concepts and reach consensus on the definitions of the main terms used
- review and learn from the existing models and methods of health impact assessment
- define appropriate principles and approaches to the implementation of health impact assessment
- test and evaluate these in a number of pilot countries and regions, and revise the suggested approaches accordingly.[3]

Canada and Australia

Canada and some Australian states have well-developed HIA programmes. In Canada, HIA has been incorporated into the legislative framework. The approach used is consistent with what has evolved in NW England and Sweden—namely that HIA should be viewed as an extension of the well-established environmental impact assessment (EIA) which links HIA to planning decisions.[4] HIA has been conducted in developing countries over a number of years. The World Health Organization and the World Bank have expressed an interest in its application to their work.

United Kingdom

The UK government is strongly committed to the principle of prospective HIA. The UK White Papers on public health strategy have referred to the requirement for health impact assessment of both national and local policies and projects.[5] The Scottish Needs Assessment Programme has produced a review of piloting the process in Scotland and also reports of two pilot studies on a housing strategy and a transport strategy.[6] Further emphasis has been given by the introduction of a new duty on local authorities to promote the economic, social, and environmental well-being of their areas, in partnership with all relevant local interests. Health impact assessment of policies and projects has also been included in the evaluation process for the government's area-based neighbourhood regeneration initiative—New Deal for Communities.[7] Most recently, HIA was recommended as good practice in the new National Service Framework for Coronary Heart Disease which set a target for all National Health Service organizations (health authorities, hospital and community trusts, and primary care groups/trusts) and Local Authorities by April 2001 to 'have a mechanism for ensuring that all new policies and all existing policies subject to review can be screened for health impacts'.[8]

The HIA process

Although HIA methods are still at an early phase in their development, initial indications are that HIA can draw attention to potential health impacts in a way which permits constructive changes to be made to project or policy proposals. This type of HIA needs to be distinguished from the established technical procedure (sometimes termed HRA or health risk assessment) employed retrospectively after chemical and other environmental incidents, and also prospectively in emergency planning.

It is important to distinguish between *procedures* and *methods* for health impact assessment:

- procedures are frameworks for commissioning and implementing HIAs
- methods are the systems for carrying them out (see Figure 1.6.1).

Managing an HIA: procedures

There are four procedures in the HIA process:

(a) screening

(b) steering group and terms of reference

(c) negotiation of favoured options

(d) implementation, monitoring, and evaluation.

(a) Screening

The issues on which selection is based are shown in the figure. Potential projects, programmes, or policies should be rapidly assessed with regard to their likely performance in relation to each

Procedures **Methods**

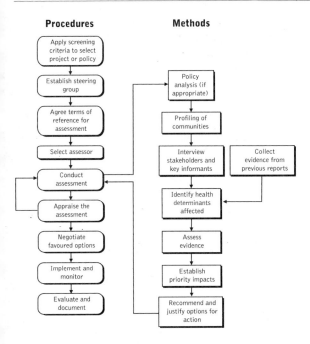

Figure 1.6.1 Stages in the HIA process. (© Scott-Samuel, Birley, and Arden.[9])

of these issues. While the procedure is necessarily crude, it can give a useful indication of how resources for HIA can be most effectively deployed. For the remainder of the description of procedures and methods, the term 'project' is used to refer to projects, programmes, or policies.

Health impact assessment screening procedure:

Economic issues

- the size of the project and of the population(s) affected
- the costs of the project, and their distribution

Outcome issues

- the nature of potential health impacts of the project
- the likely nature and extent of disruption caused to communities by the project
- the existence of potentially cumulative impacts

Epidemiological issues

- the degree of certainty (risk) of health impacts
- the likely frequency (incidence/prevalence rates) of potential health impacts
- the likely severity of potential health impacts
- the size of any probable health service impacts
- the likely consistency of 'expert' and 'community' perceptions of probability (i.e. risk), frequency, and severity of important impacts. The greater the agreement between expert and lay perceptions of important impacts, the greater the need for an HIA.

There is a general need to give greater priority to policies than to programmes, and to programmes than to projects, all other things being equal. (This is due to the broader scope—and hence potential impact—of policies as compared to programmes and to projects.)

The HIA is prospective wherever possible. Timing might be affected by planning regulations and other statutory frameworks, whether the project requires an Environmental Impact Assessment, and the relevance of the HIA to local decision making.

(b) Steering group and terms of reference

Following screening and project selection, a multi-disciplinary steering group should be established to agree the terms of reference of the HIA and to provide advice and support as it develops. Its membership should include representatives of the commissioners of the HIA, the assessors carrying it out, the project's proponents, affected communities, and other stakeholders as appropriate. Members should ideally be able to take decisions on behalf of those they represent.

(c) Negotiation of favoured options

The consideration of alternative options does not conclude the process. Even when there appear to be clear messages regarding the best way forward, it cannot be assumed that these will automatically be adopted. Achieving agreement on options for mitigating or enhancing predicted health impacts might require skilful negotiation on the part of those involved.

(d) Implementation, monitoring, and evaluation

HIA is analogous to an audit cycle in which the results of subsequent monitoring and evaluation in turn influence the continuing operation of the project. The indicators and methods proposed for monitoring will depend on the nature and content of the project, and also on the perceived importance of this stage of the assessment.

Outcome evaluation is constrained by the degree of success of the HIA; negative impacts which have been successfully avoided (or weakly positive ones which have been successfully enhanced) due to the modification of the project will clearly not be identifiable. In practice, things are rarely this perfect and it may be possible to construct and compare notional and actual outcomes relating to the proposed and actual projects. Multi-method assessments of specified outcomes (triangulation) should be undertaken where feasible, in order to increase validity.

Process evaluation involves the assessment of the HIA procedures against the terms of reference initially agreed by the Steering Group and the assessment of the extent to which agreed recommendations of the HIA were implemented.

Methods of assessing health impacts

The range of methods and of approaches to HIA should reflect the nature and complexity of the subject matter. It is important to use all methods and involve all disciplines that may contribute to the overall task:

(a) policy analysis

(b) profiling of affected areas/communities

(c) identification of potential positive and negative health impacts

(d) assessments of perceived health risks

(e) quantification and valuation of health impacts

(f) ranking the most important impacts

(g) consideration of alternative options and recommendations.

(a) Policy analysis

HIAs of policies will require initial policy analysis to determine key aspects that the HIA will need to address; this may build on or use material already available from earlier policy development work. Key aspects include:

• content and dimensions of the policy

• socio-political and policy context

• policy objectives, priorities, and intended outputs

• trade-offs and critical socio-cultural impacts which may affect its implementation.

(b) Profiling of affected areas/communities

A profile of the areas and communities likely to be affected by the project is compiled using available socio-demographic and health data and information from key informants. The profile should include an assessment of the nature and characteristics of groups whose health could be enhanced or placed at risk by the project's effects. Vulnerable and disadvantaged groups require special consideration. Public participation throughout the HIA is essential, both to ensure that local concerns are addressed and for ethical reasons of social justice (see chapter 8.2).

The process of HIA requires broad participation if a comprehensive picture of potential health impacts is to be established. The co-operation and expertise of a wide range of stakeholders and key informants will be needed, including:

- those involved in the project or who will be directly affected by it
- those who have knowledge or information of relevance to the project and its outcomes
- representative(s) of affected communities
- proponents of the project
- local or outside experts whose knowledge is relevant to the project
- relevant health professionals e.g. general practitioners, health visitors, social or community workers
- voluntary organizations.

(c) Identification of potential positive and negative health impacts

The range of potential health impacts identified in HIA is dependent on the definition of health that is employed. Consider using a socio-environmental model of health derived from the work of Lalonde[10] and Labonté.[11] Data collection involves qualitative methods including interviews, focus groups, and scenarios. We use a model of health impact assessment in which a policy, programme, or project changes the determinants of health and this, in turn, may change the health status of the affected communities.

The following table presents those determinants of health most often encountered in an HIA; wherever possible differential impacts on relevant population subgroups should be identified.

(d) Assessments of perceived health risks

Perceptions of risk are, when possible, recorded at the time of identification of potential impacts. In some instances existing evidence will permit precise assessment of risk. In many cases, however, risk assessment will be based on subjective perceptions. Assuming adequate sampling, such subjective risk data are arguably no less valid or important than are more precise technical data—particularly where sensory perceptions (such as increased noise or smell, or deterioration of outlook) are concerned.

Risk perceptions can be recorded using simple three-point scales of measurability (potential impacts are characterized as qualitative, estimable, or calculable) and of certainty of occurrence (definite, probable, or speculative). The temptation to quantify such scales should be resisted—such numbers could not be compared with validity and would carry a spurious authority.

Table 1.6.1 Key areas influencing health encountered in health impact analysis.

Categories of influences on health	Examples of specific influences (health determinants)
Personal and family environment	family structure and functioning, primary/secondary/adult education, occupation, unemployment, income, risk-taking behaviour, diet, smoking, alcohol, substance misuse, exercise, recreation, means of transport (cycle/car ownership)
Social environment	culture, peer pressures, discrimination, social support/cohesion/capital (neighbourliness, social networks/isolation), community/cultural/spiritual participation
Physical environment	air, water, housing conditions, working conditions, noise, smell, view, public safety, civic design, shops (location/range/quality), communications (road/rail), land use, waste disposal, energy, local environmental features
Public services	access to (location/disabled access/costs) and quality of primary/community/secondary health care, child care, social services, housing/leisure/employment/public transport/law and order/other health-relevant public services/non-statutory agencies and services

(e) Quantification and valuation of health impacts

It may prove possible to assess the size of quantifiable impacts at the time they are identified by informants; in others, this will require to be done separately—e.g. through reviews of previously published evidence. The same applies to valuation—though evidence on the resource implications and opportunity costs of potential impacts will often prove hard to come by. However, such data can in principle be made comparable using QALYs,* DALYs,* or other such measures (see chapter 2.6).

(f) Ranking the most important impacts

Informants should be encouraged to prioritize or rank those potential impacts that they identify. Once all the initial evidence has been collected, a priority-setting exercise should be carried out. Because of differential perceptions of risk there will rarely be complete consensus; criteria may need to be agreed so that the views of all informants are adequately reflected.

(g) Consideration of alternative options and recommendations for management of priority impacts

A series of options, to provide the optimum health impact of the project being assessed, should be defined and presented. The final result will be an agreed set of recommendations for modifying the project such that its health impacts are optimized—in the context of the many and complex constraints which invariably constitute the social, material, and political environment in which it will be undertaken.

Recommendations should cover the following issues:

- the stage(s) of project development or operation when the recommendation will be implemented
- the precise timing of implementation
- the health determinants which will be affected by implementation
- the nature of these effects and the probability that they will occur
- the agencies that will implement and fund the implementation of the recommendation
- the technical adequacy of the recommendation
- the social equity and acceptability of the recommendation
- the costs of the recommendation—direct/indirect; capital/revenue; fixed/variable; financial /economic
- how the implementation of the recommendation will be monitored.

On some occasions, the recommendation might include the option of not proceeding with the project.

Key issues in HIA

HIA is not strictly a science although it draws on a scientific knowledge base. Each HIA is uniquely located in time, space, and local conditions—though its evidence base can be evaluated, and the rigour with which procedures and methods were implemented can (and should) be assessed.

Uncertainties encountered during the undertaking of HIAs will frequently dictate the need to make assumptions: these are acceptable as long as they are stated explicitly.

HIA should take place early enough in the development of a project to permit constructive modifications to be carried out prior to its implementation, but late enough for a clear idea to have been formed as to its nature and content.

The financial and opportunity costs of undertaking health impact assessment dictate the need both to screen potential candidate projects and also to have a range of methods available according to the depth of analysis required.

Political imperatives may ultimately determine the outcome. Disagreements or power inequalities between different stakeholder factions may be similarly important.

Further resources

Birley MH (1995). *The health impact assessment of development projects.* HMSO, London.

Birley MH, Gomes M, and Davy A (1997). *Health aspects of environmental assessment.* The Environmental Division, The World Bank, Washington DC.

International Association for Impact Assessment. www.iaia.org/ (accessed 21 August 2000).

Lock K (2000). Health impact assessment. *BMJ,* **320,** 1395–8.

NHS Executive London (2000). *A short guide to health impact assessment—informing health decisions.* NHS Executive London, London. www.londonshealth.gov.uk (accessed 21 August 2000).

UK Department of Health (October 1999). *Health impact assessment: report of a methodological seminar.* www.doh.gov.uk/research/documents/rd2/health-impact.pdf (accessed 11 August 2000).

The International Health Impact Consortium has useful national and international links and an e-mail discussion group: www.liv.ac.uk/lstm/ihia.htm (accessed 29 April 2001).

Will S, Ardern K, Spencely M, and Watkins S (1994). *A prospective health impact assessment of the proposed development of a second runway at Manchester International Airport.* Written submission to the public inquiry. Manchester and Stockport Health Commissions.

References

1. Scott-Samuel A (1998). Health impact assessment—theory into practice. *JECH,* **52,** 74–5.
2. The Federation of Swedish County Councils (1998). *How can the health impact of policy decisions be assessed?* Federation of Swedish County Councils, Stockholm.
3. WHO Regional Office for Europe and the European Centre for Health Policy (December 1999). *Health impact assessment: the Gothenburg Consensus Paper.* European Centre for Health Policy, Brussels.
4. Birley MH, Boland A, Davies L, Edwards RT, Glanville H, Ison E, Millstone E, Osborn D, Scott-Samuel A, and Treweek J (1998). *Health and environmental impact assessment: an integrated approach.* Earthscan/British Medical Association, London.
5. Secretary of State for Health (1998). *Saving lives: our healthier nation.* The Stationery Office, London.
6. Scottish Needs Assessment Programme (May 2000). *HIA: piloting the process in Scotland.* Scottish Needs Assessment Programme, Glasgow.
7. UK Department of Environment, Transport and the Regions (1998). *New deal for communities.* HMSO, London.
8. UK Department of Health (March 2000). *Our healthier nation: national service framework for coronary heart disease. Chapter 1: Reducing heart disease in the population,* pp. 6,11,12, 18. Department of Health, London.

9. Scott-Samuel A, Birley MH, and Ardern K (1998). *The Merseyside guidelines for Health Impact Assessment.* The Merseyside Health Impact Assessment Steering Group. Liverpool Public Health Observatory, Liverpool.

10. Lalonde M (1974). *A new perspective on the health of Canadians.* Ministry of Supply and Services, Ottawa.

11. Labonté R (1993). *Health promotion and empowerment: practice frameworks.* Centre for Health Promotion, University of Toronto and Particip-Action, Toronto.

Part 2
Options and decisions

Introduction

People who dislike decisions should not become public health practitioners. Sometimes there appears to be only one option—a single case of meningitis necessitates some action, but what action? Even when the initial decision is easy to take, others follow which are more subtle and challenging. The first decision is whether or not there is a public health problem to be tackled, and not all problems that affect populations are appropriate problems for public health practitioners or departments alone. Often the issue has to be examined from different perspectives to understand what is actually going on. Trouble on a housing estate, for example, high levels of crime, violence and environmental decay, combined with social deprivation, flare up one hot summer's day and make local and national headlines. Obviously the health of that population is affected both in the long term and in the short term. Is this a public health problem, an economic problem, or a political problem? Or, to be more precise, what should a public health practitioner or department do?

Coping with multiple realities

The civil engineer who is told to build a bypass has a relatively simple task, although environmental protesters may prick their conscience and disturb the equanimity of a modern macro project.

The choices an engineer has to make are relatively simple, based on cost and safety. Public health options have to take into account a wide range of different types of factor such as:

- the needs of the population and the relative importance of different problems

- the evidence about the cost-effectiveness of different options

- the values of the population and the ethical basis of those values.

Choices in public health therefore have to be based upon the integration of economics, evidence, and ethics, and they are rarely easy or clear-cut, particularly because public health so often has to manage a mess.

Managing messes

Many of the great achievements of nineteenth-century public health were made on the principle that disorder and mess were the causes of disease, and anything that was offensive to the senses, to the eyes or the nose or the taste buds, was *ipso facto* harmful to health; the word 'nuisance', which we use as a relatively trivial problem today derives from the Old French '*nuire*', to harm, and the concept of the nuisance was at the heart of the nineteenth-century public health revolution. Today public health is also involved in what management theorists call 'messes'—highly complex problems with two managerial characteristics:

- there is no ideal solution, and
- every solution creates further problems.

Increasing the price of cigarettes reduces consumption but also increases smuggling; the pedestrianization of a city centre may cause problems for people with disabilities; partnerships with major supermarket chains to improve the diet may widen the health gap between rich and poor.

Decisions, decisions, decisions

The public health professional, therefore, faces decisions every day, some of which have huge consequences. There has been a large literature on clinical decision making in the last decade; in this part of the book we focus on public health decision making to help the reader make better choices.

The part begins with two chapters that identify the steps needed for turning messy issues into answerable questions. When the questions and issues are clearer, chapters 3 and 4 detail the steps needed to find and appraise the evidence that should be one part of the decision-making process. Managing knowledge is at the heart of a public health practitioner's job; chapter 5 sets out the definition and infrastructure which frame this essential task. Evidence must be combined with a firm grasp of resources, values, and ethics, all of which are tackled in the last three chapters of this part of the handbook.

JAMG

2.1 Scoping public health problems

Gabriele Bammer

What does scoping mean?

Scoping is a process that has two components:

• the identification of all the dimensions of a public health issue

• the determination of which dimensions are central to the issue at hand and which are peripheral.

Why is scoping important?

It is important to have comprehensive understanding of a problem in order to see and appreciate the insights (often of others) that are integral to its solution. The aim of scoping is to broaden the view of the problem, to move us beyond our own perspectives and to help us see the problem through other eyes. It means that the approach taken to the problem is not limited to what we know and understand, but also incorporates the knowledge and understanding of others. Scoping encourages us to take a larger view so that we determine better strategies and priorities for approaching the problem. The problem becomes central, rather than our own expertise.

Scoping involves recognizing and respecting different points of view, especially in controversial areas. Paying attention to the range of arguments usually smoothes the path to compromise. Views often soften once people feel they have been respectfully heard. In addition, 'if it is clear that all reasonable alternatives are being seriously considered, the public will usually be more satisfied with the choice among them'.[1]

Scoping has become integral to the development of environmental impact statements and the process has been best documented in this context.[1,2,3] This chapter also draws on the experience of scoping the feasibility of a controversial treatment for heroin dependence.[4]

Objectives

This chapter provides tools for seeing public health problems more broadly, for dealing with competing views, and for setting priorities for addressing the problems. This will make public health practitioners more effective in turning problems into answerable questions and in turn being able to find workable solutions which have broad-based support (see chapter 2.2).

Eight important scoping questions

There are eight important questions to ask about any 'public health problem'. The first four questions can help identify the *dimensions* of the problem, while the last four can help set *priorities*.

Identifying the dimensions:

* what do we know about the problem?
* what areas are contentious?
* which interest groups and academic disciplines have or could be expected to have a useful perspective on this problem?
* what are the political and structural aspects of the problem—the big-picture issues?

And setting priorities:

* why is this problem on the agenda now? (don't confuse the urgent with the important)
* what support and resources are likely to be available for tackling the problem?
* what parts of the problem are already well covered and where are the areas of greatest need?
* where can the most effective, strategic interventions be made?

Identifying the dimensions of the problem

Finding out what is already known about the problem

* libraries, particularly specialist libraries, with experienced librarians, are an invaluable asset (see chapter 2.3)
* the internet provides copious information, but sorting the wheat from the chaff can be a challenge. The same problems apply to requests for assistance sent out through electronic mailing lists
* people with knowledge and know-how can save enormous amounts of time and different sorts of expertise may be relevant, including content, disciplinary approaches, and understanding of interest groups
* networks can be useful for identifying experts and can also be useful in providing general orientation. For example, support groups can put a human face on a problem or people that you know can provide a useful entry point. In my case, a neighbour who was a policeman was very helpful in explaining the hierarchy in the police service, as well as identifying the appropriate people to approach.

Dealing with areas of contention

While it can be tempting to avoid areas of contention, it is generally advisable to deal with them head on and early on. That allows you to get a balanced view of the controversy and to determine the framework in which it will be handled. Trying to avoid the controversy almost certainly means that you will, wittingly or unwittingly, align yourself with one side, which can make opening dialogue with the other side more difficult.

It is important to establish what is at the bottom of the controversy—is it a clash of egos between two important players, is it simple misunderstanding resulting from poor communication, or is there a fundamental difference in values? That will tell you if the controversy can be resolved, whether a compromise is likely, or if a stance supporting one side or the other is the only outcome. It helps greatly if you can be dispassionate and genuinely open to hearing all arguments.

Dealing with controversies is assisted if you can develop personal working relationships with the parties. People usually respond positively if they are treated as partners and if they feel confident that their views are heard and taken seriously. You need to ensure that this is both done and seen to be done. Then, even if people disagree with the outcome, they can be satisfied that the decision-making process was fair and, hopefully, both they and you will have learnt from it.[1]

Bringing together people who disagree can be helpful in some situations, but can inflame passions in others. It is probably only advisable to do this if you are confident that you can mediate a productive dialogue and that the players will enter a dialogue rather than using the meeting for grandstanding and pointscoring.

Working with interest groups and disciplines

Working with interest groups and disciplines other than your own is a learning experience and will enrich your approach to the problem. Interest groups will give you an 'on-the-ground' perspective and could include people affected by the problem and those who deal with it in one way or another (treatment and other service providers, families, work-mates, etc.). They can be particularly useful in identifying areas of unmet need and can provide a 'reality check' on the value of existing information.

Different disciplines have different ways of viewing the world and integrating these should also improve relevance and generalizability. In addition, different disciplines have different technical and methodological expertise; bringing these together can enhance the rigour of your approach to the problem.

Working with interest groups and different disciplines can also break down stereotypes and help the project to avoid entrenching or legitimizing misinformation.

The world-views that you will have access to may be unfamiliar and even threatening and you will need to find people who can orient you to these different perspectives and priorities. Personal and professional networks can be invaluable. Some experts may also be prepared to fulfil this function, but do not be put off by those who do not see that as their role. They will usually be prepared to help once you have put the effort into mastering the basics.

It can be useful to have a defined role for those you consult. Possible roles are as:

• collaborator (a partner with you in helping to define the project)

• member of an advisory group (who gives advice on the project overall)

• member of a reference group (who advises on just one aspect of the project).

A defined and acknowledged role is one way of publicly recognizing the contribution made to the scoping process; you should also consider if other forms of recognition and reward are warranted.[4]

Tackling big-picture issues

The influence of government policy, advertising, and business practice on public health issues deserves the same level of attention as individual behaviour, and changes here can be more far-reaching and effective. On the one hand, you should view these perspectives as you would those of any other interest group—something that you need to respectfully take into account. On the other hand you need to recognise the power imbalance and that the key players may not see the problem under consideration as being of any consequence or may not wish to legitimize your activity by participating in it.

You should find out who the key actors are, if there is any formal level of co-ordination and what level of authority the actors and co-ordinating group carry.[5] You should certainly try to involve players who can represent big-picture issues; do not assume that they will not be interested. They may well be aware of the problem and welcome an opportunity to be involved in dealing with it. But you do need to exercise extra caution, so that they do not hijack the agenda or find ways to bog the process down.

Setting priorities—what's central and what's peripheral?

(For a practical example of priority setting in health care, see chapter 6.1.)

The first task is to identify the boundaries for the scoping. Two questions should provide useful pointers:

• why is this problem on the agenda now?

• what support and resources are likely to be available for tackling the problem?

It will often be useful to develop a clear statement of the boundaries as a first step in the scoping process, although you might need to modify that statement or seek to renegotiate support and resources as you gather more information. It may also be useful to draft a timeline for activities, so that you keep the components of the task in perspective and to avoid getting bogged down.

Once you start to get some handles on the dimensions of the problem, the boundaries will assist in setting priorities, both in further investigation of the dimensions of the problem and in deciding where to concentrate your efforts in determining an action plan. These two questions should be useful here:

- what parts of the problem are already well covered and where are the areas of greatest need?
- where can the most effective strategic interventions be made?

Two commonly-used techniques for determining priorities are face-to-face meetings and the Delphi method. Face-to-face meetings can use a highly structured technique for narrowing down a problem or can involve a less formal process where issues are identified and ranked.[6] The Delphi method is a formal process originally devised for technological forecasting, which has been adapted to a range of problems requiring judgement. It is generally undertaken by correspondence, telephone, or computer conference.[7]

Can this be tackled systematically? Yes, iterate!

An iterative, rather than a linear process, usually works best when scoping a public health issue. However, there does have to be progression rather than going round in circles; the broad direction of progression should cover the following steps:

- establish the boundaries of the scoping
- find out what is known and what the areas of disagreement are
- set some priorities for further investigation of knowledge gaps and areas of disagreement
- document the relevant issues which need to be addressed and develop plans of action for workable solutions
- prioritize plans of action
- finalize one or more of the workable solutions
- reality test.

Attempting to work through this list in a linear fashion brings with it a real danger of getting bogged down, especially when charting unfamiliar territory. The judicious use of experts is crucial in saving time and keeping momentum. The challenge is to establish what is needed to put together an understanding of the problem, what you know and don't know, and who to bring in to fill the gaps. As new players are brought into the picture, their perspectives may lead you to revisit your understandings of what is known or the areas of disagreement or the priorities. You must be open to this, but you also need a clear sense of direction, so that you are not diverted by less relevant agendas which other players may have.

Back-to-back spirals are illustrative of the process—the outward expansion of the top spiral indicates the build up of knowledge and perspectives, whereas the inward direction of the second shows the knowledge and perspectives being used to set priorities. The loops illustrate revisiting what is known, bringing in other people who might have a useful perspective and so on. As Figure 2.1.1 illustrates, the starting point may be somewhat off-centre—in other words, your own knowledge and expertise may be limited, but the action plan should address central issues.

'Reality testing' can profitably be undertaken at several points. The aim here is to find holes in the knowledge base or the arguments on which priorities are based and, from this, to highlight where further data gathering or consultation needs to be undertaken. This is where advisory and reference groups can be invaluable, as they can be asked to comment along the way. Asking people to comment on written drafts is often the most efficient use of time and you should give clear instructions about what you are seeking comments on and on timelines for feedback. Although it seems elementary, the draft should be clearly written and spell-checked, so that the readers are not diverted from the main task by sloppiness and infelicities of expression.

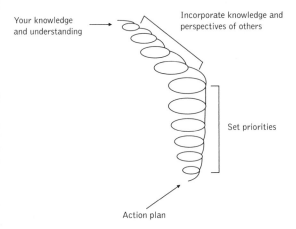

Figure 2.1.1 Broadening, aligning, and focussing perspectives.

What are the competencies needed for effective scoping?

There are no competencies specific to this area, but the following attributes are particularly important:[2,4,5]

+ integrity
+ credibility and a dispassionate approach
+ wide-ranging network of contacts, so that you know the key players or an intermediary
+ skill in facilitating meetings and interactions, including encouraging open debate and the challenging of ideas, handling negotiations and conflict
+ management skills
+ understanding of the 'cultures' of different interest groups and the ability to empathize with different concerns
+ the ability to identify which disciplines are relevant and enough knowledge about the disciplines to know what they can offer, to identify experts, and to involve experts in the problem
+ an understanding of relevant policies and other big-picture issues, their history, the key players and the political sensitivities
+ the ability to integrate a range of knowledge and expertise, to cut through to the essentials and to lead a priority-setting process.

What are the potential pitfalls in the scoping process?

It is important to realize that there are pitfalls. In particular:

+ not having enough resources to undertaken an adequate process
+ no real political commitment to understand and deal with the problem, for example when a process has been set in train for reasons of political expediency, so that the plug is pulled as soon as the political heat dies down
+ not being the right person for the job, for example if you are not interested in this process, not experienced enough to keep control, or if you hold a strong view about the problem and cannot deal with opposition respectfully
+ getting bogged down. Losing momentum and timeliness can be fatal. Beware of wallowing in factual detail, meetings without a clear purpose, and red herrings. Don't feel that you have to be on top of all the material—rely on experts who understand the interest group or disciplinary perspective
+ choosing inappropriate representatives of interest groups. Representatives must be knowledgeable and respected, (rather than from

the extreme wings of interest groups). Involving people in a process helps legitimize their point of view; you should think carefully about including fringe groups. If people who are not respected are included in the process, respected players may pull out or not participate fully

- having an inappropriate balance of interest groups or disciplines. The problem has to be seen in perspective, so that the process involves an appropriate mix of interest groups and academic disciplines, the powerful and the powerless and, for contentious issues, different points of view

- avoiding the contentious issues. Ignoring particular groups in an attempt to avoid contentious issues will often backfire, with their exclusion providing additional opportunity to further their cause or even undermining the outcomes of the process

- exhausting key players. Interest group representatives and experts from particular disciplines usually have a substantive job to do and they may get no recognition or credit for being involved in the scoping process. Use their time wisely, sparingly, and efficiently

- promoting conflict. Scoping processes that involve contentious issues usually seek to find compromise, but if the players are not chosen carefully and the process is not handled appropriately, conflict can be escalated rather than dampened down

- not showing leadership. If those in charge of the scoping process do not show leadership, the process is open to being hijacked by the more powerful participants. This can also be a factor in the promotion of conflict

- avoiding decisions. Never underestimate the temptation to not make a decision when the problem is difficult or contentious. Yield not to temptation!

- not being prepared to combat the wrath of the powerful. Many scoping processes will involve challenging entrenched power bases and provoking a reaction could well be a measure of success. Don't be naïve and do be prepared to counter these forces

- not learning from your mistakes

- not giving it a go unless there is a legitimate reason to avoid the problem, do not be put off by the difficulties.

This list of pitfalls looks daunting, but trying to solve the problem is better than avoiding it. Find experienced mentors, powerful allies, and supportive colleagues. If you don't give it a go, who will?

How will you know when you have been successful?

Once you have scoped and defined the problem, the overall markers of success are when your problem definition has:

- broad-based support

- clear and implementable steps for solution
- covmmitment from the key players and the interest groups they represent to stay involved in seeking a solution
- respect between opponents.

In specific circumstances, where a major power base has been challenged, and where the power base is seeking to protect its interests, measures of success include:

- a coalition, which includes people of influence, that will stand up to the power base and continue to fight for the solution
- openings for negotiation.

Conclusion

Scoping is a challenging process. It will use to the full your expertise and creative and political skills in public health. It is also a worthwhile investment to help maximize the impact of the limited resources of public health.

References

1. Executive Office of the President, Council on Environmental Quality (30 April 1981). *Memorandum for General Counsels, NEPA liaisons and participants in scoping.* ceq.eh.doe.gov/nepa/regs/scope/scoping.htm (accessed 16 August 2000).
2. Philippine Environmental Impact Statement System, Department of Environmental and Natural Resources (DENR) in Caraga. butuan.mozcom.com/~denr/EISsys.html (accessed 16 August 2000).
3. Purdue University, Environmental Assessment Resource Guide. pasture.ecn.purdue.edu/~agenhtml/agen521/epadir/earg/start.html (accessed 11 May 2001).
4. Bammer G (1997). Multidisciplinary policy research – an Australian experience. *Prometheus, 15,* 27–39.
5. Toth FL (1988). Policy exercises: procedures and implementation. *Simulation and Games, 19,* 256–76.
6. Emery M (1999). *Searching, the theory and practice of making cultural change.* John Benjamin Publisher, Amsterdam & Philadelphia.
7. Linstone HA and Turoff M (ed.) (1975). *The Delphi method, techniques and applications.* Addison-Wesley Publishing Co., Reading MA.

2.2 Turning public health problems into answerable questions

Ian Harvey

The scope of public health

Although public health is defined as 'the science and art of preventing disease, prolonging life and promoting health through the organized efforts of society',[1] this science and art can only be effected if the principles underpinning them are appreciated and understood:

- the emphasis on collective responsibility for health and the major role of the state in protecting and promoting the public's health
- a focus on whole populations
- an emphasis upon prevention, especially primary prevention
- a concern for the underlying socio-economic determinants of health and disease, as well as the more proximal risk factors
- a multi-disciplinary basis which incorporates quantitative and qualitative methods as appropriate
- partnership with the populations served.
  (*Adapted from Beaglehole and Bonita.*[2])

Its breadth is both its strength and its potential weakness. It grapples with the 'big issues' and so is quite different in approach and methods to individually-based health care. However, in so doing, its practitioners risk developing ideas and elaborations that tend to obscure a problem rather than to clarify it.[3]

How to avoid making issues more complex: general principles

> '*Far better an approximate answer to the right question* . . . . *than an exact answer to the wrong question*'[4].

Clear thinking is critical in public health. There are several vital steps to be taken in proceeding from the general awareness of public health problems through to taking well-targeted action:

- be aware that different groups will identify totally different public health problems affecting a given population. The extremes of view are often associated with professionals (health professionals and managers) on the one hand and consumers and communities on the other. Explore ways of collecting and prioritizing these diverse views[5]

- one of the most difficult steps in turning many public health problems into answerable questions is clearly defining what the problem is actually perceived to be. There will often be many different perceptions of this, depending on who is asked

- public health practitioners should never be afraid to use the challenging words—'why' and 'what'—both on themselves and on others. 'Why do you feel this is important?' 'What do you understand by this concept?' It can be helpful to try to write down in a few sentences the key questions that need to be addressed

- use a lateral thinking approach to properly explore what is really meant by apparently simple terms, such as 'deprivation' or 'poverty' or 'prioritize'

- before suddenly collecting or presenting data (whether quantitative or qualitative), ensure that the data will help you answer one or more of the questions you have posed. Avoid collecting 'orphan data'— data that have been collected without a clear idea of how they will be used—remembering that on occasion the act of collecting even orphan data may serve a useful wider purpose of allaying public concern

- pursue the questions that you have identified as important— avoid distracting side-issues

- remember the basic rules of traditional planning (see chapter 6.3 for alternative approaches)
  - where are we now?
  - where do we want to get to?
  - how do we get there? (both in terms of what action to take and how to get support for that action)

- remember that 'unless data are turned into stories that can be understood by all, they are not effective in any process of change'.[6]

Key steps in formulating answerable questions

Be realistic and pragmatic:

> ### Box 2.2.1
> 'As pure scientists, epidemiologists can remain tentative about the nature of associations. As public health specialists, however, judgements must be made in the absence of final proof in order to reduce the health risks to the public.'[2]

- think broadly. Recognize at the outset that intervening to modify the determinants of public health potentially embraces social, political, and environmental factors, lifestyle factors, issues of clinical effectiveness, access to clinical services, and genetics. All are legitimate public health areas

- decide first if there is a 'real' public health problem present at all. On occasion there may be an apparent rather than a real increase in disease occurrence. The most common reasons for this are:
  - pseudo-epidemics, for example, meningitis and birth defects attributable to increased ascertainment
  - changes in disease definition or coding practices
  - identification of 'at risk' populations *post hoc* after inspecting the data[7]
  - heightened awareness due to media publicity
- in some instances mass socio-genic illness can result as a spin-off of real public health problems (such as an 'epidemic' of illness in Belgium after drinking Coca-Cola believed at the time to be contaminated with dioxin).[8] Even artefactual public health problems need to be managed rigorously and account taken of differences between professional and lay approaches to risk
- what approach does the problem require?—a mainly data-based/ empirical approach or a predominantly organizational/social psychology approach? (An example of the latter would be a campaign to increase the proportion of children registered with a dentist)
- if an empirical element is helpful, should this involve quantitative data, qualitative data, or a mixture of the two? The best approach is to select methods solely on the basis of whether they are likely to produce the most valid and useful answer
- can already published data be used, or routinely available data? Will a rapid 'ethnographic' approach be useful to describe the size of the problem, for example in needs assessment? Is *ad hoc* data collection necessary, and if so what resources are required?

An example of turning an issue into a question

Suicide, especially in young men, has been identified as a growing public health problem in several countries, including the UK. The public health questions include:

Descriptive questions—to quantify the problem:

- how large is the problem?
- how great is the problem of under-ascertainment?
- what is the pattern of suicide rates subdivided by time, place, and person characteristics?
- what proportion of suicide victims have had contact with caring agencies in a defined period before the event?

Analytical questions—to identify options:

- to what degree is previous deliberate self-harm a risk marker for later suicide?

- to what extent are substance misuse, unemployment, and poor social support risk factors for suicide?

- what suicide-prevention interventions have been shown to be effective in the published literature?

- what plausible suicide-prevention measures have yet to be evaluated, and how should they be evaluated?

Managerial questions—to plan the intervention:

- which agencies need to be included in any systematic efforts to reduce suicide rates?

- which agencies will tend to be enthusiastic about such an initiative and which not?

- how can such scepticism be overcome?

Specific public health questions

- '*What is causing this public health problem?*' Here the focus is on trying to work out what the mechanism is that is causing the problem. A classic example is an outbreak of infectious disease, the archetypal vehicle for applied epidemiology. Such epidemiological detective work requires hypotheses to be developed (generated from descriptive data (e.g. time, place, and person breakdown), from the history taken from patients, and by the investigator in the light of prior knowledge). These hypotheses can then be tested, typically using either a case control or cohort study approach. Finally practical action needs to be taken—such as the closure of a food outlet, in the case of food-borne disease. Perhaps the best recent examples of this detective work have been the elucidation of the causes of such conditions as AIDS and Toxic Shock syndrome.

- '*How do we alleviate this problem? What effective action can be taken?*' A good example is the case of social class inequalities in health, which are by common consent viewed as unjust. Much energy has been devoted to describing the extent of these and many reports have been produced in the UK alone, but less is known about how to counteract these inequalities. What is required to begin to answer this question are systematic reviews of the published literature (to summarize what we already know), supplemented with further evaluative research (to fill in the many gaps). Systematic reviews are now being produced and are beginning to provide a stronger evidential basis for public health activities aimed at reducing inequalities.[9] Among the interventions identified as effective are those aimed at reducing unwanted pregnancy among teenage girls and mentoring of disadvantaged first-time mothers by experienced mothers to improve immunization uptake and enhance mothers' self-esteem.

Public health questions—scientific and socio-political

The most effective public health practitioners are both scientists and change agents. Turning issues into questions that lead to a combination of data and oratory is a key skill in public health practice. Every public health problem should therefore lead to both:

• *scientific/technical questions* (what causes lung cancer?) and
• *socio-political questions* (who are the key people who will need persuading?).

The latter can involve such techniques as SWOT analysis (Strengths, Weaknesses, Opportunities, Threats)[10] and stakeholder analysis.[11] These techniques are aimed at identifying the significant individuals and groups whose views should be taken into account and whose support should, if possible, be gained.

Being opportunistic and realistic

As a public health practitioner, you must be both scientifically astute and politically adept.

> Box 2.2.2
> 'Problem solvers often complain that they have worked out ideal solutions but that no one will use them...Real problems include not only the specified problem situation but also the 'person situation', which includes the people who have to accept and act on the solution.'[3]

A solution is not a solution if it is not possible to implement it. The same is true for a policy (see chapter 3.3).

You must keep abreast of developments at international, national, and local levels, embracing statutory and voluntary organizations, as well as the views of the media and local communities. Newly produced policies and reports often provide an opportunity to bring a favoured public health issue to the fore. Every public health problem requires some sort of analysis of who are the key people or groups to involve or inform, so that successful public health action will happen. Public health specialists often need to work with, and enlist the support of, others such as local authorities, voluntary organizations, and the private sector, as well as health services. They need also to work with other professionals, including health professionals, statisticians, behavioural scientists, and policy analysts.

Public health practitioners should be realistic enough to practice 'the art of the possible', whilst remaining imbued with a strong sense of onward progress. In other words, public health practitioners need passion as well as knowledge and skills.[12]

There are clear examples of effective public health action where perceived public health problems were successfully translated into answerable questions. They also exemplify that effective action:

• can sometimes occur for the wrong reasons

• often needs luck.

For example, Edwin Chadwick, a lawyer by training, produced his *Report on the sanitary conditions of the labouring population of Great Britain* (1842) mainly in response to concern that ill-health was putting upward financial pressure on the cost of Poor Law relief. The Public Health Act that resulted (1848) was a landmark in the development of clean water and effective sewage disposal, though it was vigorously opposed in some quarters. Chadwick did not however subscribe to the modern view that poverty can cause ill-health—he maintained that the reverse applied.[13] He also supported the 'miasma' (bad smells) theory rather than the germ theory of transmission of infection, a belief which directed his efforts—beneficially as it happens, but for the wrong reasons—towards improved hygiene. Concerns in government about the hazards posed by cholera outbreaks gave much-needed additional impetus to his controversial reforms.

Remember finally that public health action taken in response to the answer to a public health question can sometimes have counter-intuitive and unintended harmful results.

This can be minimized by:

• considering the interconnections between social factors

• being as inclusive as possible when measuring the outcome of public health interventions

• mastering the art of seeing the 'big picture' as well as the detail.

In 1927 in Stockton-on-Tees a natural experiment occurred in which the occupants of one area of poor housing were re-housed in modern accommodation whilst a control group remained in slum dwellings. Age/sex standardized death rates *increased* sharply among those re-housed. This unexpected finding was eventually traced back to a deterioration in diet among those re-housed, resulting from a reduction in disposable income, itself caused by the higher rental costs of the newer housing.[14]

Further resources

A wide range of public health problems and the approaches used to answer them are available in a *Database of Abstracts* from the reports submitted as part of the Part II examination for membership of the UK Faculty of Public Health Medicine at www.fphm.org.uk (accessed 16 August 2000).

Handy CB (1985). *Understanding organisations*. Penguin Books, London.

References

1. Acheson ED (1988). *Public health in England. Report of the Committee of Inquiry into the future development of the public health function*. HMSO, London.

2. Beaglehole R and Bonita R (1997). *Public health at the crossroads*. Cambridge University Press, Cambridge.

3. de Bono E (1971). *Lateral thinking for management*. McGraw-Hill, Maidenhead.

4. Tukey JW (1962). The future of data analysis. *Ann Math Stat*, **33**, 1–67.

5. Baum F (1995). Researching public health: behind the qualitative–quantitative methodological debate. *Soc Sci Med*, **40**, 459–68.

6. Duhl L and Hancock T (1988). *A guide to assessing healthy cities*. WHO Healthy Cities, Paper No. 3. FADL Publishers, Copenhagen.

7. Harvey I (1994). How can we determine if living close to industry harms your health? *BMJ*, **309**, 425–6.

8. Nemery B, Fischler B, Boogaerts M, and Lison D (1999). Dioxins, Coca-Cola, and mass sociogenic illness in Belgium. *Lancet*, **354**, 77.

9. Arblaster L, Entwistle V, Lambert M, Forster M, Sheldon T, and Watt I (1995). *Review of the research on the effectiveness of Health Service interventions to reduce variations in health*, (CRD Report 3). NHS Centre for Reviews and Dissemination, York.

10. Casebeer A (1993). Application of SWOT analysis. *Br J Hosp Med*, **49**, 430–1.

11. Evans D (1996). A stakeholder analysis of developments at the primary and secondary care interface. *Br J Gen Pract*, **46**, 675–7.

12. Horton R (1998). The *new* new public health of risk and radical engagement. *Lancet*, **352**, 251–2.

13. Hamlin C and Sheard S (1998). Revolutions in public health: 1848 and 1998? *Br Med J*, **317**, 587–91.

14. Holland WW and Stewart S (1998). *Public health: the vision and the challenge*. The Nuffield Trust, London.

2.3 Finding evidence

Alison Hill, Anne Brice, and Katie Enoch

Objectives

Good public health decision making depends on combining good *information* (much of it routine—see chapters 1.1 and 1.4) with good *research evidence*. The next two chapters are designed to help you find and appraise good research evidence.

Finding evidence

It can be difficult to find exactly the research evidence you need, and to know when you have found it. Developments in technology, particularly the internet, mean that you can potentially access a huge range of resources. However, if you don't have a systematic and reproducible approach to your search, it is easy to waste a large amount of time in searching, and to end up with only a small proportion of the relevant literature. In addition, you may end up with much unhelpful material. Your searching techniques need to be as sensitive as possible (to get as much of the information that you *do* need) and as specific as possible (to minimize the amount of retrieved information that you *do not* need).

The information cycle

When undertaking a search for literature it is useful to remember that the process is not a linear one, and there have to be iterations to improve your identification of relevant papers. This is depicted in Figure 2.3.1.

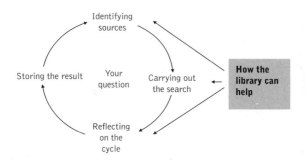

Figure 2.3.1 The information cycle.

Identifying sources of information

Evidence is published in a range of sources including books, journals, and research reports. There are between 20,000 and 30,000 biomedical journals and 17,000 new biomedical books published annually, which makes the task sound very daunting. But as long as you have a tightly defined question and are clear which sources you need to search, your task is made easier.

Useful information sources include colleagues, books, primary and secondary journals, grey literature, guidelines, the Cochrane Library, bibliographic databases, and the many resources on the internet. A detailed description of each of these sources and their advantages and disadvantages (derived from feedback sessions at workshops held with a range of health practitioners) is given on the CASP Finding the Evidence (CASPfew) web site.[1] It is not intended to be comprehensive, although the site has comprehensive, detailed, and up-to-date information on sources of evidence, and links to other web-based guides.

Protocol for selecting sources

When deciding on your search strategy, and in particular which sources you should use, it is important to use a protocol with which to plan your approach, so that your actions are reproducible (like any other quantitative research).

A sample protocol is included in Figure 2.3.2. Another useful protocol can be found at the School of Health and Related Research in Sheffield, UK (SCHARR) web site.[2]

Doing the search

When creating a search strategy it is essential to go back to your formulated question. This will help you identify relevant terms on which to base your search, and to build the blocks of your strategy. It is a good idea to start with a broad, or sensitive, search. This will find a lot of material, some of which may not be relevant. It is important not to limit or narrow the search too quickly as this may exclude vital evidence from your search results.

For example, in order to search as broadly as possible in MEDLINE* we need to know how to:

- perform a MeSH search
- perform a text word, or free-text search.

It is important to keep the search as broad as possible until you are sure that you are not excluding relevant evidence. For example, using techniques such as 'exploding' thesaurus terms, applying all subheadings, and using truncation and wild cards will help ensure that useful evidence is not excluded. The search can always be

**Search for an evidence-based clinical practice guideline,
or summaries of the best available evidence**

The UK National Electronic Library for Health (NeLH) will often be
a first portal* www.nelh.nhs.uk/

Royal Colleges may also produce guidelines
UK—www.psychiatry.ox.ac.uk/cebmh/guidelines/
US—www.ahcpr.gov/
www.psych.org/clin_res/prac_guide.html
Canada—www.cma.ca/cpgs/

As do Medical Journals
↓
Clinical Evidence, BMJ, UK
www.evidence.org/index-welcome.htm

↓

**Search for a good quality systematic review of
randomized controlled trials of the intervention**

The Cochrane Library (includes: CDSR,*/DARE)
www.update-software.com/cochrane/cochrane-frame.html

*Best Evidence (Evidence-Based Medicine, ACP Journal Club),
Evidence Based Nursing
Evidence-Based Mental Health and other evidence-based journals*
www.bmjpg.com/data/ebm.htm
www.psychiatry.ox.ac.uk/cebmh/journal/

*MEDLINE,*EMBASE,* Cinahl* or PsychLit
MEDLINE online*—www.ncbi.nlm.nih.gov/PubMed/

↓

Search for a single randomized controlled trial

*The Cochrane Library (CCTR)
Evidence-based Journals
MEDLINE, EMBASE, Cinahl, or PsychLit
and other subject specialist databases*

And now ongoing trials in the Controlled Trials Register
www.update-software.com/cochrane/cochrane-frame.html

↓

Search for the next level of evidence

*MEDLINE, EMBASE, Cinahl, or PsychLit
The Internet—gateways and guides*
cebm.jr2.ox.ac.uk/
www.cebmh.com/
libsun1.jr2.ox.ac.uk/caspfew/sources.html
www.shef.ac.uk/~scharr/ir/netting/

(All sites accessed 16 August 2000)

Figure 2.3.2 A systematic approach to searching for evidence.

refined later if the results are not as expected. As indexing quality is variable, it is important to build a search strategy using a combination of MeSH terms and text words, and combine the results using Boolean logic 'operators' such as 'AND' and 'OR' and 'NOT'.

Searching for quality

There are different ways of narrowing a search, or increasing its specificity, and to get the best results this should be done in a number of steps, systematically excluding the least useful articles, for instance by restricting to high quality studies, or by using different combinations of terms.

Using search field suffixes

Knowing which abbreviations your particular version of MEDLINE database uses is invaluable in finding evidence. This applies to the situation where you know the approximate reference (e.g. you could use smith-j.au in CD-Ovid), or where you are searching for a particular word in a title (syntax = .ti) or the abstract (syntax = .ab). There are good guides to help with these skills in more detail.[3]

Using search filters

Search filters are tried and tested literature search strategies that provide a more effective way of limiting your search to high quality evidence appropriate to your type of question. They can be used to identify systematic review and randomized controlled trial literature on MEDLINE, and in other databases. There are also methodological search filters which will help you retrieve sound clinical studies that deal with:

- diagnosis
- prognosis
- therapy
- aetiology
- guidelines
- treatment outcomes
- evidence-based health care methods.

They can be stored on your computer or floppy disk to be run against your subject search in whichever software you use (e.g. Silver Platter Information Ltd., Ovid Technologies).

You can find out more about these filters at libsun1.jr2.ox.ac.uk/caspfew/filters.

Conclusion

Remember that searching for evidence is a research methodology in itself. The actual process should be made explicit each time it is performed. Like any methodology, it should be reliable: repeating the process should give the same results. It is therefore very important to be explicit each time it is performed. You will never be perfect, but at least you can be explicit.

Further resources

Searching literature improves with practice. There are good exercises to work through (either on your own or with an experienced librarian) in: Greenhalgh T (1997). *How to read a paper—the basics of evidence based medicine.* BMJ Books, London.

CASP and HCLU (1999). *Evidence-based health care: a computer aided learning resource.* Update Software, England.

CASP and HCLU (1999). *Evidence-based health care: an open learning resource for healthcare professionals.* Update Software, England.

For more help on searching techniques contact your local health librarian, or look at a demonstration of some basic techniques, using some of the learning materials held at libsun1.jr2.ox.ac.uk/caspfew (accessed 16 August 2000).

References

1. CASPfew. libsun1.jr2.ox.ac.uk/caspfew/sources.html (accessed 16 August 2000).
2. School of Health and Related Research, Sheffield, UK (SCHARR). www.shef.ac.uk/uni/academic/R-Z/scharr/ir/proto.html (accessed 16 August 2000).
3. Greenhalgh T (1997). *How to read a paper—the basics of evidence based medicine.* BMJ Books, London.

2.4 **Appraising research evidence**

Alison Hill, Anne Brice, and Katie Enock

Introduction

There is a wealth of public health research available, but its quality is variable. To act on unreliable evidence can easily result in harm or wasted resources (or both) at an individual and a population level. It is therefore essential to appraise research evidence carefully before making decisions to act. Evidence is never perfect, but it is an important public health task to be as explicit as possible when justifying decisions on the basis of evidence, resources, and values.

Methods

Critical appraisal provides a systematic approach to appraising evidence. When critically appraising a paper it is too easy to be very critical of the methods. Think of the classical meaning of the word 'critical' in terms of 'critique', or 'to find value in' rather than 'criticize—to find fault'. Trying to think how you might have done the research better will help you understand the constraints that many researchers are working within. The essence of critical appraisal is to find in the evidence anything of value that will help you make a better decision.

In any critical appraisal, the most important four questions, regardless of methodology are:

1. *Why did they start*? What is the issue/question?

2. *What did they do*? Were the right methods chosen for the question, and were the methods performed correctly? (internal validity)

3. *What did they find*? What are the results, can you trust them, and how exactly do you communicate them?

4. *What does it mean*? Are the results relevant to your problem? (external validity).

In order to establish these four things, you have to appraise the research design and methodology, the quality of the data, and the analysis and interpretation placed on the findings.

The general rule is not to assume that any aspect of a research study is sound. Unless you have established that the quality markers you are looking for (for instance, a clear description of the design of the study) are present, it is safer to assume that the research is not sound. Indeed, when groups or people practise critical appraisal skills as part of a teaching session they almost invariably find problems with the study being appraised. In public health practice, the question is whether the methodology is good *enough* or if the relevance is close *enough*.

Public health practice is increasingly involved with secondary research (i.e. where the unit of analysis is other research). Therefore, we have concentrated on systematic reviews as an example of evidence.

The following check-list provides a guide for assessing the quality of a systematic review. In making decisions based on the best evidence, the gold standard is the systematic review of research trials, with a numerical meta-analysis in addition if it is appropriate. (For many public health interventions you may not find any randomized controlled trials, but the check-list is also appropriate for systematic reviews of other types of controlled trials.)

The questions in Box 2.4.1 are copyrighted to CASP (permission granted through authorship).

Box 2.4.1 **A critical appraisal check-list for a systematic review**[1]

(a) Are the results of the review valid?

1. **Screening question: Did the review address a clearly focused issue?**
   An issue can be 'focused' in terms of:
   – the population studied
   – the intervention given
   – the outcomes considered.

   Learning points: It is important to be clear about the focus of the question, to confirm that the review is useful to you and will help to inform your question. Unfocused reviews cannot provide you with reliable answers. If it is unfocused don't continue with the appraisal.

2. **Screening question: Did the review include the right type of studies?**
   These would:
   – address the review's question
   – have an appropriate study design (e.g. RCTs for interventions).

   Learning points: Included studies should closely match up with Question 1 in terms of population, intervention, and outcomes. A clear statement of the inclusion criteria makes it less likely that the authors only cite studies that support their prior hypothesis.

Box 2.4.1 (continued)

If you are not confident of the answers to these questions, you may not want to waste time reading further.

3. **Detailed questions: Did the reviewers try to identify all relevant studies?**
   Look for:

   – *which bibliographic databases were used*

   – *follow up from reference lists*

   – *personal contact with experts*

   – *search for unpublished as well as published studies*

   – *search for non-English language studies.*

   Learning points: You need to feel confident that the authors looked hard enough to find all studies, both published and unpublished, that met their inclusion criteria. More than one source should be used. A thorough search will reduce the risks of:

   (i) random error which might occur because of small numbers in the trials

   (ii) systematic error from:
   – publication bias (this often occurs because trials showing no effect or negative effects are often not published)

   – retrieval bias (this occurs when trials that are not published in widely read and easy-to-access journals are missed).

4. **Did the reviewers assess the quality of the included studies?**
   A clear, pre-determined strategy should be used to determine which studies are included.
   Look for:

   – *a scoring system*

   – *more than one assessor.*

   Learning points: This question is important because studies with weaker designs will be less valid and can overestimate effects. It asks if the authors assessed the validity of the studies in detail. This should ideally be undertaken by two independent reviewers.

5. **If the results of the review have been combined, was it reasonable to do so?**
Consider whether:

– *the results of all the included studies are clearly displayed*

– *the results of the different studies are similar* (look for tests of heterogeneity)

– *the reasons for any variations in results are discussed.*

Learning points: It is important to consider whether it was acceptable to combine the primary studies and the reviewers need to convince us that they are combining like with like.
Look at the graphs and tables, to see if different studies are finding similar results, or studies which are using different methodologies are finding similar results.
Think about variations due to differences in populations, intervention/exposure, or outcomes, to study methods, or to chance.

(b) What are the main results of the review?

6. **What is the overall result of the review?**
Consider:

– *how the results are expressed (e.g. odds ratio, relative risk, etc.)*

– *what the results are.*

Learning point: What do the results mean? Are they statistically significant as well as significant in terms of practice?

7. **Could these results be due to chance?**
Look for tests of statistical significance (p-values) and confidence intervals (CIs).

Learning points: The confidence interval (CI) will indicate how precise the results are: a very wide CI will indicate uncertainty in results. If the CI goes over the line of no difference then the results are not statistically significant. When reading the results, go to the results section looking for each outcome. Sometimes authors will write up the abstract to show their best results which might not be their main outcomes.

Box 2.4.1 (continued)

(C) Will the results help locally?

8. **Can the results be applied to the local population?**
   Consider whether:

   – *the population sample covered by the review could be sufficiently different from your population to cause concern*

   – *your local setting is likely to differ much from that of the review.*

   Learning points: It is important to consider if there are any differences which would make it impossible to apply this to the local population.

9. **Were all important outcomes considered?**
   Consider outcomes from the point of view of the:

   – *individual*

   – *policy makers and practitioners*

   – *family / carers*

   – *wider community.*

   Learning points: Studies are not able to look at all the outcomes in which we may be interested. Consider if the authors have answered their question and whether an important outcome has been missed.

10. **Should policy and practice change as a result of the evidence contained in this review?**
    Trials are not able to look at all the outcomes in which you may be interested. It is unlikely that a cost analysis will be included in the study, so reflect on the value of the new intervention, its likely cost implications, and the benefits or potential harm (see chapter 2.6).

Box 2.4.2 **Checklist for appraising cohort studies**

(a) Are the results of the study valid?

Screening Questions

1. Did the study address a clearly focused issue?

2. Did the authors use an appropriate method to answer their question?

Detailed Questions

3. Was the cohort recruited in an acceptable way?
HINT: Look for selection bias

4. Was the exposure accurately measured to minimize bias?
HINT: Look for measurement or classification bias

5. Was the outcome accurately measured to minimize bias?
HINT: Look for measurement or classification bias

6. (i) Have the authors taken account of the important confounding factors in the design and/or in their analysis?

   (ii) Are there any other important confounding factors that the authors should have accounted for?

7. (i) Was the follow up of subjects complete enough?

   (ii) Was the follow up of subjects long enough?

(b) What are the results?

8. How precise are the results?
   How precise is the estimate of risk?

9. Do you believe the results?

(c) Will the results help locally?

10. Can the results be applied to the local population?

11. Do the results of this study fit with other available evidence?

Critically appraising other types of studies

Box 2.4.2 is a checklist for a cohort study. If you want to see this and other checklists in more detail with the hints, they are available on the CASP website www.casp.org.uk The Evidence Based Medicine

Working Group, a group of clinicians at MacMaster University, Hamilton, Canada, and colleagues across North America, have created a set of guides, published in the Journal of the American Medical Association.[2]

References for these are available at the School of Health and Related Research (SCHARR) *Netting the Evidence* website in the UK (www.shef.ac.uk/~scharr/ir/userg.html, accessed 16 August 2000).

A check-list for critically appraising guidelines is available from St George's Hospital Medical School in the UK www.sghms.ac.uk/phs/hceu/nhsguide.htm (accessed 16 August 2000).

Further resources

CASP and HCLU (1999). *Evidence-based health care: a computer aided learning resource*. Update Software, England.

CASP and HCLU (1999). *Evidence-based health care: an open learning resource for healthcare professionals*. Update Software, England.

Gray JAM (1997). *Evidence-based healthcare: how to make health policy and management decisions*. Churchill Livingstone, London.

Greenhalgh T (1997). *How to read a paper: the basics of evidence based medicine*. BMJ Books, London.

Sackett DL, Richardson WS, Rosenberg W, and Haynes RB (1997). *Evidence-based medicine: how to practice and teach EBM*. Churchill Livingstone, London.

References

1. Adapted from: Oxman AD, Guyatt GH, *et al.* (1994). Users' guides to the medical literature. VI: How to use an overview. *JAMA*, **272** (**17**), 1367–71.
2. Oxman AD, Sackett DL, and Guyatt G (1993). Users' guides to the medical literature. I. How to get started. The Evidence-Based Medicine Working Group. *JAMA*, **270**, 2093–5.

2.5 Managing public health information and knowledge

Iain Buchan, Larry Chambers, and Muir Gray

Introduction

Public health departments rarely have the human and financial resources commensurate with their task of improving the health of populations through the organized efforts of society. Public health practitioners usually work in relatively small organizations without direct control over (although with potential for considerable influence on) the resources of those organizations that do determine the health of populations directly. Their departments are, however, rich in information and knowledge and as such have the potential of becoming exemplars of the modern knowledge-based enterprises.

Objectives

After reading this chapter, you should:

- appreciate the added value that public health practitioners can bring to public health organizations through the efficient management of knowledge
- understand and begin to develop the skills needed to achieve this influence and added value.

Organizations rich in knowledge

We are now in the knowledge era. Companies that manage knowledge well grow to dominate over those companies that focus on twentieth-century oil-based, or nineteenth-century steel-based products. Companies are now valued according to their intangible as well as their tangible assets, with the quote value of a company being much greater than the sum total of its buildings and stock (the traditional valuation).

The new knowledge-based organizations are appraised on their intangible assets, notably by:

- the amount of knowledge they have
- how well they manage that knowledge
- the expertise of their staff
- the quality of their relationships with the people they serve
- their constant drive for improvement.

Terminology in knowledge management

The application of formal knowledge management has grown with advances in computing, and with this comes some commonly-used terms such as data, information, and knowledge (see chapters 1.1 and 1.4):

* *data* are discrete, objective facts about events
* *information* is data transformed (contextualized, categorized, corrected, calculated, condensed) into a message, and can thus be thought of as data intended to make a difference
* *knowledge* is a fluid mix of experience, values, contextual information, and expert insight that provides a framework for evaluating and incorporating new experiences and information.[1]

There is however much debate over such definitions of information, knowledge, experience, intuition, and wisdom. Even more hotly debated are the definition of, and basic principles for, managing knowledge. The term 'knowledge management' means widely different things to different people; however, there is a consensus that knowledge management is defined as the degree to which the potential value of both tacit and explicit knowledge are realized by an organization or individual.

Types of knowledge

In such an information-rich world as public health, it is important to develop a sense of the different types of knowledge. One important distinction is between 'explicit' knowledge and 'tacit' knowledge (see Table 2.5.1).

Table 2.5.1 Types of knowledge: explicit vs. tacit knowledge.

Explicit knowledge	Tacit knowledge
Usually based on research	Usually based on experience
Written	Often unwritten
Facts or evidence-based guidelines	Know-how
Generalizable	Often relevant only to the organization in which it was developed
Highly regarded by academics	Highly regarded by practitioners

Explicit knowledge

Explicit knowledge is derived from the analysis of specially collected data, i.e. research or the analysis of routinely collected data. Examples:

* a Cochrane Review
* an article in the *American Journal of Public Health*
* the Annual Report of a Director of Public Health
* a government report
* Last's *Dictionary of epidemiology*

- the web site of the International Society of Health Technology Assessment
- a study of the cancer registration rates in different populations
- an analysis of smoking trends in a population.

Tacit knowledge

Tacit knowledge, sometimes called know-how, is a type of knowledge that is often unwritten, although the drive to improve the training of public health practitioners has increased the pressure to write down and codify tacit knowledge. However, tacit knowledge is not particularly generalizable even when written down and is different from explicit knowledge. Examples of tacit knowledge are:

- how to manage a meningitis contact tracing emergency
- handling the press and developing a proactive rather than reactive strategy when there is bad news
- investigating a clinical complaint
- handling a sexual harassment claim by a staff member.

Much tacit knowledge is used in running organizations and is particularly useful when events are uncommon, for it may be that everyone involved on the previous occasion of, for example, a radiation scare, has left the department. Tacit knowledge can help the public health practitioner or team to be seen as credible and to be effective. Much of this book is concerned with making tacit knowledge explicit, for example:

- working with 'hard to reach' populations
- tackling deprivation and inequality.

It is hard to generalize about these types of activities in the way that one can generalize about the effects of beta blockers, but there is undoubtedly knowledge that is available to help the person responsible for this type of challenge, and that tacit knowledge is increasingly the knowledge that public health practitioners and teams need and use.

Improving knowledge management in public health

To improve knowledge management in public health, teams and individuals must:

(a) develop and lead an organization's capacity for managing knowledge—(example: a hyper-linked public health organization)

(b) develop the individual's capacity for managing knowledge

(c) inform and involve the public.

(a) Developing and leading an organization's capacity for managing knowledge

If public health departments and teams are to be effective, they have to manage knowledge effectively. In this way, they can make the other resources which are available to them really work.

The leader of a team or organization has to emphasize the importance of knowledge and its management, making it clear when to use tacit knowledge or explicit knowledge, or when to simply give an opinion.

A checklist of questions that anyone, especially a head of department, should ask of any knowledge on which a decision is taken is set out below:

- what is the issue/question of interest?
- what is the evidence to justify the assertions and conclusions of this report? (e.g. references)
- are we clearly distinguishing between evidence, values, and opinion?
- what are the consequences for decision making?

Applying this analysis routinely is the foundation for an organization open to new knowledge. It will only come from effective leadership of teams with the importance of knowledge at the forefront.

The importance of leadership in managing public health knowledge (see chapter 7.1.)

Leadership from public health practitioners within organizations is important if the organization is to:

- create a culture in which knowledge is valued, managed, and used effectively
- develop simple, effective systems for knowledge management, ensuring that the team has access to evidence and communicates the best current knowledge both internally and externally
- ensure organizational structures do not hinder effective knowledge management.

An important part of this process is to identify someone to be specifically responsible for knowledge management, called, increasingly in large commercial organizations, the Chief Knowledge Officer.[2] This person should be a member of the senior management team, and have sufficient authority to:

- strongly influence the flow of knowledge into the organization, deciding what sources should be promoted and what should not
- decide where that knowledge is directed and that the new relevant information is brought to the attention of the executive team and the Chief Executive

- ensure that knowledge flows within the organization where and when it is needed

- ensure that knowledge available to the public is of adequate quality and that the methods used to produce that knowledge are explicit and evidence-based

- be responsible for the navigation scheme, presentation, and key content of organizational intranet and public-facing internet web sites.

The knowledge-aware and knowledge-skilled team

The importance of teams in public health endeavours cannot be overstated (see chapter 8.1). Within a department it is often useful to create a team consisting of epidemiologists and other experts who assist public health practitioners by:

- collecting data (especially from different sources)

- identifying trends

- identifying hypotheses worthy of further research

- forecasting

- disseminating and advocacy

- supporting local public health practitioners' skills development in health monitoring.

Such teams are bridging entities connecting community health monitoring across organizations and communities. All communities have an abundance of health-related data which are greatly under-used because of inadequate pan-community health monitoring systems to make the data available to the right people at the right time and in a form that is easy to understand.

These teams can cover populations of any size from 100,000 or less to the whole population of a country. In 1999, population health monitoring in the UK was given a new lease of life by the introduction of Public Health Observatories in England, which allowed a reappraisal of the functions of regional and national health intelligence units. In order to help achieve the twin aims of the 1999 UK Department of Health White Paper *Saving Lives*[3] (to improve health, and to reduce health inequalities), it called for such a 'Public Health Observatory' to be established in each of the eight NHS regions of England.

'In order to strengthen the availability and use of information about health at local level we will ensure that there is a Public Health Observatory in each NHS region of the country. These observatories will be closely linked with universities to help bring an academic rigour to their work.

Their main tasks will be to support local bodies by:

- monitoring health and disease trends and highlighting areas for action

- identifying gaps in health information
- advising on methods for health and health inequality impact assessments drawing together information from different sources in new ways to improve health
- carrying out projects to highlight particular health issues
- evaluating progress by local agencies in improving health and cutting inequality
- looking ahead to give early warning of future public health problems.'[4]

Example: Building a hyper-linked organization—a public health observatory

In their classic study of knowledge-creating organizations, Nonaka and Takeuchi[5] ran a hypertext organization. Many other names are now applied to this type of organization, e.g. the learning organization, the virtual organization, and the web-based organization. Characteristics of this type of organizational approach are:

- the organization has a hierarchy, but the teams are not watertight compartments, simply labour pools looking after people with the same skill mix
- the organization organizes its work through a series of finite projects, objectives, and outcomes
- project and programme teams are composed of people from different labour pools
- every member of the organization is clear about their role and how much time they are spending on different projects and programmes
- the project and programme leaders are accountable for the work of the project teams and have to bid for resources to the executive team
- each labour pool, each project, and each programme has its own internal web site
- central filing is kept to a minimum, with the number of filing cabinets being progressively reduced.

The organization thus develops systems to manage projects and programmes and ensures that they are adequately integrated and co-ordinated. The skills that the individuals and teams require to achieve this are:

- data (and data-set) collection, collation, and analysis (analysis of past and future trends, early warning mechanisms)
- critical appraisal of local, national, and international research evidence
- research and evaluation skills
- problem-oriented and focused report writing
- leadership and management skills.

Primary responsibility for the health of the population in the United Kingdom remains with the health authorities, whose populations range from 500,000 to around a million. However, it was recognized that there were insufficient resources for each of those health authorities to develop a comprehensive health intelligence unit, although they continue to have prime responsibility for monitoring the health of their populations. Accordingly eight Regional Public Health Observatories and a national Observatory were set up.

The Observatory is responsible not only for community health monitoring but also for managing public health knowledge. The combination of local health monitoring and knowledge derived from the scientific literature is essential.

(b) Developing the skills of individuals

It is essential that individuals are competent in the use of all the relevant information technologies, and that of course is a fast-moving target.

All public health practitioners should be able to:

* keep up to date with information through an explicit 'general scanning' and 'specific searching' policy
* find and search electronic databases
* manipulate data electronically in databases and spreadsheets
* use internet-based technologies (e-mail, listservers, web sites)
* manage references to numerical and written evidence in the appropriate written and electronic format (searching, finding, downloading, manipulating, sorting, citing . . .)
* word process, and paper or web publish concise reports using data, evidence, and good communication skills in order to achieve change efficiently.

The ability to do these tasks, and to learn new tasks as technology allows, enables public health teams to contribute to their organization's objectives in a focused and efficient way.

(c) Public information and involvement

The need for accountability and openness is now clearly accepted, and public health departments should play a leading part in promoting these principles. Public websites can be used for openly and transparently sharing news, agendas, minutes, and other materials for supporting public health decision making e.g. in the local implementation of a national initiative. Each public health department needs to have a responsible and enterprising approach to public information.

Conclusion

Data, information, and knowledge are the raw ingredients of effective public health action. Generating, finding, storing, converting, and using them to make better decisions is at the heart of public health action. The ability to do this in electronic ways, with virtual teams, over wider geographical areas, emphasizes the need to stay abreast, not only of the ever-increasing information sources we have access to, but also of the rapidly expanding skill base needed to use them efficiently.

Further resources

Dancy J and Sosa E (ed.) (1993). *A companion to epistemology*. Blackwell, Oxford.

Department of Health (1998). *Communicating about risk to public health*. HMSO, London. www.doh.gov.uk/pointers.htm (accessed 17 August 2000).

Eysenbach G, *et al.* (1998). Towards quality management of medical information on the Internet: evaluation, labelling, and filtering of information. *BMJ*, **317**, 1496–1502.

Gibbons M, *et al.* (1994). *The new production of knowledge*. Sage, London.

Haines A and Donald A (1998). *Getting research findings into practice*. BMJ Books, London.

Smith MA and Kollock P (ed.) (1999). *Communities in cyberspace*. Routledge, London.

Warner HR *et al.* (1997). *Knowledge engineering in health informatics*. Springer-Verlag, New York.

Weed LL and Weed L (1999). Opening the black box of clinical judgement. *BMJ*, **319(7220)**, 1279. (Data supplement/complete version on *eBMJ*.)

References

1. Davenport TH and Prusak L (1998). *Working knowledge: how organizations manage what they know*. Harvard Business School Press, Boston.
2. Gray JAM (1998). Where's the chief knowledge officer? To manage the most precious resource of all. *BMJ*, **317**, 832–40.
3. Department of Health (1999). *Saving Lives: our healthier nation*. Department of Health, London. www.official-documents.co.uk/document/cm43/4386/4386.htm (accessed 21 August 2000).
4. Department of Health (1999). *Saving Lives: our healthier nation*, chapter 11, paragraph 11.30. Department of Health, London. www.official-documents. co.uk/document/cm43/4386/4386-11.htm (accessed 21 August 2000).
5. Nonaka I and Takeuchi H (1995). *The knowledge-creating company: how Japanese companies create the dynamics of innovation*. Oxford University Press, Oxford.

The complexity of modern medicine exceeds the limitations of the unaided human mind.

David Eddy

2.6 Economic evaluation — the science of making choices

John Appleby and Peter Brambleby

Introduction

Most professional activity involves making choices. This can be particularly challenging in protecting and promoting health and preventing disease as:

- the outcomes can threaten quality of life and life itself
- the resources are not unlimited
- the evidence base is not perfect.

Objectives

This chapter explains the underlying thinking, and describes some of the more frequently used techniques in economic evaluation and when to apply them. It will help the reader:

- to understand the terminology of economic evaluation
- to apply the concepts of economic evaluation when they appear in management situations
- to be able to pose better questions when important choices are apparent and when the help of a professional health economist is involved.

What is economic evaluation?

The practitioner often has to make, or advise others on making, choices such as:

- deciding whether or not to introduce a new intervention or service
- how one could go about comparing four bids for new money when only two of the bids could be funded
- the best way to go about deciding how to take money out of a service.

Whether one is involved with the planning or the delivery of health care, the job involves many seemingly complex choices. Whether it is a publicly funded system (such as the UK National Health Service (NHS)), or a public/private mixture, there is the added dimension of having to be accountable for stewardship of public resources.

Box 2.6.1

Health economics is a discipline that aims to make systematic the analysis, and addressing of, issues of scarcity and choice in health care.

Despite its name, economics is not primarily about 'making economies' or even about money. Money is just one type of resource (others include people, time, buildings). Costs can be tangible, such as journeys to hospital, or intangible, such as pain. An economic approach to an issue or problem is equally concerned with effectiveness and benefits, for example, as it is with resources and costs.

Where there is scarcity, there is choice. The choices are in two areas, to be tackled in the right order:

• the first questions would relate to *outcomes*

• only after that, to *costs*.

Much of economic appraisal is concerned with the relationship between costs and outcomes. The steps often follow this pattern:

1. What are we trying to achieve?

2. What are the different ways of achieving this (options)?

3. Do these options work at all?

4. If so, how do they compare with each other, taking adverse effects into account as well as benefits?

5. What costs are involved for each option, taking not only NHS factors into consideration, but others such as costs to the patient?

Similarly, if a service might be stopped or reduced, the considerations are:

1. What are we trying to achieve?

2. What are the different ways of achieving this? (options)

3. What benefits will be lost with each option?

4. What resources will be released with each option?

5. How might these resources be used, and the outcomes realized, in comparison with the outcomes of the original service?

Health economics provides a means of handling these decisions. It can be regarded as an overall way of thinking (a shared perspective on problem-solving that decision makers find useful) and as a particular set of techniques.

Health economics as a way of thinking

Health economics is not a substitute for thought, but a way of organizing it.[1] Nor is it a technical fix that tells you precisely what to do.[2] The approach is;

• *utilitarian*—trying to get the greatest good for the greatest number

and concerned with:

• *efficiency*—getting the greatest outcome from a fixed amount of resource.

Although these are the health economist's starting point, they need not necessarily be adopted as the only criteria to guide decisions. The gulf between that which is possible and that which can be afforded (by the individual or the state), and the inevitability of having to choose, is the starting point for economic appraisal. Health economics recognizes the existence of trade-offs inherent in any system. Choice involves sacrifice. It is perfectly legitimate to trade off some efficiency for the sake of other considerations such as equity— the willingness to give a protected 'fair share' to a particular group in society even if that does not maximize total outcomes for the population as a whole. It serves to emphasize that choices are not free—there is an *opportunity cost** (benefit foregone) once resources are committed. In other words, once resources have been committed, the real cost is not the monetary value but the best alternative use to which that resource could have been put. Just like epidemiology and sociology, it is concerned with whole populations and not just individuals (see 'Trading off dimensions of quality' in chapter 5.1).

Economic evaluations

Economic evaluations deal with the relationships between costs and outcomes when choices have to be made between competing options. Sometimes, though rarely, the outcomes are the same and the issue is simply one of which option consumes least resources, taking all costs into consideration. In this situation the appropriate tool is *cost-minimization analysis*.

More often, the costs and outcomes are both different, but the units in which the outcomes are measured are the same (typically 'natural units', like years of life added for choices between cancer treatments, peak expiratory flow rates for choices between asthma treatments, or successful live births in choices between infertility treatments). In such cases the appropriate tool is *cost-effectiveness analysis*.

Sometimes the choice is between very different types of outcome, measured in different units, and with different costs. An example would be deciding whether to put some additional resources into cancer care, orthopaedics, or diabetes. The issue is one of finding a common set of units such as quality-adjusted life-years (QALYs*) or disability-adjusted life-years (DALYs*) to allow a 'cost per QALY' or 'cost per DALY' comparison on a like-for-like basis. The term given to appraisals that convert different sorts of outcome into these common 'utility' units is *cost–utility analysis*.

Sometimes it is simply a question of weighing up whether the costs of a new intervention outweigh the benefits or not, and whether it should go ahead at all. Costs and benefits are both ascribed a monetary value in order to make the comparison. This is called *'cost–benefit analysis'*.* (Note that 'cost–benefit analysis' has a precise meaning and is not a blanket term for all comparisons of costs and outcomes—a better phrase to describe these techniques collectively is *'economic appraisal'*.)

The tools for addressing these situations are dealt with in Box 2.6.2.

Box 2.6.2 **Forms of economic evaluation**

Cost-minimization analysis: When the outcomes (the benefits) of alternative interventions are the same in terms of volume and type, the cheapest programme should be chosen on the grounds of efficiency—e.g. choosing between a branded and a generic drug.

Cost-effectiveness analysis: When the volume (but not the type) of outcomes of alternative programmes are *different*, then the efficient choice is that programme which costs least to produce a unit of outcome (such as a life saved)—e.g. choosing between two interventions of different cost and effectiveness which both prolong life in people with breast cancer.

Cost–utility analysis: When the type (and perhaps the volume) of outcomes from alternative programmes are *not* the same, then a 'common outcome currency' (such as a quality-adjusted life-year (QALY) or disability-adjusted life-year (DALY)) is used as a measure of benefit and to enable comparisons between programmes to be made. Choice of programme will then depend on the cost of producing a unit of the chosen currency (e.g. the cost per QALY), e.g. choosing between hip replacements, coronary artery bypass grafts, and haemodialysis for the next time period's investment.

Cost–benefit analysis: The preceding evaluative methods all leave the outcome/benefit side of the equation in 'natural' units (lives saved, QALYs, etc.). Cost–benefit analysis places monetary values on these benefits (to enable comparison with the monetary units used to measure costs). This analysis compares 'doing something' with 'doing nothing' (as opposed to 'doing something' vs. 'doing something else') e.g. advising the Highways Authority on whether or not to invest in crash barriers along a ten-mile stretch of road to avoid road traffic deaths and injuries.

Additional concepts

This is a simplification of the decision-guiding process. A health economist will also apply an annual percentage '*discounting*' to costs and benefits which fall at some time in the future to give them all a present-day value (this could be in the order of, for instance, 6% per annum). A benefit in the future is valued less highly than a benefit today (hence the value of a benefit only available at some time in the future is 'discounted'). This is of enormous public health importance, as the level we arbitrarily choose very much dictates the likelihood of any public health investment where the benefit is not realized for many years.

A '*sensitivity analysis*' would also be done to several values rather than single-point estimates, since data on costs and outcomes are seldom precise. This is done to check how much the estimates (and particularly a range of estimates) affect the final outcome.

Priority setting through programme budgeting and marginal analysis

A pioneer of this technique was Professor Alain Enthoven, who took it from its application to the American Armed Forces and applied it to health care planning (or purchasing) at population level. He endorsed its use in the UK National Health Service in his 1999 Rock Carling Fellowship review.[3] An entire issue of *Health Policy*[4] was devoted to articles on this topic.

Table 2.6.1 Programme budgeting and marginal analysis.

Action	Comment
Define health care programmes	Break down the priority-setting process into more manageable programmes (e.g. client groups, specialities, disease groups) and define health care objectives and outputs for each
Establish programme management groups	Management groups (clinicians, managers, user representatives) are responsible for priority setting within their programme
Estimate programme budgets	Identify current spending on, and broad outputs from, each programme. Often we know how much is spent on, say, nurses, but not on hip replacements
Define sub-programmes of care	Identify further breakdowns in programmes, with estimates of spending and defined objectives and outputs

Focus on marginal change	Most priority setting concerns changes to existing services (i.e. changes at the margin). Therefore, most attention can be paid to changes within rather than between programmes. However, do not be afraid to look horizontally at the entire programme for a district, spread across several hospitals, and examine marginal changes in the whole programme
Identify incremental and decremental 'wish lists'	Given extra (fewer) resources, what services should be expanded (reduced) for the greatest benefit of (causing least distress to) patients?
Cost the wish lists	How much would it cost (to health services and patients) to implement incremental and decremental wish lists?
Examine relative benefits generated by changes in spending	What would be implemented from the wish lists if specific amounts of money were made available or taken away?
Consider equity implications	The steps above focus on efficiency—getting more health care/healthiness for each unit of resource—but who is to benefit?
Consult	Out of necessity, 'point estimates' of cost and outcome are used, but in reality confidence limits are wide and overlapping. Do not let the veneer of scientific precision blind you to the underlying value judgements. The process to this point is about clarifying and organizing thought. It is imperative to check the assumptions with those most affected
Choose where to invest and where to disinvest	Having identified new patterns of spending based on clinical and economic evidence, decisions need to be taken to implement changes—managers earn their pay!

(Source: adapted from Mooney, et al.[5])

Is *health* economics different from conventional economics?

From the conventional point of view of economics, health care is unusual.[6] Standard economic ideas of supply and demand are often difficult to square with the reality of how health care systems actually function. In virtually all countries, demand for health care is mediated through a medical professional—consumers are not sovereign as in a typical market model. Patients need the help of a clinician to identify what their state of health really is, what their health care needs are and what interventions are appropriate to address them. This is known as the *agency role* of the health professions.

Both supply and demand for health care, especially secondary health care, are heavily regulated and managed. Complex insurance markets—run by the state, independent sector or a mixture of the two—have grown up in response to the inherent uncertainties of illness and the costs of treatments. Governments can play a significant part in health care regulation, from setting rules about practitioner qualifications through to resource allocation, standard setting, and direct control of provision.

The importance of the margin

Another important concept in health economics is that of the '*margin*'—loosely defined as the cost of the *next* (or one additional) unit of input or output. The importance of this is that in health care many choices are made about relatively small incremental changes in service (either to increase or decrease) rather than whole-scale strategic shifts. The issue is: 'What is the extra cost over and above what we pay now, and what is the extra benefit?' (The reverse applies for disinvestment decisions: 'What resources do we release and what benefits do we lose?')

A related concept is the '*stepped cost*':

Example:

Suppose a cardiac surgery unit is built, staffed, and equipped to deal with 900 patients a year and funded accordingly. This would mean all the costs—'fixed costs' (things like buildings), 'semi-fixed costs' (things like staff salaries), and 'variable costs' (things like drugs) were covered. Suppose that with this complement of personnel and beds it could actually cope with a further 50 patients. The additional (marginal) cost of each extra patient up to 50 would be relatively small, and chiefly reflect the 'variable costs'. But a point would come when, to accommodate just one more patient (over and above the extra 50), extra staff would have to be taken on or a new ward built—that would be a substantial 'stepped cost'. To see the relevance of this, imagine you were a health care purchaser with 200 extra patients requiring cardiac surgery and three cardiac centres within reasonable travel time for your population. It would be in everyone's interest to try to spread that additional workload between all three centres if that enabled them to work closer to capacity, but if that were not possible, then to look at a strategic stepped development at just one.

The same applies to benefits. Suppose an immunization programme reaches only 80% of the child population. An additional £50,000 might enable a further 10% to be reached, but the addition of a yet another £50,000 on top of that might only enable a further 5% to be reached. In common parlance this is 'the law of diminishing returns' but to the economist it is 'diminishing marginal benefit'.

The important points to remember are that *average* cost and benefit (*total* cost divided by *total* benefit) can differ substantially from *marginal* cost and benefit—marginal cost and marginal benefit do not increase (or decrease) in a smooth linear fashion.

Ethics and equity

The ethical stance of health economics is sometimes questioned by clinicians because the utilitarian approach can be at odds with the 'Hippocratic' ethic of doing the very best for the individual in a trusting doctor–patient relationship. (Economics is not known as the 'dismal science' for nothing!) But an economist would justify the pursuit of efficiency on the grounds that the true cost of inefficiency is borne in terms of pain, disability, and premature death by those waiting for treatment. In a publicly funded health care system, where policy making, funding, and provision are all controlled largely by the state, the primary objective of trying to ensure the greatest good for the greatest number is legitimate. One could extend this and argue that it is better to have a system where everyone gets access to a service which meets basic standards, even if those are not the very best possible, if the alternative means that some should go without altogether (see chapter 2.8).

Efficiency (technical vs. allocative)

In general terms, health care policy makers and those who 'commission' are primarily concerned with '*allocative efficiency*'—trying to maximize the population health gain from a fixed allocation of resources. (One is trying to reach a position where no one waiting for treatment has a greater ability to benefit than anyone who is already being treated.)

Health care 'providers' are more often concerned with '*technical efficiency*'—achieving a desired objective at least cost. Many of the objectives are set for them—numbers to be treated, waiting times, and so on.

In an attempt to address both types of efficiency the UK NHS in the 1990s experimented with a market model whereby the funds were held by 'purchasers' and devolved, ostensibly according to population need, to 'providers' who deliver the care. This was an attempt to harness 'market forces' to drive up quality and drive out inefficiency. Although introduced by a Conservative administration, the Labour administration which followed it in 1997 perpetuated many elements of the model, especially the separation of purchasing and providing roles. For a lucid analysis of the strengths and weaknesses of the market models in the NHS, see Enthoven, 1999.[3] For an evaluation of the evidence on the UK NHS internal market, see Legrand.[7]

Conclusion

Everyone concerned with health care can benefit from a familiarity with the health economist's way of thinking, language, and some of the tools. Health economics gives a structured approach to decision making in health care where need appears almost limitless, resources are always scarce, and therefore choices are inevitable. It is not a formulaic approach that bypasses critical appraisal, but it can greatly improve the rigour and transparency of the decision-making process.

References

1. Drummond MF, O'Brien BJ, Stoddard GL, and Torrance GW (1997). *Methods for the economic evaluation of health care programmes*, (2nd edn). Oxford University Press, Oxford.
2. Robinson R (1993). *Economic evaluation and health care*. A series of six articles in the *BMJ*: What does it mean? *BMJ*, **307**, 670–3; Costs and cost minimisation analysis. *BMJ*, **307**, 726–8; Cost effectiveness analysis. *BMJ*, **307**, 793–5; Cost utility analysis. *BMJ*, **307**, 859–62; Cost benefit analysis. *BMJ*, **307**, 924–6; The policy context. *BMJ*, **307**, 994–6.
3. Enthoven A (1999). Rock Carling Fellowship 1999. *In pursuit of an improving National Health Service*. The Nuffield Trust, London.
4. Programme budgeting and marginal analysis. An entire issue of *Health Policy* (Vol. 33, 1995) was devoted to this subject.
5. Mooney G, Gerard K, Donaldson C, and Farrar S (1992). *Priority setting in purchasing: some practical guidelines*. Research Paper 6. National Association of Health Authorities and Trusts (NAHAT), Birmingham.
6. McGuire A, Henderson J, and Mooney G (1988). *The economics of health care: an introductory text*. Routledge, London.
7. LeGrand J, Mays N, and Mulligan J (1998). *Learning from the NHS Internal market: a review of the evidence*. King's Fund, London.

2.7 **Values in public health**

Nick Steel

Objectives

Reading this chapter will:

- enable you to explain different approaches to measuring values in public health
- help you appreciate how combining an understanding of both scientific evidence and values can help make better decisions.

This chapter links economic evaluation (chapter 2.6) with ethics (chapter 2.8).

Definitions

- knowledge is ascertained by observation and experiment, critically tested and systematized
- values are moral principles or standards of behaviour; what we consider important about the way we live
- utility is the desirability of a particular outcome.

Why is it important to understand the relationship between values and public health science?

The development of a more open and explicit approach to decision making (e.g. evidence-based health care*) shows that professional behaviour is influenced by personal values. Science and values are inseparable. The challenge is to clarify the values and combine them with the science in a way that allows us to make better decisions (see chapter 2.8).

Two complementary approaches to combining science and values

It can be helpful to consider two complementary approaches to combining science and values in public health decision making:

- the *first* approach is to measure the desirability of a particular outcome (utility) in order to try to make quantitative comparisons between alternatives. Examples are decision analysis (Box 2.7.1) and quality-adjusted life-years (QALYs) and disability-adjusted life-years (DALYs) (Box 2.7.2)
- the *second* approach is holistic, placing science within the context of society's values (moral principles). The broad effects of public health decisions are considered.

Box 2.7.1 **Decision analysis**

(See chapter 5.3.)

Decision analysis quantifies the effects of the different options in a decision.[1] It combines scientific information with valuations of the benefits and burdens of the options. The analysis is usually expressed as a decision tree. For each decision in the tree, the probability of each outcome is weighted by the value of the outcome. The probability should be based on the best research available. Values are expressed as a number between 0 and 1. For example, if a person would tolerate a 20% chance of dying to *avoid* a particular outcome, then that outcome has a value of 0.8 (80%) attached to it. A variety of methods have been developed to measure values (see above). Values will change over time and according to how people are asked about them. They will be different for people with a real health problem than for a sample of the general population who might consider an illness more theoretically.

Box 2.7.2 **QALYs* and DALYs***

QALYs are years of healthy life lived. Scientific information on life expectancy is weighted with the utility of different health states. They are used as an outcome measure in cost–utility analysis (see chapter 2.6).

DALYs are years of healthy life lost. They use disability (rather than utility) weights, and are a measure of the burden of disease on a defined population.[2] The key choices are about:

- the potential years of life lost as a result of a death at a given age
- the relative value of a year of healthy life lived at different ages
- the discount rate, to allow for the greater value of human life and health in the present than the future
- the disability weights used to convert life lived with a disability to a common measure with premature death.

Measuring values

Values can be quantified by measuring preferences for health outcomes with techniques such as the standard gamble, the time trade-off, and visual analogue scales.[3] Because this is time-consuming and complex, it can be simpler to use a pre-scored multi-attribute health status classification system. Three such systems are Quality of Well-Being, Health Utilities Index, and EuroQol.[3] These include aspects of health such as pain, disability, mood, self-care, social activities, and work.

Decision analysis can be used to provide guidelines for managing similar groups of patients. The analysis is run using a selection of probabilities and values within a reasonable range for:

- the estimated probability of each outcome used in the analysis
- the estimated incidence of side effects
- the values used
- any financial cost estimates.

Treatment can then be tailored when required by matching the guidelines to the characteristics of the patient or population.[4]

The strength of decision analysis is that the values on which the decisions are based are explicit, and can be varied. The weakness lies in trying to replace the uncertainties, mysteries, and doubts that are human values by a number between 0 and 1. Using decision analysis to make decisions about groups of people may create ethical dilemmas if inequalities are increased as a result. For example, those with poor health may have low expectations, and put a low value on an intervention to improve their health. In contrast, a healthier group may have higher expectations and put a high value on an intervention to give them a relatively small health gain. A decision that incorporated these expressed values would risk increasing inequalities between the two groups.

The use of QALYs is limited by concerns over the validity of single indices of quality of life and over the effect on equity when QALYs are used to prioritize services.[3] The use of DALYs is limited by the assumption that the lives of disabled people have less value than those of people without disabilities.

Developing a holistic approach

Before applying the results of a decision analysis or cost–utility study, or any scientific evidence, the wider implications need to be considered. The perspectives of different groups in society need to be considered. Whose values are being considered? In public health decision making, most people can be considered to belong to one of three main groups:

- *professional or technocrat* (often termed 'technical')
- *public* (often termed 'user')
- *politician* (often termed 'funder').

Different perspectives lead people to draw different conclusions from the same evidence. No evidence is truly objective: all evidence is value-laden. Hence it is rarely possible to change someone's behaviour by defeating them with logic. Exploring assumptions nearly always improves the quality of decisions and their acceptability to diverse groups.

This broader approach can be fostered by reading widely. George Eliot's *Middlemarch*[5] is an example of a well-known novel that explores the impact of values on scientific progress. Robert Pirsig's *Zen and the art of motorcycle maintenance*[6] is an entertaining search for the indefinable quality that comes before the division of the world into science and values. The New York University School of Medicine Database of Literature and Medicine is one source of suitable texts.[7]

Accepting that uncertainty and variation are inevitable will foster a broader approach to decisions. Stephen Jay Gould wrote about the inevitability of uncertainty after he was diagnosed with mesothelioma and discovered the low median survival time from the disease: 'variation is the hard reality, not a set of imperfect measures for a central tendency. Means and medians are the abstractions'.[8]

Tasks to consider when combining science and values in making decisions

- be explicit about the nature of the problem, the choices available, and the relevant outcomes (especially the outcomes as valued by different [sorts of] people)
- collaborate with all those involved with the issue within your organization and outside it to incorporate as wide a range of perspectives as possible
- appraise the validity and relevance of the scientific evidence
- identify whose perspective is used to tell the story and present the evidence
- ask what has been left out
- think laterally to generate new ideas and challenge assumptions[9]
- think about the language and images used and the effect they have on the meaning
- identify which events are under human control and which are governed by chance
- distinguish the probabilities of outcomes from the values and be as precise as possible about each
- ascertain who appraised the value of outcomes, and how they did it
- be explicit about assumptions and uncertainties
- consider a sensitivity analysis to explore how varying the values and probabilities changes the decision.

Engaging other people

JK Galbraith claimed that the denigration of value judgement is one of the devices by which the scientific establishment maintains its misconceptions. One way to engage other people is to give examples of work that failed due to the denigration of value judgement, or succeeded where the contribution of both science and values was clear. The success or failure of evidence and guideline implementation are often suitable examples (see chapters 6.9 and 6.10).

Potential pitfalls

Decisions about treatment options are particularly sensitive to values when:

- the possible outcomes are greatly different (e.g. death or disability)
- treatments have greatly different probabilities and types of complications
- choices are made between short-term and long-term outcomes
- an individual or group involved is particularly risk-averse
- an individual or group considers some possible outcomes particularly important.[10]

Over-confidence in either science or values is another potential pitfall. It can lead to 'group-think', when a group making a decision looks at too few alternatives and becomes very selective in the sort of facts it sees and asks for.

Dogma, myths, and fallacies

Combining values with science has been criticized for devaluing objective knowledge. In fact, it merely recognizes that all knowledge is subjective, and the important skill is to understand whose perspective is being used, and how it affects the results. How people act is determined by an interaction between what they value and what they construe as reality. With the same information and alternatives, different people make different choices. Better choices are made when different values are explored and acknowledged as a central part of the public health task.

Conclusion

Health measures should always take account of relevant values where possible. An appreciation and acknowledgement of both the scientific base *and* value base will contribute to better, more sustainable decisions concerning the health of a population. It may be difficult to measure the success of combining science and values, but the benefits will be clear to all involved, both in terms of process and outcome.

References

1. Weinstein MC, Fineberg HV, Elstein AS, Frazier HS, Neuhauser D, Neutra RR, *et al.* (1980). *Clinical decision analysis.* WB Saunders Co., Philadelphia.
2. The World Bank (1993). *World development report 1993.* Oxford University Press, New York.
3. Drummond MF, O'Brien B, Stoddart GL, and Torrance GW (1997). *Methods for the economic evaluation of health care programmes,* (2nd edn). Oxford University Press, Oxford.
4. Lilford RJ, Pauker SG, Braunholtz DA, and Chard J (1998). Decision analysis and the implementation of research findings. *BMJ,* **317**, 405–9.
5. George Eliot (1999). *Middlemarch.* Oxford University Press, Oxford.
6. Pirsig RM (1991). *Zen and the art of motorcycle maintenance.* Vintage Press, New York.
7. New York School of Medicine. endeavor.med.nyu.edu/lit-med (accessed 17 August 2000).
8. Gould SJ (1998). The median isn't the message. In *Narrative based medicine,* (ed. T Greenhalgh and B Hurwitz), pp. 29–33. BMJ Books, London.
9. De Bono E (1990). *Lateral thinking.* Penguin Books, Harmondsworth.
10. Kassirer JP (1994). Incorporating patients' preferences into medical decisions. *N Engl J Med,* **330**, 1895–6.

2.8 **Ethics in public health**

Stuart Donnan

Objectives

By reading this chapter you will be able to appreciate more clearly the moral and ethical dimensions of public health analysis and action, and be aware of some of the ways in which these dimensions can be addressed.

Several other chapters and parts cover related material, not always distinguishing it as 'ethical' because it is so fundamental to the public health endeavour. (One particular chapter deals with the practical issues and ethical dilemmas of prioritizing; and the ways in which they can be addressed (see chapter 6.1.1).)

Background

A 1999 *BMJ* editorial entitled 'Fluoridation of water supplies: debate on the ethics must be informed by sound science'[1] encapsulates many of the important ethical issues in public health:

* *what should we be doing?*—in terms of personal liberty, what is the right of a society to medicate or intervene at a whole population level?

* *for whom should we be doing it, and at what cost/risk to others?*—where is the boundary for restricting the liberty of (or even increasing the risk of harm to) some people in order to promote the health of others?[†]

* *who should decide and how?*—to what extent, and how, should public health actions take account of public opinion?

Four important questions:

1. What are you trying to do?
2. Why are you doing it?
3. Who should decide?
4. How should it be decided?

---

† Some examples may appear simple: e.g. it is generally thought acceptable to restrict the liberty of drivers who live with epilepsy. However, to where should this boundary of restricting individual liberty extend? People who would benefit most from some public health interventions (e.g. deprived children might benefit from drinking water fluoridation) are not necessarily those who would be put at most risk by the same population intervention (people with high intakes of fluoride from other sources).

Principles

We are accustomed to the notion of evidence-based medicine where the 'right' treatment or 'right' decision is based on evidence. This implies that, somewhere, there is an objective, value-free answer. This is rarely true, even in a relatively simple clinical decision (e.g. concerning the effectiveness of a particular intervention on a defined population to produce a desired outcome) (see chapter 2.7). In public health practice, the 'right' decision almost always has an ethical, as well as a scientific dimension. Beauchamp and Childress[2] have expounded what have come to be called the 'four principles' of ethical debate and behaviour (see below). Downie and Calman in the United Kingdom have contributed to the same debate.[3,4]

The 'four principles' of ethical debate and behaviour

1. *Autonomy*: the right to individual self determination.

2. *Beneficence*: the doing of good.

3. *Non-maleficence*: the avoidance of doing harm.

4. *Justice*: equity, fairness.

From a population perspective, *justice* could be construed as subsuming *beneficence, non-maleficence,* (both related to what we might call effectiveness) and *utility* (equivalent to 'maximizing health gains for populations' in the shared ethical principles for all working in health proposed by the Tavistock Group[5]). This principle of justice and equity is held in a delicate balance with *autonomy*.

Just as the different (and often competing) dimensions of 'quality' assume importance when considered from different perspectives (see chapter 5.1), so the different (and often competing) ethical dimensions vie for importance. Nowhere is this more obvious than the balance of autonomy and individualism: Downie and Calman's[3] overarching ethical principle in a public health context is that of promoting equity.

It may appear, therefore, that some sacrifice may need to be borne in some parts of a population for the greater good. However, before his untimely death, Jonathan Mann pointed out that in public health circles, although there is often an unspoken sense that concerns over individual human rights[‡] are inherently confrontational,[6]

[‡] There are some basic dogmas or beliefs which are more or less universal or global (certainly they are labelled that way). The axiom often called the 'golden rule' (treat others as you would wish to be treated yourself) appears in some form in almost all philosophical and religious traditions around the world. Article I of the Universal Declaration of Human Rights uses the words 'dignity' and 'rights' as the basis for human relationships. (*Article I of the Universal Declaration of Human Rights*: 'All human beings are born free and equal in dignity and rights. They are endowed with reason and conscience and should act towards one another in a spirit of brotherhood.')

not all decisions necessarily involve some people with sacrifice. Discrimination toward HIV-infected people and people with AIDS is ultimately counter-productive—when infected people were deprived of employment, education, or ability to travel, the consequence was that participation in prevention programmes diminished, resulting in loss to all.

The importance of ethical analysis in public health

The history of public health is of:

* *paternalism*—with 'experts' deciding what should be done to protect communities. (In practice, this has often been to protect more affluent sections from poorer sections of the community.) Paternalism is based on certain moral and political views. For instance, at what stage are there too many public health professionals being anti-smoking crusaders and health fascists?[7]

* *utilitarianism*—the greatest good for the greatest number (Edwin Chadwick was secretary to Jeremy Bentham who, in turn, was a student of John Stuart Mill).

The ethics of public health—both 'the public health' as a phenomenon and 'public health' as an activity for professionals and others—cannot be anything but the ethics of political activity and decision making. The Ottawa Charter for Health Promotion[8] includes social justice and equity among the fundamental conditions and resources for health (with peace, shelter, education, food, income, a stable ecosystem, and sustainable resources). Beauchamp[9] goes so far as to propose *public health as social justice*.

Public health and ethics are even more closely connected in the words of John Kenneth Galbraith, who actually uses the expression 'the good society' rather than 'the healthy society'.[10]

Ethics in health has mostly focused on individuals. The population dimension has, from the earliest days, been treated as 'politics'. However, it concerns similar issues and values. Consequently, in order to do their job, public health practitioners need to be not just ethically and politically aware, but also competent in ethical and political analysis and action.

Tasks and approaches

The important challenges for public health practitioners are therefore to:

* identify and address ethical issues, not only from a traditionally individual approach, but also from a population approach

* achieve the right balance between the rights of individuals and of populations.

Such a balanced approach should avoid an over-ideological approach to decision making. Some decisions will need an individually-based approach where individual autonomy takes precedent. Conversely, other situations involve decisions where the population perspective, or 'common good' is to the fore. For instance, screening programmes are based on the the notion that the population health is improved at the expense of anxiety (false positives) and false reassurance (false negatives) for many individuals[11] (see chapter 4.7).

Defining the 'common good' involves different ethical issues from different perspectives:[12]

- *medical*: the 'prevention paradox' where public health and health promotion interventions have less immediate results for individuals and generate less public and political support
- *behavioural*: conflict between individual rights and state utilitarianism
- *socio-environmental*: an 'empowered' relationship between the state and communities to create health-promoting conditions.

Many activists would contend that, rather than agonize about what is 'just', we should focus on obvious injustices or inequities. However, this still begs the questions:

- who should decide what is just?
- how is this decided?

The importance of participative decision making

An essential ethical part of public health practice is that of involving people with the making of those decisions that have a significant ethical dimension. This is based on Galbraith's assertion that 'the prime essential for achieving the good society is a more nearly perfect expression of democratic will—genuine, inclusive'.[10] Ethical principles in public health have no meaning at all, and are certainly no warrant for action, if they are not the values and principles of the players and recipients in the public health field. Inequity and inequality can only be properly defined by including those on the receiving end.

It is important to be aware of the range of mechanisms to involve the values, views, and wishes of a wide range of people (see chapter 8.2). This includes:

- citizens' juries
- user consultation
- panels
- focus groups*
- questionnaire surveys
- opinion surveys[13]

For instance, while all UK governments want to sustain the NHS, they struggle to engage the public in deciding how to trade universal access (free at the point of delivery), comprehensiveness, and high quality, all within current resources.[14]

Politicians are unwilling to lead on rationing because it would involve them (rather than the health professionals) taking the criticism and blame. Public health practitioners often find themselves taking the lead in informing people and shaping opinion (see chapter 6.1). This new, benign paternalism[15] nevertheless brings with it a heavy responsibility for being open and, in particular, being patient and tolerant when the public thinks differently from the professionals and the politicians.

Downie and Calman[3] ask, 'How do we know that our principles are true, rather than a matter of taste, or opinion, or Western prejudice?' We should work with the principles which we have genuinely elicited from—and have come to share with—the communities we work with (rather than with any principles intrinsically associated with being public health practitioners). We can only know about success and failures, in both our analysis and our actions, if we are in touch with the people whose health is the object of the exercise— they are the ones who know about inequities and inequalities and dis-utilities and exclusion.

Successes and failures and how to distinguish them

Prioritization of public services within a limited budget is often used as the litmus test of how a society makes difficult decisions. Two of the best known examples are from Oregon, USA, and from New Zealand:

• The well-known prioritization exercise in Oregon did not succeed in involving the public in its decision making.[16] (Most of the public consultations were populated by professionals.)

• The New Zealand prioritization exercise used a Delphi process among professionals.[17] (These were not successes if measured by participation.)

Conclusion

The challenge is to get '...needed goods distributed to needy people in proportion to their neediness...to get all this right, or to get it roughly right, is to map out the entire social world'.[18] However, the public health practitioner must remember that they are engaged in an ethical and not simply a technical mission:

'...the central ethical dilemma in public health (is) the conflict between the rights of the individual and the responsibilities of the society for all its members.'[19]

Remember:

* most issues in public health have an ethical dimension
* the important dilemmas are usually between the rights of individuals and of populations, and between different subgroups within populations
* it is important to avoid ideological approaches to ethical decision making; at least be open and clear about the different ethical dimensions and how they interrelate
* be clear about exactly what you are trying to achieve, for what reason, for whom, and how
* even if you can not guarantee the decisions are right, you *can* guarantee the rationale is clear, and the process is explicit
* handling ethical issues well involves genuine participative decision making
* be patient.

Further resources

Beauchamp DE and Steinbock B (1999). *New ethics for the public's health*. Oxford University Press, Oxford.

References

1. Coggon D and Cooper C (1999). Fluoridation of water supplies: debate on ethics must be informed by sound science. *BMJ*, **319**, 269–70.
2. Beauchamp TL and Childress JF (1994). *Principles of biomedical ethics*, (4th edn). Oxford University Press, New York.
3. Downie RS and Calman KC (1994). *Healthy respect: ethics in health care*, (2nd edn). Oxford University Press, Oxford.
4. Calman KC and Downie RS (1997). Ethical principles and ethical issues in public health. In *Oxford textbook of public health*, Vol. 1, (3rd edn), ch. 23. Oxford University Press, Oxford.
5. Tavistock Group (1999). Shared ethical principles for everybody in health care. *BMJ*, **318**, 248–51.
6. Mann J (1997). Medicine and public health; ethics and human rights. *Hastings Center Reports*, **27**(3), 6–13.
7. Skrabanek P (1994). *The death of humane medicine and the rise of coercive healthism*. Social Affairs Unit, London.
8. World Health Organization (1986). *Ottawa charter for health promotion*, Report on the 1st International Conference on Health Promotion. WHO, Geneva.
9. Beauchamp DE (1976). Exploring new ethics for public health. *J Health Politics, Policy and Law*, **1**, 338–54.
10. Galbraith JK (1996). *The good society: the humane agenda*. Houghton Mifflin, Boston.
11. Shickle D and Chadwick R (1994). The ethics of screening: is screeningitis an incurable disease? *J Med Ethics*, **20**, 12–8.
12. Labonte R (1998). Health promotion and the common good: towards a politics of practice. *Critical Public Health*, **2**, 107–29.

13. Jordan J, Donswell T, Harrison S, Lilford RJ, and Mort M (1998). Whose priorities? Listening to users and the public. *BMJ*, **316**, 1668–70.

14. Smith R (1999). Stumbling into rationing. *BMJ*, **319**, 936.

15. *Paternalism or partnership.* Editorial and a series of papers in the *British Medical Journal* of 18 September 1999 (vol. 319, pp 719 and ff.).

16. Honigsbaum F (1991). *Who shall live? Who shall die?—Oregon's health financing proposals.* King's Fund College Papers 4. King's Fund, London.

17. Hadorn DC and Holmes AC (1997). The New Zealand priority criteria project—Part 1, Overview. *BMJ*, **314**, 131–4.

18. Walzer M (1983). *Spheres of justice—a defence of pluralism and equality.* Blackwell, Oxford.

19. Horner J (2000). The virtuous public health physician. *Pub Hlth Med*, **22**, 48–53.

The only freedom which deserves its name, is that of pursuing our own good in our own way, so long as we do not attempt to deprive others of theirs, or impede their efforts to obtain it.

Mill JS 1806–73

The only purpose for which power can be rightfully exercised over any member of a civilised community against his will, is to prevent harm to others.

Mill JS 1806–73

Part 3
Policy

Introduction

Policy is 'a course of action or principle adopted or proposed by a government, party, business, or individual'.[1]

In this part we consider approaches to influencing policy, from the micro-environment of the public health practitioner's own team or organization, through to the international arena. At each of these levels, policies can have powerful effects on health, and public health practitioners need to be armed with the skills and insights necessary to safeguard and improve health by improving policy. Without the coherent framework that good policy offers, the actions of organizations can become fragmented and different initiatives can easily undermine each other.

Science and logic may help to identify public health problems and potential solutions, but emotion and power relationships determine whether anything is done about them. Turning analysis into policy requires a range of specific skills. At the organizational level, personal skills and relationships are clearly important, and thoughtful approaches to them can help, as Koh illustrates in chapter 3.1.

Good policy is designed for successful implementation, and one approach to focusing attention on the progress of policy implementation is to set targets. In chapter 3.2, Frommer, *et al.* provide an overview and examples, highlighting the methodological skills, local knowledge, communication skills, and understanding of the process of government that is needed to translate centrally set targets into local action.

In chapter 3.3, Anderson and Hussey provide a thorough guide to understanding policy and policy making at governmental level, with examples from the USA and the UK. The US political system at federal level is characterized by a relatively weak executive branch of government, often in policy making competition with different groupings in Congress. With expensive and frequent elections, interest groups, the media, and public opinion are openly acknowledged as central to the policy making agenda. They distinguish between policy as a statement and policy making as a process. Anderson and Hussey also emphasize how much policy can change during the implementation process, and how important evaluation of the end results of policy is to making further progress.

In countries with a measure of democracy, public opinion and the actions of interest groups become ever more important. Harnessing public opinion and engaging in public debate is therefore one of the major challenges of contemporary public health. As Wall points out in chapter 3.4, scientists are still mostly content with the traditional modes of journal publication, but public health practitioners should accept the challenge of 'taking the message to the mainstream'.

Much of the public discourse on health issues is abbreviated by the media into simplified notions of what each issue is really about. To public health practitioners, gun control is about saving lives, but to the gun lobby, opposing gun control is about limiting the power of the state and preserving the freedom of the individual. As Chapman makes clear in chapter 3.5, such framing of issues in the media is critical to how they are dealt with, and understanding this process, and responding directly to an adverse framing of an issue, can be critical to influencing policy and politicians.

Public health action is influenced by governments at many different levels, from regional or constituent states, to national and supranational legislative institutions like the European Union. Global companies and global organizations can now have major influences on 'local' public health problems, and practitioners must now both think and act locally and globally, as Lang and Caraher explain in chapter 3.6.

In an age in which people are encouraged to think of themselves as individuals and consumers, the collective institutions of government and business influence ever more aspects of health. These institutions are themselves held together by links at every level from the local to the global. In the global village, public opinion and the media can be critical to getting public health issues onto the policy agenda, and keeping them there. In analysing the opportunities to influence policy at the various levels, our contributors have returned to the same major themes: the importance of recognizing the task of influencing policy as a specific challenge of public health practice, as a challenge that requires an understanding of the policy making process and the adoption of specific attitudes and skills. At most levels above the local, getting public health issues into the mainstream of public debate and influencing public opinion are seen as a major challenge to public health practitioners.

Further resources

Spasoff RA (1999). *Epidemiologic methods for health policy*. Oxford University Press, Oxford.

References

1. *The new Oxford dictionary of English* (1998). Oxford University Press, Oxford.

DM

3.1 Shaping your organization's policy

Yi Mien Koh

Introduction

One of the key functions of a public health professional is to influence and shape policy decisions at all levels for the benefit of the public's health. The ability of you and your team to shape policy is largely dictated by the influence you have within your organization. In particular, your ability to drive forward health-related policy will depend on the way you use and develop your power through your communication, negotiation, and conflict-handling skills.

Objectives

After studying this chapter you will be better able to:

- understand what influences how policies are made in organizations
- examine the role of power in organizations
- appreciate the way power is managed through personal behaviour
- improve your skills in managing conflict
- understand the impact change has on you and others
- develop your own ability to influence policy making.

Organizations and policies

A policy is a plan or course of action that a person, team, or organization takes, or proposes to take. It makes explicit the principles that will be used when faced with an opportunity, challenge, or problem. Policies can be triggered by internal or external factors. Internal factors include new people in senior posts, the introduction of new systems, changes in organizational structures, or the identification of problems leading to action being needed. External factors can include new government policies cascading down for local implementation, changes in technology, and changes in local, national, or global economic or political conditions.

In order to influence policy in your organization, you need to understand both the current situation and the preceding events. In particular, you need to understand:

- the rationale of the prevailing policies—what they are intended to achieve
- the actual consequences of the policies—what they actually achieve

* the origins of these policies—both in terms of organizations and of people

* the forces that have shaped, encouraged (and inhibited) both their ratification and implementation.

Any significant change in policy, or revision of old policies, implies changes to the ways people and organizations work. Change is rarely universally welcomed; some people are likely to resist it, often for personal reasons as much as for more ideological reasons. Either way, policy changes are heavily influenced by power relationships within groups of people.

Power as a source of influence

Power can be defined as the capacity to get others to do things they might not otherwise do. Effective management requires the appropriate use of power. Within an organization, the power and influence of an individual or team depends on how valuable they are perceived to be, usually by other powerful people. Your value, or the value of your team, to the organization will be determined by your perceived ability to contribute to the organization's goals. Similarly, your value to any other individual or team in the organization depends on how valuable you are to their goals (whether or not these equate to the organization's goals).

Maintaining and increasing your power in an organization in order to allow you to shape policy therefore means being highly attuned to the organization's objectives, and to the objectives of other influential people within it. In order to maintain your policy-shaping ability, you need to evolve, being highly sensitive to influential people. (In contrast, revolution nearly always involves looking in other directions for support.) Lastly, the degree of power you have depends on how much power others have—power is relative.

In order to understand the power, influence, and policy-shaping abilities of those around you, it can be helpful to appreciate how power is manifested. French and Raven[1] identified different power types:

* *resource power (reward power)*—the person with this power has control of the resources valued by the potential recipient, and has the power to reward those that comply with his request

* *position power (also known as legislative power)*—occupancy of the role or position entitles you to all the rights of that role in the organization

* *coercive power*—having the ability to punish, for example the withdrawal of privileges or imposed penalties

* *personal power*—this is also called charisma or referent power. This power resides in the person and in their personality. Although enhanced by a position or by expert status, it is tied to

the individual rather than the position. Charisma refers to the near-magical ability of some individuals to influence others

- *expert power*—this is a power that is vested in someone because of his or her acknowledged expertise—a public health professional in an organization usually has expert power, but only if they develop their expertise and use it effectively and appropriately

- *negative power*—this power is the capacity to stop things happening. It is probably more appropriately described as the negative use of power, so called when the domain of power is regarded as disruptive and illegitimate.

These types of power are important if you wish to be influential. They will help you identify your own sources of power which you may be under-using, or of which you may be unaware. The list may also help you identify those sources of power which you need to develop in order to achieve effective public health change.

Power, politics, and political behaviour

The use of power is a political process. Put another way, politics is the use of different sorts of power to shape policy and achieve desired ends. The appropriate use of power requires appropriate use of political process, and vice versa. Although many people are understandably suspicious about the political process, politics is a highly necessary and effective way of achieving change. It is important not to become over-cynical about the political process.

Remember, politics can:

- be organizational rather than self focused
- be well-intentioned rather than ill-intentioned
- be supportive rather than destructive, and
- support organizational change rather than individual interest.

Political behaviour to shape policy is largely governed by:

- knowing what you are trying to achieve (see chapter 7.1)
- the methods and the skills you are going to use in order to achieve it
- the ability to interact well with your surroundings.

Being aware and being open

The ability to interact well with your surroundings depends on a vitally important set of skills: being aware (sensing and processing incoming information) and being appropriately open with others (processing and transmitting outgoing information). In summary:

- the degree of awareness you have of what is happening around you (listening skills, your skills whilst 'on receive')

- the degree of openness with which you interact with others (your skills whilst 'on transmit').

  This is shown in Figure 3.3.1 below:

	Open communication	**Closed communication**
High awareness of what is happening around you	a Aware — open communication	b Aware — closed communication
Low awareness of what is happening around you	c Unaware — open communication	d Unaware — closed communication

Figure 3.1.1 Being aware, and being open (adapted from Baddeley and James.[2])

(a) Aware–open communication (left upper quadrant)

These people believe that different interests can be satisfied. They believe in their personal power to achieve change, and in collaboration to gain support. They are usually aware of the purpose and interested in the direction. They can cope with being disliked, have good interpersonal skills and have high levels of self knowledge. They think before they speak, are assertive, tactful, plan actions, and check gossip or rumour. They are aware of others' viewpoints, take account of other people personally, and publicly value their contribution. They know how the informal processes work, are non-defensive, learn from mistakes, and reflect on events. They can make procedures work for them. Often there is a sense of loyalty to the immediate team and a capacity for friendship. These people need to recognize, however, that not all game players will collaborate. This group may not recognize when personal goals become more important.

(b) Aware–closed communication (right upper quadrant)

These people believe in their personal power to achieve and in their personal vision and responsibility. They risk seeing organizations as principally political playgrounds and organizational goals as secondary to their own personal goals. They often think before speaking, are often aggressive but well masked, with a charming appearance. They check gossip and rumour and are aware of others' viewpoints.

The main problem with such individuals is that they get diverted from organizational goals. They fail to recognize their impact on others and often achieve only limited change.

(c) Unaware–open communication (left lower quadrant)

These people believe in expert and position power—you are powerful if you are right. Characteristics include tending to rely on authority, sticking to etiquette for organizational and professional rules, taking things literally, having capacity for friendship, being open, and seeing things in black or white. They have strong sense of loyalty, and try to avoid conflict but tend to get involved unwittingly. These behaviours are limiting because the individuals do not appreciate political purpose, they don't network and thus don't know how to get support.

(d) Unaware–closed communication (right lower quadrant)

These individuals believe that they can't personally make a difference and that nothing ever really changes. They see managing change as someone else's responsibility. These people see things in black and white. They often lack interpersonal skills, don't recognize 'directions', and don't appreciate political purpose. Often they are concerned with their own feelings rather than those of others and lack the skills to develop partnerships.

The ideal goal is to have everyone in the top left quadrant. That may not be achievable, but you can start by understanding yourself, and improving your political awareness, by working through the framework below. In order to make this diagram useful, ask yourself the following questions:

- where is my influence and power?
- what do I need to do to start influencing more effectively as in the top left quadrant?
- where do key people sit in the matrix?
- what can I do to encourage others to manage their relationship with me in the top left quadrant?
- what can I do to manage relationships with people who will not operate in the top left quadrant?

Managing conflict

Conflicts are bound to arise when new policies are being developed or implemented. Conflicts arise because we all want different things (both in terms of process and outcome), especially at times of change. Individuals will make every effort to get as much as possible out of a changing situation. To enable the policy change to be accepted successfully, you also need to consider putting effort into giving what other people want. When conflict arises, it is possible to observe (and adopt) any of the following behavioural characteristics (sometimes in combination):

(a) Competing

You put a lot of effort into getting what you want and get your way. This does not achieve others' goals and ends up with a win/lose approach. This style leads to other people becoming competitive too.

(b) Avoiding

This style is used when you are unassertive and unco-operative: you simply avoid the issue—which can be useful when you think the time is not right, but can often be because you prefer an unsatisfactory situation to a possibly more satisfactory situation which involves conflict. The lesson is to know when conflict is necessary and when it is counter-productive. Unfortunately some people like conflict for the sake of it . . .

(c) Accommodating

This style is used when you are willing to give in to others. You can use this to build banks of favours on things that are not that important to you, but more important to others. Too much accommodating, however, can make you ineffective. This style is co-operative but not always assertive.

(d) Collaborating

This style is high on the assertive–co-operation spectrum. You need to be acutely aware of the needs and desires of others, as well as your own self-interest. By managing everyone's self-interest you may be in a good position to remove threat and gain more support.

(e) Compromising

This style involves both parties ending up with some of their interests met.

Successful management skills require you to be assertive, and to be able to see things from the other person's point of view. Key personal skills to be developed include presenting your arguments clearly; using questions effectively, listening actively, and perceiving other people's behaviour accurately.

Summary

Understanding your environment and the power that is wielded within this environment is essential in order to shape organizational policy. Having now understood the roles politics and conflict play in organizational change, you can consult at least two other related chapters elsewhere in this guide:

* develop a high level of self-awareness, and self development (see chapter 7.7)
* lead other people (see chapter 7.1).

Conclusion

Few public health practitioners hold formal positions that come with great power to shape their organizations, but most have the potential for considerable influence. Improving your effectiveness in influencing organizational policy is built on understanding power, politics, leadership, and the management of change. Understanding these concepts and skills should help you learn to engage in organizational politics and policy making in a positive and more effective way.

Further resources

Goleman D (2000). Leadership that gets results. *Harvard Business Review*, 78(2), 78–90.

References

1. French JP and Raven B (1986). The bases of social power. In *Group dynamics: research and theory*, (3rd edn), (ed. D Cartwright and AF Zander). Harper and Row, New York.
2. Baddeley S and James K (1987). Owl, fox, donkey or sheep: political skills for managers. *Management Education and Development*, 18(1), 3–19.

3.2 Translating goals and targets into public health action

Michael Frommer, Stephen Leeder, George Rubin, and Michelle Tjhin

Introduction

Governments in many countries responded to the World Health Organization's Alma Ata declaration of Health for All by the Year 2000[1] by setting health goals and targets and taking action to implement them. Surprisingly, the setting of explicit national and international objectives for health has only recently become a major theme of health policy. Few instances can be found before the 1950s. Early examples, such as the objectives of American public health efforts in the 1950s and 1960s to reduce infant mortality rates and improve tuberculosis control, were more implicit than explicit.[2] The 1966 World Health Organization resolution to eradicate smallpox by 31 December 1976[3] is a more explicit example. It is also a highly impressive illustration of the potential public health impact of a goal, linked with an expressed target, leading to political commitment and effective programmes of action.

Objectives

In this chapter we show how goals and targets can be applied in practice to enhance the effectiveness of public health services. Our use of 'goal', 'target', and related terms is explained in Box 3.2.1.

A health *goal* may refer to health status; prevalence or incidence of, or mortality from, a particular condition; diagnostic or treatment processes; social, personal, or environmental risk factors; processes to modify risk factors or outcomes; or any other social dimension connected with health. Goals may be relevant to a whole population or to particular groups within it.

Targets provide a measure of what could be achieved with effective intervention. Targets usually express the intended occurrence of the phenomenon at a future date, and this future value is often published together with a baseline figure. A goal may be related to or expressed in terms of one or more targets. Targets are usually expressed in terms of indicators.

Targets should be SMART:

- Specific
- Measurable

Box 3.2.1 **Explanation of terms**

Goal

A goal is a general statement of intent or aspiration. It refers to outcomes that are considered to be achievable with current knowledge and resources[4] e.g. 'reduce the incidence of, and mortality from, melanoma'.

Target

A target specifies a measurable positive change in a health-related phenomenon that could occur within a given period of time, in a particular population, if steps are taken to achieve the desired change; e.g. to reduce melanoma incidence to 32 new cases per 100,000 men in Australia by 2000.

Indicator

An indicator is a measure that reflects, directly or indirectly, the occurrence of a health-related phenomenon, some aspect of a health-related phenomenon, or a process that could influence the occurrence of a health-related phenomenon.

* Achievable
* Relevant/Realistic
* Timed.

Health *indicators* may be classified as reflecting health status; the outcomes of particular interventions; risk factors; or processes. Note however that this terminology is not universal, and terms can vary between countries.

Translating national goals into local targets and indicators

The *primary task* of the health service is to reconcile the broad national goals and targets with the health needs of your region's population. This involves:

* developing a local plan which reflects the national approach, while emphasizing the effective interventions relevant to the goals
* implementing the plans
* monitoring progress.

Regional efforts to contribute to national goals and targets should concentrate on interventions for which there is evidence of effectiveness. Monitoring systems that can track locally important health indicators as well as progress towards national targets are an essential part of the response.

The health service should be opportunistic and creative in pursuing additional resources that are likely to accompany national and regional political commitment to goals and targets. These resources (funds and intellectual capacity) can be used for regional priorities that mirror the national priorities, and (if framed shrewdly) can also provide spin-off support for other regional priorities.

Developing a local plan

Developing a plan for local implementation of the national goals and targets involves seven steps.

1. **Situation analysis,** which entails:
   - getting a clear and detailed understanding of national and regional expectations associated with the publication of the national goals and targets
   - reviewing the epidemiology of health problems at a regional level which relates to the national goals and targets, and the availability of data about these problems
   - reviewing current regional objectives and programmes relevant to the national goals and targets
   - comparing the epidemiological profile, availability of data, and relevant current programmes with the regional picture
   - listing leading regional health problems which are not covered by the national goals and targets.

2. **Consultation** with professional and managerial colleagues and the community. Effective consultation is crucial both for the validity of the plan and for its subsequent implementation, and must begin at the start of the development of the plan. Implementation of the plan will be a complex process, with individuals in the health service or the community standing to lose or gain from some of your recommendations. Your consultation process should both identify barriers to the implementation of the plan and lay the groundwork for lowering or removing them.

3. **Review of published information** to find and/or evaluate interventions that are likely to work in solving the problems identified in the situation analysis.

4. **Assessment of the feasibility, acceptability, costs, and benefits** of these interventions if they were applied in the region (or their benefits and opportunity costs, if they are already being applied).

5. **Estimate of resources** needed to carry out the plan. This should be accompanied by estimates of known available resources and additional resources needed.

6. **Formulation of recommendations for action,** with timetable and allocation of responsibilities. This will include the setting of local targets, discussed in more detail below. Local targets will often differ from national targets. This should not cause a problem if the reasons are stated and justified.

7. **Preparation of a planning document.** This must:

   • persuade your own executives to make a commitment to your recommendations

   • provide national and regional authorities with evidence that your region is responding positively to their policy agenda.

The document should contain the following, with an explanation of the rationale, resource implications, timetable, and line of responsibility for each recommendation (see chapter 8.4):

• a list of new actions to be started (new interventions or new programmes which are supported by evidence or other strong rationale)

• a list of existing interventions or programmes to be stopped (because there is evidence that they do not work)

• a list of existing interventions to be maintained, either at their current level or with some enhancement or diminution.

In addition to these lists of specific actions, the document should provide:

• a summary of costs, available resources, and additional resources needed for implementation of the plan

• a description of how the health service should monitor both the implementation of the plan and its consequences for the health of the region's population. This should include a specification of indicators and local targets, which should correspond to or supplement, but not replace, the indicators published for the national targets.

Setting local targets

The setting of regional or local targets is important because it helps to establish appropriate local expectations, taking account of:

• baseline local rates of health problems (your initial situation analysis should tell you whether and how much these differ from national rates)

• evidence of the likely magnitude of the effect of proposed interventions

• the local feasibility of these interventions.

The setting of local targets for melanoma in your region serves as an example. Melanoma was selected as a 'priority cancer' in Australia because of:

• the burden of illness and the number of person-years of life lost
• the potential for prevention and the potential benefits of early detection
• the fact that its incidence has increased (although the increase may have been due partly to improved and earlier detection).

The goal is to 'reduce the incidence of and mortality from melanoma'.

Melanoma is the fourth most common cancer nationally, and the third most common cancer in your region. From your previous epidemiological surveillance using data from your region's cancer registry (see chapter 1.3), you already know that the incidence in your region is 40% higher than the regional incidence. This might reflect the coastal subtropical setting of the region, and the skin characteristics of much of the population. Risk factors for melanoma include exposure to sunlight (ultraviolet radiation), especially intermittent exposure and childhood exposure, sensitivity of the skin to sunlight, and family history of melanoma.

Reduction in the incidence of melanoma is likely to occur in the longer term through a combination of personal protection from sunlight and environmental changes. Reduction in melanoma mortality is likely to follow from prevention and early detection. Programmes to promote prevention and early detection—aimed at the general community, educational institutions, workplaces, and the health professions—are already in progress in your region.

National and regional data on the occurrence of melanoma are given in Box 3.2.2. 'What are the issues in setting local targets for melanoma?'

Key issues are:

1. *The high baseline incidence.* This may lead you to expect a greater *reduction* than the national targets project, but a *higher local target incidence* than the national target incidence (as shown in Box 3.2.2, the original national target incidence is unlikely to be achieved).

2. *The long latent period.* Although you may have been running prevention programmes for some time, their effect on melanoma incidence is unlikely to be detectable for many years. Enhancement of these programmes in tune with the national goals and targets will take even longer to be detectable.

3. The need, therefore, to focus on *targets* that reflect process change (e.g. changes in interventions) and risk factor change (environmental—e.g. shaded areas, and behavioural—e.g. reduction in exposure to sunlight).

Box 3.2.2 **'What are the issues in setting local targets for melanoma?'**

Melanoma is the fourth most common cancer in Australia. The 1994 Australia-wide incidence was 42.9 new cases per 100,000 population in men, and 32.4 in women. There were 3,694 new cases in total.

Melanoma is the third most common cancer in the state of New South Wales. The 1994 NSW incidence was 45.1 new cases per 100,000 population in men, and 30.6 in women.

National melanoma death rates in 1996 were 6.7 per 100,000 population in men, and 3.0 in women.

National projections indicate a rising incidence (to 49.1 per 100,000 in men and 35.9 in women in 1999), with a widening gap between male and female rates.

The figures cited above are all age-adjusted using the Australian population as at 30 June 1991 as the standard population.

The year 2000 Australian incidence target for melanoma, published in 1994 from a 1988 baseline, was 32.4 new cases per 100,000 in men, and 27.6 in women. In view of subsequent trends and the 1999 projections given above, these rates are most unlikely to be achieved.

Data taken from the Australian Institute of Health and Welfare, 1998, Public Health Division, Sydney, NSW, 1997 and the Commonwealth Department of Human Services and Health, 1994.

4. *Linkage* of these targets with particular groups in the region's population. Your knowledge of the local population (coupled with input from your consultation process) will help you to specify groups in which particular interventions are important and likely to be effective. These might include certain occupational groups with intermittent high levels of sun exposure, or communities with high proportions of children and young people. Special process and risk factor change targets can be set for such groups. Tangible progress (or lack of progress) towards them can be monitored relatively easily, and the lessons be reported and applied elsewhere.

5. *Surgical treatment indicators.* Given the regional focus on melanoma, you might expect regional services for the early detection of melanoma to be as effective as those in the major centres. Early detection relies on community awareness of its importance, prompt and appropriate referral from primary care services, and competent surgical and pathology services. With existing or enhanced programmes in these areas, your proposed target for early detection (the proportion of melanomas with less than

a critical thickness at the time of diagnosis) could be the same as, or more stringent than, the national targets.[5]

6. *Mortality*. Regional targets for overall melanoma mortality should reflect the high baseline incidence, although, with effective early detection, case fatality rates should be similar to those in the best centres.

In setting local targets, it is important to recognize the heterogeneity of the population, not only because of variations in baseline occurrence of diseases or risk factors among groups within a population, but also because of the varying responsiveness of particular groups to specific interventions. For some conditions, variations in baseline rates are enormous. For example, the prevalence of type 2 diabetes in many Aboriginal communities is up to ten times that of the rest of the Australian population, with diabetes affecting almost half of the adults in these communities. The setting of targets for diabetes control in these communities—and the interventions which might lead to the achievement of the targets—requires not only a detailed knowledge of the medical opportunities for diabetes control, but also a deep understanding of Aboriginal social values and community processes.

In setting targets generally, disease modelling aimed at estimating what change in incidence could be achieved by plausible changes in risk exposure, can help in setting targets. Can-Trol is an example of such a model, which was used in developing cancer objectives in the USA.[6]

The hazards of setting targets

When realistic targets are set, based on an understanding of the intervention evidence, they can catalyse local action to achieve the desired health goals. Unfortunately, targets are sometimes set in an irrational political or managerial atmosphere, and appear to be used on occasions to deflect attention or seek populist advantage. In such circumstances, the chosen targets are often arbitrary. Targets should be realistic: it is important not to set either impossible or very easy targets.

As time and effort moves on to implementation and monitoring of progress, failure to achieve targets can lead to disappointment or disillusion, even when much good work has been done and a worthwhile proportion of the heath goal had been achieved. Sometimes failure to fully achieve targets is used in efforts to discredit the goals themselves, as has happened from time to time in the political debate over efforts to reduce poverty.

A good evidence base, and a collaborative and inclusive approach to setting targets, as well as regular review and updating of targets and indicators, are all necessary in the successful achievement of goals.

Conclusion

As a public health practitioner you can make a major contribution to the implementation of national health goals and targets at a local or regional level. You can bring:

- methodological skills: the ability to search literature databases and appraise published evidence for and against particular interventions, and the methodological skills and experience in epidemiology, population health surveillance, health needs assessment, public health programme development, implementation and evaluation, and health economics

- local knowledge: first-hand personal and epidemiological knowledge of the local population and the local environment (political, social, and physical), and knowledge of, and possible responsibility for, local programmes (existing, planned, and possible) which are likely to have a bearing on the goals and targets

- communication skills: which enable you to persuade others (such as members of the regional executive) to initiate, support, and sustain effective programmes, or cease ineffective interventions.

In addition to your knowledge, skills, and experience, you can also bring a crucial understanding of government processes. You therefore know when and how to persist with well-argued public health recommendations in the face of varying budget cycles and the continuous structural changes that affect all health systems. You also know how to identify opportunities when they arise, and you are ready to adjust your recommendations in response to new opportunities.

Further resources

European Journal of Public Health. Supplement 2000.

van Herten LM and van de Water H (1999). New global Health for All targets. *BMJ*, **319(7211)**, 700–3.

McKee M and Fulop N (2000). On target for health? *BMJ*, **320(7231)**, 327–8.

Our Healthier Nation, (1998), ch.4. HMSO, London.

Public Health Division (1997). *The health of the people of New South Wales— report of the Chief Health Officer*. NSW Health Department, Sydney.

References

1. World Health Organization (WHO) (1978). *Alma Ata 1978: primary health care*, Health For All series, No. 1. WHO, Geneva.
2. Breslow L (1987). Setting objectives for public health. *Annual Review of Public Health*, **8**, 289–307.
3. World Health Organization (WHO) (1971). *Handbook of resolutions and decisions of the World Health Assembly and the Executive Board*. WHO, Geneva.
4. Commonwealth Department of Human Services and Health (1994). *Better health outcomes for Australians. National goals, targets and strategies for*

better health outcomes into the next century. Australian Government Publishing Service, Canberra.

5. Nutbeam D, Wise M, Bauman A, Harris E, and Leeder S (1994). *Goals and targets for Australia's health in the year 2000 and beyond.* Australian Government Publishing Service, Canberra.

6. Eddy DM (1986). Setting priorities for cancer control programs. *J Natl Cancer Inst*, **76**, 187–99.

3.3 Influencing government policy: a framework

Gerard Anderson and Peter Sotir Hussey

Introduction

Influencing government policy requires an understanding of what public policy is, how public policy is developed, and what levers are available to influence the policy making process. While countries differ in the details of their policy making arrangements, the broad themes set out below are relevant in most Western democracies.

The national policy process is important to public health professionals because much of the funding of public health activities comes from national sources. In addition, policy makers establish regulations, administer programmes, and influence many activities relevant to the health of their populations.

Objectives

This chapter will help you:

• understand the nature and steps involved in national policy process
• understand the available levers and skills needed to influence policy.

Public policy and the policy making process

> Box 3.3.1
> **Public policy** is what the government chooses to do or not to do about perceived problems, and **policy making** is the process by which the government decides what will be done about perceived problems.

Political scientists have summarized the policy making process in four stages. The four stages are shown in Figure 3.3.1.

1. Agenda setting

Agenda setting occurs when policy makers identify a problem and develop broad goals to address it. In health care, examples of potential problems include rising health expenditures, an unexpected increase in infant mortality, or an unexpected increase in the prevalence of a disease (e.g. AIDS). Health care issues such as these must compete against other policy issues (such as national defence) to become

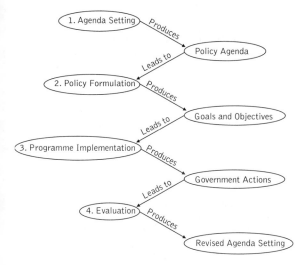

Figure 3.3.1 The policy making process.

national priorities, and specific health issues must compete for attention with other health issues. Policy makers can focus on only a limited number of problems at any one time.

A considerable amount of effort is required to place an issue on the forefront of the policy making agenda. The following factors can help *place an issue on the political agenda*:

- the greater the number of people who perceive that the problem exists
- the greater the perceived severity of the problem
- the more immediate and novel the problem is perceived to be
- the more likely it is to affect an individual personally.

Public interest alone does not guarantee that an issue will be placed on the public agenda, however. To be placed on the public agenda, policy makers must *consider the issue within the purview of government action* and deserving of public attention. Many policy issues that have long-term consequences or only minor consequences for an individual are unlikely to become one of the two or three most pressing health care policy concerns. Unfortunately, many traditional public health issues fall into this category.

Many different approaches are used to place an issue at the forefront of the public policy agenda. One method is to try to influence public opinion. This can be done through the media, personal appeals by public officials and celebrities, public awareness advertising campaigns, and many other approaches. Public opinion has its greatest impact on government decision making when people feel strongly about clear-cut preferences. Although government policy tends to coincide with public opinion, this may not always be the case, particularly when a well-organized interest group intervenes or public apathy is evident. Special interests can have a particularly important role on technical issues or issues than involve only a few people.

In health care, there is an unequal distribution of information; doctors and other health professionals have specialized knowledge. As a result, individuals must often place their trust in health care professionals. These health professionals who hold and control information have considerable leverage over public opinion.

> ## Box 3.3.2
> As a major source of political information, *the media* help shape the public's perception of reality. These perceptions, in turn, constitute a basis for the public's political activity.

The *media* can have a strong influence on public opinion. Interest groups, politicians, and others are all trying to influence how the media frame issues and reports the news. Political leaders and news people are often mutually dependent. Politicians rely on the media to provide them with information and to convey their message to the public. The media, in turn, rely heavily on public officials for information they use as the basis for their reporting (see chapters 3.5 and 7.4).

Interest groups attempt to influence the agenda-setting process to foster their own particular interests. They provide information and financial resources, mobilize voters, and use other techniques to influence the agenda-setting process. The influence of individual interest groups depends on such factors as the nature of the group's membership, its financial and leadership resources, its prestige and status, and government structure, rules, and procedures.

Political parties serve as linkages or intermediaries between the citizens and their government.

'A Party is a body of men united, for promoting by their endeavors the national interest, upon some particular principle in which they are all agreed.'

Edmund Burke, 1770

Officially and unofficially they have a major role in agenda setting. Party leaders have major roles in determining the agenda of the party in advance of an election and then balancing the conflicting priorities of various interest groups between elections.

2. Policy formulation

Once it is widely recognized that a problem requires government attention, policy makers must develop a policy agenda that in turn will lead to policy formulation.

Policy formulation involves developing alternative proposals and then collecting, analysing, and communicating the information necessary to assess the alternatives and begin to persuade people to support one proposal or another. Policy formulation involves compromising and bargaining in order to satisfy various interests and build a coalition of support.

Next, specific policies have to be adopted. Known by political scientists as legitimization, government policy must conform to the public's perception of the proper way to do things.

Box 3.3.3

In the United States, the benefits of *incrementalism* were most apparent in the Clinton administration's proposal to reform the health care system. Introduced as a fundamental reform of the health care system with numerous provisions that altered nearly every aspect of the health care financing and delivery system, it had the effect of alienating nearly every constituency group on some issue. Following its defeat, the Clinton administration emphasized incremental health care reform. Hillary Rodham Clinton, one of the major architects of the proposal, recently declared herself a member of the 'school of smaller steps' in the area of health care policy. (*Washington Post, 9 July 1999, p. A4*)

Frequently, previous policies of the government are good predictors of future policies, since people tend to prefer incremental changes over major changes.

Policy formulation involves many of the same components as agenda setting. Information is assembled, arguments developed, and alternatives shaped towards winning the approval of policy makers. The media, interest groups, political parties, government agencies, and other organizations are involved in policy formulation.

The level of support for policy change generally declines as the process progresses towards greater specificity.

Once the policy has been formulated, statements of government policies and programmes are promulgated. These can be laws, regulations, resource allocation decisions, court decisions, etc. Equally important, the government can decide that the best alternative is inaction.

Few government policies are self-implementing. Once a policy has been formulated and promulgated, it must be *implemented*. Even the most brilliantly crafted law, executive order, or court decision will fail to meet the designer's goals if it is poorly implemented.

3. Implementation

Implementation involves three activities directed towards putting a policy into effect. The three activities required for implementation are:

(a) interpretation

(b) organization

(c) application.

(a) **Interpretation** requires the translation of the programmatic language into acceptable and feasible administrative directives. Administrators need to discern the policy-makers' intent and fill in the details about how the goals will be accomplished. In many instances, legislation or court decisions are purposefully left somewhat vague to allow administrators wide latitude to respond to changing conditions and conflicting demands.

An example of how implementation can affect the outcome is the 1990 reform of the British National Health Service. Margaret Thatcher's Conservative government enacted fundamental reform of the health care system in 1990. One of the reforms attempted to create an 'internal market' by separating the purchasing and provision of health services. The Secretary of Health held the ultimate responsibility for the implementation of the policy, and a wide range of political and bureaucratic actors had a role in decision making. The parties affected by restructuring appealed to political officials to delay or cancel implementation of elements of the reform that ran counter to their interests. In the end, the desired effects of the 'internal market' were tempered by government control.

(b) **Organization** requires the establishment of administrative units and methods necessary to put a programme into effect. Resources (money, buildings, staff, equipment) are required to implement a programme.

(c) **Application** requires the services to be routinely administered. As described here, interpretation, organization, and application may appear to be rather dull and routine. However, the manner in which policies are implemented can dramatically affect the success or failure of a programme.

4. Policy evaluation

The last step is *evaluation*. The policy is evaluated to determine how well it was implemented, whether its goals were achieved, and what impact was achieved. The results of these assessments can result in a programme being maintained, expanded, changed, or even terminated. The general public, providers, and special interests provide input into the evaluation process. Sometimes the input is anecdotes, while in other instances it is a formal evaluation of a government programme. After the formal or informal evaluation, the policy making process is repeated, beginning with the formulation of a revised policy agenda based upon the evaluation.

Policy makers do not always encourage evaluation of their policies. For example, the Conservative government did not sponsor an evaluation of its 1990 overhaul of the NHS, suspecting that those who called for evaluation intended to slow down or derail the reforms. In addition, few independent organizations had the resources to carry out their own evaluation.[1]

Where is policy made?

As the layout of this section suggests, health and health care policy is made at national, regional, and local levels. Countries have different views of where policy should be decided. Some countries prefer more of their decision making to occur at the national level, while other countries have a more decentralized structure. Within countries, different functions are performed at different levels of government.

Tasks and skills in influencing policy

There are many different ways to influence policy. The four steps in the policy making process were described earlier. A different set of skills and actions are required for each step. Efforts to change policy are more likely to succeed if individuals and/or organizations, each with some of the necessary skills, co-operate.

What technical and managerial tasks need to be completed to implement a policy?

Political tasks

- define a public health issue
- develop broad goals
- place the specific issue on the broad policy agenda
- develop a strategy for moving issue to front of the policy agenda
- media coverage, advertising, public awareness campaign, lobbying
- develop specific policies
- evaluate alternative policies and formulate one specific policy
- modify policy in order to make it acceptable for implementation
- implement the policy
- evaluate the policy.

Managerial tasks

- identify key players on the issue (potential allies and opponents)
- build a coalition of support
- determine state of public opinion and identify ways to change it
- identify obstacles to implementation of a policy
- compromise and bargain to produce a widely acceptable policy
- determine the appropriate timing for attempting the implementation of the policy.

Each task requires a different set of skills:

- *agenda setting* requires a visionary with charisma and determination to accept frequent rejection as his or her own issue does not become one of the central issues
- *policy formulation* requires knowledge of specific programmes and how one programme interacts with another programme. It requires someone with a good overview of all the relevant government programmes and an ability to place a policy initiative into a larger context. Policy formulation requires someone who is skilled at compromise and coalition building
- *policy implementation* requires specific knowledge of the government programme that will administer the new policy, or the ability to establish and organize a new programme. It requires skills in persuading existing managers to do a task differently
- *policy evaluation* requires a set of analytic skills and some policy sense. To be successful, the evaluation must not only identify what went wrong, but also make suggestions for improvement.

What are the key determinants of success and what are the pitfalls?

As described above, incremental change is easier to bring about than major change. Two preconditions for major health care policy change are:

- the timing of policy initiatives is critical. Many factors, including those outside the health care arena, can add up to create a 'window of opportunity' for new policy
- the factors favouring policy change must be sufficient to overcome or temper resistance by the affected parties.

There are potential pitfalls at every point in the policy making process. The more 'clearance points' that must be passed, the greater the chance that a policy will be derailed. Different political systems have different 'clearance points', but at some point in the process, affected interests must be accommodated.

Opposition to policies can come in different forms. Interest groups are one form, but other forms of opposition may be more subtle.

For example, implementation of a new policy could be delegated to an agency opposed to it, an interest group in opposition could be granted a formal role in the implementation process, or officials involved in the implementation process could delay the process or make token efforts at implementation.

Health policy and the policy making process: an example

This chapter concludes with an example of a health policy issue that has been near the forefront of the national policy agenda in the United States—regulation of managed care organizations to ensure the protection of patients' rights. This example highlights:

• how an issue finds its way onto the policy agenda

• how policies are formulated in response.

Agenda setting

Doctors have been strong proponents of policies regulating managed care. Since the rapid proliferation of managed care in the United States in the 1990s, doctors have faced decreasing autonomy and increased financial risk.[2] Organizations representing doctors, including the American Medical Association, have lobbied for policies regulating managed care. In addition, doctors have tried to influence the general public, who rely on their doctors for much of their health care information.

The media have helped shape anti-managed care sentiment by publishing many negative, anecdotal stories with examples of managed care bad practices.[3]

The entertainment industry has also contributed to public anti-managed care sentiment. The most prominent example is the film *As Good as it Gets*, in which the lead character (portrayed by actress Helen Hunt) complained vehemently about her son being denied treatment by a managed care organization.

The managed care industry has spent millions of dollars lobbying against the proposed legislation and on advertisements designed to sway public opinion. Business groups have acted similarly. These groups argue that new regulations would increase costs, leading to higher premiums and ultimately to higher numbers of uninsured Americans.

Policy formulation

The states were the first to act on legislation regulating the managed care industry.[4] All 50 states have passed such laws, but the provisions of the laws vary from state to state. Regulation of the insurance industry has historically been performed by the states, but state laws do not apply to companies who self-insure, or assume the risk of health insurance for their own employees. Most large companies self-insure; these companies are governed by federal law (Employment Retirement Income Security Act, 1974).

The Executive Branch of the federal government acted on patient protection legislation, after the issue failed to progress in Congress. President Clinton signed an Executive Memorandum in February 1998 implementing patients' rights protection provisions in federal health plans, covering 85 million Americans.

Congress has now passed legislation in the House of Representatives and the Senate (as of October 1999). Since the two versions of legislation differ substantially, the two branches of Congress must work out the differences before submitting the legislation to the President.

Conclusion

Understanding the policy making process is a prerequisite to influencing it. To achieve policy change, a wide range of skills is needed, usually necessitating co-operation between groups of individuals or organizations. Both political and technical skills are needed to pass the 'clearance points' on the way to policy change.

Further reading

Downs A (1957). *An economic theory of democracy*. Harper and Row, New York.

Kingdon J (1995). *Agendas, alternatives, and public policies*. Harper Collins, New York.

Redman E (2001). *The dance of legislation*. University of Washington Press, Washington.

Walt G (1994). *Health policy*. Zed Books and Witwatersrand University Press, London.

References

1. Le Grand J (1999). Competition, co-operation, or control? Tales from the British National Health Service. *Health Affairs*, **18**(3), 27–39.
2. Bodenheimer T (1990). The American Health Care System: physicians and the changing medical marketplace. *NEJM*, **340**(7), 2369–72.
3. Brodie M, Brady LA, and Altman DE (1998). Media coverage of managed care: is there a negative bias? *Health Affairs*, **17**(1), 9–25.
4. Anderson GF (1998). State regulation of managed care: the impact on children. *Future Child*, 8(2), 76–92.

3.4 Influencing government policy: a national view

Patrick Wall

Introduction

Public health professionals should take every opportunity to influence government agendas to improve population health. They must provide decision makers with a better understanding of issues, to enable them to choose a course of action that will achieve the most desirable outcome in terms of health gain. Policies on the provision of effective health services are important, but policies in many other sectors also affect public health. Therefore it is important to introduce public health considerations into all areas of policy at all levels of government.

Objectives

This chapter explores five important issues about influencing national policy:

1. Being an advocate for the public, and providing leadership
2. Harnessing public opinion
3. Developing an authoritative source of public health advice
4. Taking the message into the mainstream of public debate
5. Lobbying for legislative support for public health policies

1. Public health professionals as advocates for the public

Public health practitioners must always adopt a robust approach and engage other professionals, politicians, and the public to ensure the maximum gain for the public's health. Public health practitioners must be advocates for the public and come into the ring in the pursuit of health gain. They must assert leadership if they are to have an impact in population health improvement.

2. Harnessing public opinion

Politicians are more often influenced by the opinions of their voters than by scientifically-derived evidence provided for decision making. Therefore public education and public awareness are essential; it is important not to underestimate the public's capacity to understand the issues. A combination of the soundbite media culture and the Internet means that the public have access to vast amounts of information, much of which may be incorrect. Public health practitioners have a role to provide accurate and well 'framed' information for the public to raise the level of debate and influence public opinion (see chapters 3.3, 3.5, and 7.4). To introduce public health considerations into all policy decisions requires partnership and ownership and cannot be achieved without consulting with, and participation of, all relevant groups in the planning and implementation of sustainable policies. Policy development can be undertaken at the level, either national or local, at which the public health issue occurs. Involvement of local communities to drive issues can be an effective strategy e.g. the Healthy Cities movement.

3. Developing an authoritative source of public health advice

There are many mechanisms for introducing public health issues into the government's decision making process. The ideal would be the development of an authoritative source for public health advice. This source should be independent of political or business interests, with the protection of citizens' health paramount, and provide advice based on the best science available. This advice should be made public so that if the government chooses to ignore it, they will be challenged to justify the alternative approaches adopted. To ensure maximum health gain, public health advice must be integrated into all decisions and requires co-operation among government agencies at national, regional, and local level and with other sectors such as business, industry, non-government agencies, and professional groups.

Unfortunately, although a lot is talked about the intersectoral approach to public health, the ideal model does not exist. Several approaches are being used and have the potential for further development. The UK Department of Health attempts to separate public health from the development and administration of health services. To develop an effective intersectoral approach to improving the population's health requires influence at the cabinet decision making level.

The profile and role of the chief medical officer to governments is important and he/she should be the public's champion.[1] One of their objectives should be to create and develop government responsibility at all levels to respond to the public health issues of concern to the citizens. The chief medical officer can influence individuals to play a role in protecting their own health and the health of society both by their behaviour and their support for health-enhancing policies.

Scientific advisory committees, working groups, and task forces convened to address particular areas of concern can be effective if they are not politicized and if their advice is published. The public health practitioners need to engender strong political commitment to implement the advice provided.

In some countries, charitable foundations support independent groups and reports that can be powerfully influential on government. The UK's Rowntree Foundation and the USA's Johnson Foundation and Commonwealth Fund are examples.

Pronouncements by professional groups like a National Medical Association or an Association of Public Health can have a great impact on influencing public opinion.

4. Taking the message into the mainstream

Most scientists are still content to present their data at scientific conferences and publish in peer-reviewed journals. Their audience is therefore largely their colleagues, who are often already convinced of the public health message. Greater efforts have to be made to take the message out into the mainstream. Public health professionals must use every opportunity to disseminate the messages to the wider public using all the available media modalities; TV, radio, broadsheet and tabloid newspapers, magazines, internet, etc. Effective communication of the key issues is essential and the public health message needs to be marketed to the public at large, like any other product (see chapter 7.4).

In some countries, interest and lobby groups are in the forefront of calling for government reforms to aspects of policy affecting public health. Public health practitioners must play a proactive role in fostering public understanding of the public heath implications of government decisions to drive change in the appropriate direction.

The development of party manifestos prior to elections provides a great opportunity to introduce a public health dimension across all policies. Public health practitioners can introduce the issues into the public domain to ensure party advisors pick them up. A government failing to deliver on pre-election promises will be brought to task by the media and the opposition.

Economic evaluation can assist in the setting of priorities in the development of policies. Economic analysis can be highly effective in discouraging excessively expensive or wasteful policies, or in advancing cost-effective programmes (see chapter 2.6).

5. Legislative support for public health policies

Health promotion needs to be broader than risk communication and needs to be backed up by legislative commitment to protect the public's health whether in areas such as:

(a) tobacco control policy

(b) transport policy

(c) environmental protection

(d) diet and nutrition

(e) food safety

(f) poverty and ill-health

(g) health care.

Legislative support demonstrates government commitment and provides those who implement the policy with legal guidance and authority.

(a) Tobacco control policy

Tobacco use is the primary cause of preventable disease in most developed countries and effective tobacco control programmes and policies are imperative. Educational programmes for the public and clinics to help smokers stop need to be coupled with taxes on tobacco and with making it illegal to sell tobacco to under-age individuals, to smoke in public places, and to advertise tobacco. California has demonstrated that by a concerted approach combining voluntary and enforced compliance, smoking can become a socially unacceptable habit.[2] (see chapter 9.6).

(b) Transport policies

There must be public health input into transport policies. Use of safety belts, control of speeding, drink driving, and vehicle emissions all impact on the public's health. Policies should be developed to reduce car use by restricting vehicle access to cities during certain times or unless there are four or more passengers (as an incentive to encourage car-pooling), and to promote cycling, walking, and public transport. Public health practitioners have a role to communicate the benefits of health policies to the public. Success will be more likely when the approach is acceptable to both policy makers and the population.

(c) Environmental protection

Industrial and domestic waste coupled with vehicle and industrial emissions are products of our ever-growing consumer society. The challenge is finding a balance between economic growth and maintenance of a healthy environment. Protection of the environment by controlling pollution and waste management is a shared responsibility between government, industry, and the population at large. All decisions should be open and transparent and clashes of interest need to be acknowledged and addressed (see chapter 4.4).

(d) Diet and public health

The relationship between diet and public health is well known, yet obesity continues to be a growing problem in all developed countries. A subset of the population has extreme difficulty in controlling weight and may require medical assistance. However, for the majority, the adoption of a healthy lifestyle and a balanced diet is a personal choice (although for some, resource constraints are an important influence on choosing diets). The links between the consumption of saturated fats and cardiovascular disease, and salt and hypertension are well established, and the potential benefits of diet in reducing the risk of cancer are emerging. The public are being bombarded with promotional material from food companies and pharmaceutical companies on what they should and should not be eating. Obesity must be regarded as a health issue not an aesthetic or cosmetic issue, and public health practitioners have a role in promoting healthy eating and drinking. Government policies with regard to nutritional content, fortification of foods with vitamins and minerals, removal of salt, and comprehensive labelling are essential to enable consumers to make informed choices.

(e) Food safety

The food industry is required to produce and sell safe food, free from harmful pathogens and residues, and this requirement must be underpinned by comprehensive legislation that is rigidly enforced. With the increasing mass production of food, pursuit of profit must not take precedence over public health. Policies regarding food safety must be developed with the primary objective of consumer protection and independent food safety agencies with this remit are the way forward. Responsibility for policing the food chain rests with many government agencies, and a co-ordinated intersectoral approach is needed if an effective inspection service is to operate from farm to fork. Because of the increasing global distribution of food, food safety policies will require co-ordination between countries in order to be effective and to ensure consistency of approach. The BSE debacle damaged consumer confidence in the ability and commitment of the regulatory agencies to protect their health. It also raises questions about the effectiveness of public health advocates in this case (see chapter 3.6).

(f) Poverty and ill-health

Of the many social and cultural factors with an impact on health, the most important is poverty. Education, health, and social services may be less accessible to the poor, thereby increasing their vulnerability. They may not have the opportunity to afford healthier lifestyles. Various sectoral policies can reduce the growing disparity in health status between the rich and poor in society. Often underprivileged and minority groups do not have access to information in an appropriate format and public health practitioners can have an important role as an advocate for these groups. The provision of appropriate education and training is important, as is the mobilization and involvement of communities and groups behind a cause or issue (see chapters 4.1 and 6.7).

(g) Health care

Rapid scientific breakthroughs are dramatically enhancing our understanding of health and disease and are making possible entirely new modalities of prevention and treatment. However, the health care resource budget is finite, and to ensure maximum health gain, equitable health care delivery systems based on clinical need (rather than ability to pay) must be developed. Public health practitioners should strive to achieve a pragmatic balance between primary, secondary, and tertiary care. To assist this the public health issues should be regularly debated if the decision making process is not to be unduly influenced by individual high-profile hardship cases. For effective public health policies to be supported by the public the benefits should be apparent in both the short and the long term (e.g. policy for cancer prevention should include improved access to the cancer specialist centres). (See parts 5 and 6.)

Conclusion

To influence public health policy, the key issues must be introduced into the public domain in a format that is comprehensible to both the public and politicians. The media helps form public opinion and public opinion influences the elected representatives who formulate and approve policy. Public health professionals need to forego their conservative approach and respond to the media's insatiable appetite for information, and use it to drive change. This involves the use of a wide range of analytic and political skills, described in this and other chapters.

Further resources

Ham C (1999). *Health policy in Britain*, (4th edn). Macmillan, London.

Ling T (ed.) (1998). *Reforming health care by consent: involving those who matter*. Radcliffe Medical Press, Oxford.

Ritsatakis A, Barnes R, Dekker E, Harrington P, Kokko S, and Makara P (ed.) (2000). *Exploring health policy development in Europe*. WHO Regional Publications, European series, No. 86. World Health Organization, Copenhagen.

Walt G (1994). *Health policy: an introduction to process and power*. Witwatersrand University Press, Johannesburg.

References

1. Calman K (1998). Lessons from Whitehall, *BMJ*, **317**, 1718–20.
2. Pierce JP, Gilpin EA, Emery SL, *et al.* (1998). Has the California tobacco control program reduced smoking? *JAMA*, **280**(10), 893–9.

3.5 Using media advocacy to shape policy

Simon Chapman

Introduction

The media are peerless as a means of engaging large numbers of people, including those with influence, in public health debates. If a public health issue is ignored by the news media, or if the media choose to frame its meaning from the perspectives of those working against the interests of public health, it is highly unlikely that sought-after political, public, or funding support will follow. There are few if any examples of robust public health policy or well-funded programmes that have not been preceded and sustained by wide-spread and supportive news coverage. As a veteran reporter of 40 years experience with the *Wall Street Journal* said:

> 'Well-done investigative reporting produces public outrage (or policy maker outrage) that forces new regulations and laws or tougher enforcement of existing ones. Ten-thousand-watt klieg lights turned on a situation focuses the minds of policy makers very fast'.[1]

Objectives

The objective of this chapter is to help readers understand:

- how public health issues are dealt with by the media
- how framing of an issue can be crucial to its success in changing policy
- how practitioners can prepare themselves to deal with the adverse framing of a public health issue.

Framing

A core skill found in effective media advocates is that they appear to audiences to have an instinct for framing their concerns in ways that make their issues instantly comprehensible in terms of wider discourses that reach beyond the manifest or overt subject of their concerns. For example, while few people may comprehend the complexities of the tobacco litigation now rampant in the USA, people do understand from years of negative press reportage about the tobacco industry[2] that the cases are being fought about allegations of negligence, cover-up, and deceit. Such dimensions or sub-texts allow audiences who may not have detailed knowledge or awareness about the particulars of a given issue to identify that here is something similar to an issue they *do* understand. Sub-texts serve to link topics to familiar, wider socio-political discourses so that coverage of particular events is decoded by audiences as instances of more general themes or types of story. In this way, much news is not instructively seen as news, but as 'olds'—essentially the retelling of age-old stories, only with new casts, circumstances, infectious agents, and so on. For example, the ongoing news saga about doping in sport and anabolic steroid use, is essentially the retelling of the myth of Narcissus—a moral tale about the dangers of vanity, inflected to involve another widely understood sub-text: that cheats should not prosper. Effective public health advocates must learn to think about their issues in such terms, rather than assume that news media have intrinsic interest in specific issues like cancer, infection, injury, and so on.[3,4]

There is no 'objective reality' that any platform of public health policy can be said to be *really* about. The often heated nature of news discourse about public health issues testifies to the essentially contested nature of advocacy. To injury prevention specialists, compulsory bicycle helmets might mean reduced brain injury and deaths; to indifferent parents their meaning might be framed more in terms of additional expense; and to fashion-conscious youth, the intrusion of a paternalistic state on their ability to dress as they please and thumb their nose at danger. Reality is always a socially constructed notion.

The emphasis or 'framing' that is placed around particular events or issues that seeks to define *what this issue is really about* will represent but one of many competing meanings that jostle for public dominance. While health interests may frame the meaning of a Bill to introduce proof of immunization in terms of the protection of children's health, people who oppose immunization may choose to describe the Bill in terms of the encroachment of the 'nanny state', 'compulsory medication', and other negative metaphors.[5]

> 'Politics is largely about the problem of competing interest groups seeking to advance multiple definitions of the same events.'

Politics, *and therefore the progression of public health policy*, is largely about the problem of competing interest groups seeking to advance multiple definitions of the same events. In public health, policy advocacy is ultimately the process by which advocates for different positions and values seek to define what is at issue for the public, media gatekeepers, and policy makers and legislators. For example: are compulsory fences for backyard swimming pools:[6]

- a blight on garden aesthetics and evidence of Big Brother, regulatory bureaucracy stepping ever closer into our personal lives?

- the use of a sledgehammer to crack a walnut (i.e. with any given pool having a very low probability of 'hosting' a drowning, should every pool owner—particularly those with no children—bear the cost of installing a fence?)

- a safety net to prevent drowning, the leading cause of death in 1–5 year olds in Australia?

An example: gun deaths

Gun control provides a good example of the role of 'framing' in the media handling of an issue, and in the progress of efforts to change policy.

Are gun deaths:

- the occasional, unfortunate 'blood price' communities with liberal gun laws pay for the freedom to defend their homes from malevolent intruders?
- perpetrated by criminals and the mentally ill who are beyond the reach of law?
- preventable carnage, capable of reduction as with any other public health problem?

When a lone gunman shot 35 people dead at Port Arthur, Australia, in April 1996, within a month, all political parties united in support of the Australian Prime Minister's call for semi-automatic rifles and shotguns to be banned, for all guns to be registered, for self-defence to be explicitly excluded as a legitimate reason to own a gun, and for gun ownership to be limited to only those who satisfied a limited number of reasons to own a gun. Australian gun control advocates had promoted these policies for years and Port Arthur was a watershed event that overnight made gun law reform politically compelling.

Both before and after Port Arthur, the gun lobby sought to define gun control in ways that would minimize political interest in its implementation. The task for gun control advocates, of course, was to do the opposite.

Over the years, we had collected many examples of their key arguments and in hindsight, came to see that we had subjected these to a process of analysis amenable for use in media advocacy planning. Rather than responding off-the-cuff to gun lobby efforts to frame gun control as misguided folly, hundreds of media opportunities were disciplined by strategic attempts at repeatedly framing the debate[7] to achieve particular objectives.

Planning attempts to reframe debates

A prepared and disciplined response to debates of public health issues depends on dealing with the following questions:

- what was our public health objective?
- what frame put around this objective would most neatly and clearly define what was at issue?
- what symbols, metaphors, or visual images could be referenced that would trigger this frame in audiences?

- what 'soundbites' (typically, about seven seconds of speech or two to three sentences in newsprint) could encapsulate the essence of the frame?

Table 3.5.1 illustrates two examples of how this process is an adaptation of an approach suggested by Charlotte Ryan[8] and subsequently applied by the Berkeley Media Studies Group to the study of the way that gun control is debated in the US press. Gun lobby 'definitions' of what was at issue are shown, together with a strategy to reframe the issues encompassing the four questions listed above.

Table 3.5.1 Two worked examples for framing media advocacy.

Gun lobby position 1: 'Why don't you ban knives, axes and baseball bats too?'	
Public health objective	To communicate that guns are especially dangerous because they are so effective at killing. They kill and injure many more than other weapons, so they merit special restrictions
Frame	Guns as ultra-lethal
Symbol, visual image or metaphor	—When a gun is available during an argument, it's like throwing petrol on a fire —Fist fight vs. gun fight —With guns, minor altercations can lead to death
Soundbite	—Gun + criminal intent = 17 dead (Dunblane); gun + criminal intent = 35 dead (Port Arthur); but machete + criminal intent = 7 injured (Wolverhampton) —Guns are a permanent solution to a temporary problem —I've never heard of a *drive-by stabbing*
Gun lobby position 2: 'Guns don't kill people, people kill people'	
Public health objective	To refocus on the lethality of guns
Frame	—To pull guns back inside the frame defining directions for solutions —Guns as controllable, people as less controllable
Symbol, visual image or metaphor	A violent/disturbed/upset person with an ultra-lethal means of expressing anger
Soundbite	—People kill—guns make it possible —This is like saying . . . bare wires don't kill, electricians do —Guns don't die—people do!

Conclusion

Media debates of public health and other issues are characterized by the use of simplified 'sub-texts' of what the issues are 'really' about.

This 'framing' of issues provides opposing sides in debates with metaphors and images to use, to advance their own views and oppose the views of others. Politics, and therefore the progression of public health policy, is largely about competing interest groups seeking to advance multiple definitions of the same events.

A prepared and disciplined response to debates of public health issues is possible and depends on identifying and using the symbols that would trigger the desired 'frame' in audiences and using the right 'soundbite' to encapsulate the essence of that frame.

References

1. Otten AL (1992). The influence of the mass media on health policy. *Health Affairs*, **Winter 1992**, 111–18.
2. Christophides N, Dominello A, and Chapman S (1999). The new pariahs: how the tobacco industry are depicted in the Australian press. *Aust NZ J Public Health*, **23**, 233–9.
3. Wallack L, Dorfman L, Jernigan D, and Themba M (1993). *Media advocacy and public health. Power for prevention.* Sage, Newbury Park.
4. Chapman S and Lupton D (1994). *The fight for public health: principles and practice of media advocacy.* BMJ Books, London.
5. Leask J and Chapman S (1998). 'An attempt to swindle nature': press reportage of anti immunisation, Australia 1993–97. *Aust NZ J Public Health*, **22**, 17–26.
6. Carey V, Chapman S, and Gaffney D (1994). Children's lives or garden aesthetics? A case study in public health advocacy. *Aust J Public Health*, **18**, 25–32.
7. Chapman S (1998). *Over our dead bodies: Port Arthur and Australia's fight for gun control.* Pluto, Sydney.
8. Ryan C (1991). *Prime time activism.* South End Press, Boston.

Every great movement must experience three stages: ridicule, discussion, adoption.

Mill JS 1806–73

3.6 Influencing internationa! policy

Tim Lang and Martin Caraher

Introduction

Why bother about the international when public health and ill-health is manifest locally? Addressing the international dimensions of public health might arguably be a luxury—something one would like to do, if only there were enough time. One could argue that international affairs are best left to bodies such as the World Health Organization (WHO) or UNICEF, the UN Children's Fund. This chapter argues that although these views may be common, they are also flawed.

Far from being an optional extra, it is now essential in public health always to ask the international questions. This might have been a luxury in the past—though we doubt it—but it is definitely essential in the modern age. Environmentalists have long subscribed to the view that citizens have to 'think globally and act locally'. Now, even this is inadequate: twenty-first-century public health professionals not only have to think *but act* internationally, even as we think and work locally.

Objectives

This chapter aims to help readers identify and understand:

- why public health practitioners should think and work both globally and locally
- what can be done to advance public health at the international level and what levers exist to influence international public health policy
- the need for translation of international policy into local action.

What are the reasons for needing an international focus?

There are five important reasons for needing an international focus:

(a) diseases are not confined by national boundaries

(b) the lifestyle and social causes of disease are spreading internationally

(c) increasing numbers of people are travelling internationally

(d) more goods of all types are travelling internationally

(e) the institutions for addressing transnational problems are often poorly resourced and/or poorly organized to cope with public health challenges.

(a) Diseases know no boundaries

National borders, like most boundaries, are social constructs. Communicable diseases have a tendency to travel, within and between countries. There is nothing new about this, with a long history including the medieval plagues and the spread of virulent influenza strains, notably just after World War I. The role of public health bodies has always included the monitoring of how diseases spread and providing an early warning system.

(b) Non-communicable diseases also cross borders

For example, diet-related diseases are spreading globally through lifestyle and social changes. Obesity and coronary heart disease (CHD) and some food-related cancers (e.g. bowel)[1] are on the increase in developing countries, where the more affluent social groups are tending towards a more 'Western' lifestyle—eating different foods, taking less exercise, and not just aspiring to, but achieving, Western patterns of consumption. In developing countries obesity now exists alongside more traditional problems of under-nutrition.

(c) People are travelling increasing distances (and more rapidly) out of choice

An estimated 600 million people are international tourists each year. It has been estimated that these tourists run an estimated 20–50% risk of contracting a food-borne illness.[2] The very act of travel can also be a significant contribution to environmental damage, air transport being associated with atmospheric pollution.

(d) Goods increasingly travel

The removal of barriers to trade at a global level, through the General Agreement of Tariffs and Trade (GATT), has significantly accelerated this trend. There are different patterns for different commodities, but in the case of food, for example, rich consumer societies are increasingly able to source elements of their diet globally. They can eat foods 'out of season' and buy other people's land and food space. This can have a tremendous impact within poorer countries—leading to a situation where food is exported when there is need locally (something that also happened in the Irish Famine in the nineteenth century). Generally, a revolution in the food trade has meant that more food comes longer distances: the so-called 'food miles' effect.[3,4] A mass food system increases the chance of problems when there is a breakdown in health controls.

(e) Public health professionals have to think and work internationally...

... because they cannot always assume that the political and institutional frameworks for addressing the 'transnationalization'* of health patterns are either resourced enough or modernized to keep abreast of these economic, social, and cultural changes. Public health institutions tend to be locally and nationally focused and based, partly due to funding and tax-collection systems, while economic and social changes tend to be driven internationally. The main drivers of globalization tend to be economic and commercial. There has been considerable change in economic rules at the regional (continental) and world level, whereas public health interventions tend only to receive modernization when there is a crisis. Risks to health are a 'threat' while trade is perceived as an 'opportunity'.[5] Despite spending most of the 1980s and 1990s dismantling public health trade barriers, the BSE crisis taught the European Union the need for stronger public health measures. It has now set up a Rapid Alert System to that effect.[6] The crisis showed that public health lacked a voice and sufficient influence, compared with trade.

In summary, the internationalization of life and culture means that health professionals also have to think and work internationally. This does not mean dropping local or national work. Whatever the work, public health protection and promotion requires action on four levels simultaneously: the local, national, regional, and global. If any one is missing, the health jigsaw is incomplete.

What can be done about the international dimension of public health?

Achieving health promoting change at the international level requires:

(a) *identifying causes*: identifying the underlying causes of ill-health

(b) *identifying interventions*: identifying the necessary public health interventions

(c) *arguing for action*: arguing for action and winning policy support and resources, while dealing with ideological and other barriers.

(a) Identify the causes

The traditional public health response—to isolate sources of ill-health and to control their source—is difficult if a problem is international. The modern world is highly complex and isolating causes of changing health patterns takes time and skill. The impact of economic restructuring can take decades to betray a health effect. 'Westernization' of diets and lifestyles, for instance, showed up in new patterns of diabetes in India[7] and cancers in the developing world.[8]

It is easy to focus on symptoms rather than causes, as can happen in the case of obesity or the treatment of communicable diseases such as HIV/AIDS. There is a need to refocus on what Wilkinson[9] calls the determinants of health. For example, the food system (combined with a reduction in exercise levels) and the food we eat contributes to obesity. Concentrating on altering individual behaviour ought to be accompanied, perhaps pre-empted, by a refocus 'upstream'.[10] What forces promote excessive consumption? What stops people taking exercise?

The classic model of public health intervention is to search for the single cause of a health problem. Thus Dr John Snow is celebrated for his action to contain a cholera outbreak. He removed the pump handle at Broad Street pump in London (albeit after the peak of the epidemic), which stopped the citizenry drinking any more water from what he suspected was the source of disease. This classical model of public health intervention does not fit international public health reality. Ironically, at the same time as Snow's actions, Dr William Duncan, Medical Officer of Health in Liverpool, had a more difficult time. Liverpool's water was from deep wells (not likely to be contaminated) and at least some of its outbreaks were almost definitely associated with immigration, flies, and poor housing, harder to tackle than a pump handle. If Snow's action is the classical model, Duncan's problems remind us not just that life can also be complex but that the international is manifest before our eyes. Duncan argued: tackle the social causes of ill-health and health will improve.

(b) Identify and promote public health interventions

The use of regulation to protect public health has been politically unfashionable within the dominant neo-liberal model of economics. Regulation has been demoted in favour of a consumer-driven model, where individuals are encouraged to make their own decisions and to take responsibility for their own health. In this respect, twentieth-century globalization highlights a choice of approaches for public health, one primarily individual-focused, and the other population-oriented.[11]

Food policy is a good example of where these public policy choices for health have become clear in recent years. Tensions over food standards and information given to consumers have led to questions about whether market mechanisms can be relied upon to protect public health. The social and moral questions stem directly from changes in the food economy. Health costs are 'externalized' and not reflected in the cost paid for food by consumers at the checkout till. This is represented schematically in Table 3.6.1, where the economic neo-liberal model based on free trade and choice is contrasted with an ecological model of public health.

In practice, it is hard to develop appropriate public health responses to global phenomena, especially at a local or regional level.

Table 3.6.1 Two approaches to public health action.

Policy agenda	Neo-liberal model	'New' public health or ecological model
Relationship to general economy (health/wealth nexus)	Trickle down theory; allow for inequalities; based on markets	Reduce inequality by state action provides health safety net
Economic direction for health policy	Individual risk insurance	Social insurance including primary care and public health services
Morality	Individual responsibility/ self-protection	Societal responsibility based on a citizenship model
Health accountancy/ costs	Costs of ill-health not included in price of goods	Costs internalized where possible
Approach to the state	Keep it minimal; avoid 'paternalistic approach'	Potential corrective lever on the imbalance between individual and social forces
Consultation with the end user	As consumer	As citizen having a stake in the public health
Approach to problems	Target 'at risk' groups; focus on the end consumer	Population-wide; review entire chain of ill-health creation

We are experiencing an epidemic of obesity and diabetes. How are local and national public health approaches supposed to deal with such global phenomena? It means tackling powerful food interests, advertising and lifestyle appeals, governments, and much more. Can public health proponents really take this on? Or must they just deal with the symptoms?

(c) Argue for action

Once an international problem is recognized, public health professions can argue for action. This does not mean, necessarily, that they will win policy or political support for their work, but it helps. The global campaign to address AIDS/HIV is an illustration. Even governments that adopted a censorious moral stance (blaming 'lax' social mores for the spread of sexually transmitted diseases) were ultimately persuaded of the need to act. Global health action can be naked self-interest.[12]

There is a rich public health tradition of global action. The eradication of smallpox, for instance, took years and required formidable co-ordination, funds, and, above all, political backing. Unless professionals have access to the full international picture of disease and of the determinants of (ill) health, there is always a danger that they will expend considerable amounts of time and money treating symptoms rather than preventing causes.

What global policy levers do we have?

Many institutions operate on a global level. Table 3.6.2 summarizes these. Some are official governmental; others are non-governmental and commercial.

The world bodies concerned with health have adopted a number of conventions and agreements. The Convention on the Rights of the Child was adopted on 20 November 1989 and based upon Article 49 of the UN Charter. It provides a basis for international action to ensure, for example, good food and education; precursors to health. The WHO Code on Breastfeeding, agreed by UNICEF and the WHO in 1990, has the goal that 'all women should be enabled to practise exclusive breastfeeding and all infants should be fed exclusively on breast-milk from birth to 4–6 months'. It committed national governments to implementing a wide range of policies such as taking action on the marketing of breast-feeding supplements and to promote breast-feeding for instance in hospitals.[13] Although agreed, it has met difficulty in practice, in part due to failure of governments, hospitals, and services to implement it, and in part due to systematic attacks by business. Companies making breast-milk substitutes have looked to developing countries as new markets, subject to fewer controls than developed economies.

The International Conference on Nutrition provides an example of a global commitment, this time by national governments, to monitor the food security of 'at risk' social groups.[14] Another is the WHO European Region's 51 member states, who by signing the Health for All 21 Programme have committed themselves to a regional policy approach to public health. Twenty-one targets are set for the twenty-first century.[15] Such actions build on the 1978 Alma-Ata Declaration on Primary Health Care.[16] This committed Governments to strengthen and reorient health services towards primary care and 'to respond to current and anticipated health conditions, socio-economic circumstances and needs of the people . . . '[17]

In other words, there are conventions and international agreements that can justify public health action. The problem, however, is that they often seem remote and practitioners may not know about them. A health visitor trying to promote breast-feeding, in the face of a local hospital flouting the WHO/UNICEF Code on Marketing of breast-milk substitutes, might get personal satisfaction from knowing that she is right to do so, but lack levers to get her management to put their own house in order.

Considerable education within the public health world may be needed to shake up local complacency. Vested interests and power blocs are always strong. So alliances are needed, inside and outside

Table 3.6.2 Global institutions involved in health.

Remit	Examples of organization/bodies
Public health	World Health Organization (WHO), World Bank, Food and Agriculture Organisation (FAO)
Children and health	UNICEF—UN Children's Emergency Fund
Global economic bodies with health impact	World Bank, International Monetary Fund (IMF), UN Conference on Trade and Development (UNCTAD), World Trade Organisation (WTO), World Intellectual Property Organisation (WIPO), Organisation for Economic Co-operation and Development (OECD)
Intergovernmental agreements with a health impact	Bio-safety Convention, International Conference on Nutrition, Basel Convention on hazardous waste
Emergency aid	World Food Programme, International Committee of the Red Cross/Crescent, non-governmental organizations
Environmental health	Global Panel on Climate Change, UN Conference on Environment and Development (UNCED), International Maritime Organisation
Commercial interests	International Chamber of Commerce, Transnational Corporations, International Federation of Pharmaceutical Manufacturers Associations
Regional bodies with health role	European Union, Regional Offices of WHO and FAO
Trade Associations	International Hospitals Federation
Networks to promote public health ([WHO] indicates WHO support)	Healthy Cities Network [WHO], International Baby Food Action Network (IBFAN), Local Agenda 21 network, Pesticides Action Network, Tobacco Free Initiative [WHO]
Professional associations	International Union for Health Promotion and Education
Non-governmental organizations	Greenpeace, Friends of the Earth, Oxfam, Médecins sans Frontieres, Médecins du Monde, World Federation of Public Health Associations

the place of work. Health impact assessments offer a way forward for public health workers at a local level to build in a global public health perspective (see chapters 1.6 and 4.4).

What all this entails is a need to move beyond health education and health promotion to adopting a global population perspective and a view of health that acknowledges transnational influences on health. Too often an international perspective in health is no more than an appeal to campaign. NGO work shows how effective this can be. Campaigns on genetically modified foods or pesticides have been highly effective in debating and encouraging preventive action. Public health, as Snow and Duncan knew, requires material and political, not just attitudinal, change. Policy development should be premised on the notion of consultation and alliances, but there has to be action, not just promises.

Conclusion

If a global perspective teaches us that the cause of problems may be complex, it also shows us that public health cannot be achieved by individual action. Alliances are essential, across sectors as well as regions.

The international dimension to public health teaches the following:

- good public health combines the local, national, regional, and global approaches
- the international dimension makes action more complex but realistic
- health impact is never local or global but both
- international health institutions exist but need strengthening
- partnerships and alliances are essential in tackling the forces of ill-health.

Further resources

Birley MH, Boland A, Davies L, Edwards RT, Glanville H, Ison E, Millstone E, Osborn D, Scott-Samuel A, and Treweek J (1998). *Health and environmental impact assessment: an integrated approach.* Earthscan/British Medical Association, London.

Bradshaw YW and Wallace M (1996). *Global inequalities.* Pine Forge Press, Thousand Oaks CA.

Drewnowski A and Popkin BM (1997). The nutrition transition: new trends in the global diet. *Nutrition Reviews,* **55**(2), 31–43.

Egger G and Swinburn B (1997). An 'ecological' approach to the obesity pandemic. *BMJ,* **315,** 477–80.

Environmental Health Commission (1997). *Agendas for change.* Chartered Institute of Environmental Health, London.

Howson CP, Fineberg HV, and Bloom BR (1998). The pursuit of global health: the relevance of engagement for developed countries. *Lancet,* **351**(9102), 586–90.

Labonte R (1998). Healthy public policy and the World Trade Organisation: a proposal for an international health presence in future world trade/investment talks, *Health Promotion International,* **13**(3), 245–56.

Lang T (1996). Food security: does it conflict with globalisation? *Development,* **4,** 45–50.

Lang T and Heasman M (2000). *Food wars.* Earthscan, London.

Soros G (1998). *The crisis of global capitalism: open society endangered.* Little, Brown and Company, London.

Weil O, McKee M, Brodin M, and Oberlé D (1999). *Priorities for public health action in the European Union*. Société Francaise de Santé Publique, Vandoeuvre-les-Nancy.

WHO (1999). *Health for All in the twenty-first century*. World Health Organization, Copenhagen.

References

1. WCRF (1997). *Food, nutrition and the prevention of cancer*, ch. 9. World Cancer Research Fund/American Institute for Cancer Research, Washington DC.

2. Kaeferstein FK, Motarjemi Y, and Bettcher DW (1997). Foodborne disease control: a transnational challenge. *Emerging Infectious Diseases*, **3**, 503–10.

3. Paxton A (1994). *The food miles report*. Sustainable Agriculture, Food and Environment (SAFE) Alliance, London.

4. Sustain (1999). *Food miles—still on the road to ruin?* An assessment of the debate over the unnecessary transport of food, five years on from the first report. Sustainable Agriculture, Food and Environment (SAFE) Alliance, London.

5. Unwin N, Alberti G, Aspray T, Edwards R, Mbanya JC, Sobngwi E, Mugusi F, Rashid S, Setel P, and Whiting D (1998). Economic globalisation and its effect on health. *BMJ*, **316**, 1401–2.

6. CEC (2000). *White Paper on food safety*. Commission of the European Communities, Brussels.

7. Ramachandran A (1998). Epidemiology of non-insulin-dependent diabetes mellitus in India. In *Nutrition and chronic disease: an Asian perspective*, (ed. P Shetty and C Gopalan), pp. 38–41. Smith-Gordon, London.

8. WCRF (1997). *Food, nutrition and the prevention of cancer*. World Cancer Research Fund/American Institute for Cancer Research, Washington DC.

9. Wilkinson R (1996). *Unhealthy societies: the afflictions of inequality*. Routledge, London.

10. McKinlay JB (1993). The promotion of health through planned socio-political change: challenges for research and policy. *Social Science and Medicine*, **36**(2), 109–17.

11. Sram I and Ashton J (1998). Millennium Report to Sir Edwin Chadwick. *BMJ*, **317**, 592–6.

12. Navarro V (1999). Health and equity in the world in the era of 'globalisation'. *Int J Health Services*, **29**(2), 215–26.

13. WHO/UNICEF (1990). *Breastfeeding in the 1990s: a global initiative (The Innoceni Declaration)*. World Health Organisation, Geneva.

14. FAO/WHO (1992). *International Conference on Nutrition*. Food and Agriculture Organisation, Rome.

15. World Health Organization Regional Office for Europe (1998). *21 Targets for the 21st century—a public health guide to the targets to the Health for All policy for the European Region*. WHO, Copenhagen.

16. World Health Organization (1978). *Alma-Ata: primary health care*. Health for All Series No. 1. WHO, Geneva.

17. World Health Organization (1998). *World Health Declaration*, paragraph lll. WHO, Geneva.

Deaths, data, and decisive oratory change policy.

Part 4
Direct action

Introduction

Public health is too often seen as an abstract subject with well-meaning practitioners wrestling with fearsome but nebulous giants such as poverty, social deprivation, inequality, and the global tobacco industry. This is indeed part of the agenda of public health—the contribution of the practitioner in such areas can usually only be indirect, exerted by the influence they have on national or global policy makers (see part 3).

However, practitioners are also directly responsible for a wide range of public health services and are aware as any clinician of the benefit that a successful intervention can produce. Equally, they know the fear and apprehension which is felt when something goes wrong with controlling an outbreak, managing a screening programme, or handling a public health disaster.

Public health, unlike clinical practice, is often a thankless job. Practitioners do not receive letters of thanks or gifts from grateful members of the public. When things are working well in public health, no one says thank you; but as soon as they start to go wrong, the press can turn on public health with energy and hostility.

Taking decisions and taking action

The practitioner who is directly responsible for services has firstly to make decisions, often with imperfect information (see part 2). Having taken a decision to deliver a pubic health service in a particular way, the same practitioner is usually responsible for implementing it. On some occasions it is possible for the practitioner to do this by mobilizing resources for which they are directly accountable. If so, they should be asking the perennial ten questions:

The ten things to consider when you are asked to take action about a specific problem:

1. Is this issue really a problem?

2. If so, does the proposed action really address this problem?

3. If so, are *you* the best person to address it?

4. If so, is *now* the best time to do it?

5. If so, who else will be involved and how?

6. What are the resources available?

7. What are the likely costs involved?

8. What are the opportunities?

9. What are the barriers?

10. How will you know if you are being (or have been) successful?

Life is rarely this simple—even if answers are available to these questions, very few issues can be addressed meaningfully without the involvement of others; persuasion and advocacy are required to bring the resources and power of others to bear.

Where the buck stops

If a policy goes wrong, it is possible to blame many factors other than the public health practitioners. However, when a service fails, for example when a second youngster dies of meningitis, the public health practitioner and team need to account for the actions taken or not taken. This may sound alarming, but many people become public health practitioners, not to escape clinical decision making, but to take equally difficult decisions and to take action to make a difference on a bigger canvas.

Such actions have made a significant contribution to the public's health. It is claimed that, of the 30 extra years of life expectancy gained in the twentieth century, 25 of these years were attributed to advances in public health.[1]

Of all the achievements made, the ten great public health achievements of the twentieth century in the United States are claimed to be:[2]

- vaccination
- motor-vehicle safety
- safer workplaces
- control of infectious diseases
- decline in deaths from coronary heart diseases and stroke
- safer and healthier foods
- healthier mothers and babies
- family planning
- fluoridation of drinking water
- recognition of tobacco as a health hazard.

In this part of the handbook ways in which public health takes direct action to improve the health of populations are described; for each of them the public health practitioner will be held accountable. Important ways of taking direct action range from reaching and empowering communities, through to societal efforts to protect and sustain the environment in general and the workplace in particular. Specific public health tasks such as screening, outbreak management, and handling disasters are broken down into specific tasks and competencies. Part 4 includes chapters on working with many diverse groups of people, from community development workers to 'hard to reach' populations. Finally, there is a chapter on how public health practitioners can use their practical skills as political activists to effect change.

References

1. Bunker JP, Frazier HS, and Mosteller F (1994). Improving health: measuring effects of medical care. *Milbank Quarterly*, **72**, 225–58.
2. Ten great public health achievements—United States, 1900–1999. *MMWR Weekly*, 1999, **48**(**12**), 241–3. www.cdc.gov/epop/mmwr/preview/mmwrhtml/00056796 .htm (accessed 21 August 2000).

JAMG

Public health is where the action isn't.

Muir Gray

4.1 Facilitating community action

Anna Donald

Objectives

After reading this chapter you will understand the social determinants of health and the principles on which community action to address problems in the social environment can be undertaken.

Background

Social interventions at a community or population level are powerful ways of improving the health of individuals because they are the most powerful determinants of health (Table 4.1.1).

Table 4.1.1 Size of effect on health following universal access to health and social services. Standardized mortality ratios for social classes, men aged 20–64 years, England and Wales, 1951.

Social Classes	I	II	III	IV	V
From the Decennial Supplement (1941–51)	98	98	101	94	118
As adjusted by Registrar General (1959)	86	92	101	104	118

(Reproduced (with permission) from Blane, Brunner, and Wilkinson[1])

In 1951, three years after universal health and social protection was introduced in Britain, the age-old relationship between income and mortality changed (so much so that in 1959 the Registrar General altered the figures by removing company directors from social class I and putting them in social class II—a change that was only rectified in 1999).[1]

Being in a lower social class or having few years in formal education is much more dangerous to one's health than having high cholesterol or exercising little.[2] In most rich countries, all lifestyle factors such as smoking, excess drinking, and obesity combine to explain about one-third of differences in health outcomes. Most of the remaining difference is explained by differences in exposure to social factors, such as parental occupation, education, income, housing and transport, and political stability.[3]

How do social factors affect health?

Most social factors seem to affect health by affecting the degree to which people are able to control their actions in different spheres of life (work, home, leisure); how many physical hazards they are exposed to; and the degree of social support they enjoy. At a biological level, social factors seem to affect the human body in a cumulative fashion through neuro-endocrine, immunological, and haemostatic mechanisms, although further research is needed to identify which of them are most important.[4]

For example, people who are unemployed or who only have a few years of schooling are more likely to be depressed, and in turn are three to five times more likely to have a heart attack.[5] Those with poorly insulated houses are more likely to be cold, which in turn is a potent risk factor for cardiac events.[6]

Secondly, a poor social environment adversely affects health by making it more likely that people will smoke, drink, and eat to excess and be exposed to environmental hazards. For example, mortality rates in Russia have risen exponentially since the collapse of a stable (albeit unpopular) legal and political system, at least in part mediated through excess drinking, as well as through exposure to cold and violence.[7] In Western countries, buildings and domestic structures are associated with about half of childhood accidents.[8]

For policy purposes, it is more powerful to analyse social rather than biological factors because social factors are generally more amenable to change and their improvement is likely to have greater and more lasting results. They can be analysed using two frameworks:

(a) Effects across the life course

Longitudinal studies have found that individuals are particularly susceptible to the effects of certain factors at different times in their lives. Although poverty and poor living standards exacerbate all of them, foetuses and babies are particularly susceptible to poor nutrition; children to parental depression, poor housing, and unsafe play areas; adolescents to social isolation; adults to unemployment and low-paid jobs; and elderly people to social isolation, cold, and pollution.[9]

(b) Cross-sectional analysis

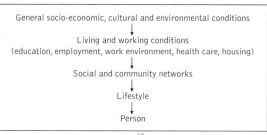

General socio-economic, cultural and environmental conditions
↓
Living and working conditions
(education, employment, work environment, health care, housing)
↓
Social and community networks
↓
Lifestyle
↓
Person

(Adapted from Drever and Whitehead[10])

Figure 4.1.1 Social factors influencing health.

At any particular life stage, people are exposed to social factors operating at different levels. From the broadest level to the most person specific level, these factors are shown in Figure 4.1.1.

Why is the social environment a public health issue?

The social environment is a public health issue because of the size of its effect on health as well as the impact that public health workers can make. Of all health professionals, public health workers are probably in the strongest position to change social factors, as they can help to reform institutions and laws that organize the social environment at a population level, rather than being restricted to treating individuals.

What can be done to improve the social environment at the community level?

1. Choose a model for change.
2. Prepare with data:
   (a) identify the main problems
   (b) assess the size and scope of each problem
   (c) assess available resources and costs.
3. Prioritize options.
4. Plan each strategy: describe tasks and barriers.
5. Evaluate.
6. Build loyalty and trust.

Table 4.1.2 describes interventions that research and routine statistics have found effective in improving social factors. How to put these into practice? At a community level, it helps to plan using steps common to any change management process:

Table 4.1.2 Examples of effective interventions to improve social risk factors (adapted from Acheson[11]).

Exposure	Intervention	Examples of outcomes
Poverty	Redistributive mechanisms, such as taxes and subsidies; Day care centres and pre-school programmes; Parental (especially maternal) education; Family planning programmes and access to contraception for adolescents and young adults; Media campaign to increase uptake of benefits; Local employment programmes	Improved all-cause mortality and morbidity

Psychosocial stress	Better job control; Crime-reduction policies, including community policing programmes and lighting of public walkways	Reduced cardiac events and all-cause mortality
Poor nutrition	Interactive health education; Surplus food schemes; Local food co-operatives; Business partnerships to make quality food available in low-income areas; Smoke reduction programmes	Reduced cardiac events in adulthood; Reduced cancer incidence
Parental depression	Mother-baby education units; Maternal education; Parental social support: home visits at critical periods	Reduced mental health disorders; Reduced child accidents; Reduced all-cause mortality
Poor housing	Smoke alarms; Insulation and heating subsidies; Planning to link housing with social networks and access to goods and services	Reduced death from fires; Reduced cardiac events; Reduced depression and all-cause mortality
Crime	Community policing programmes	Reduced stress; Reduced cardiac and all-cause mortality
Poor transport policies	Safe, maintained walking and cycling paths; Improved public transport; Child safety interventions (e.g. traffic calming devices); Subsidized public transport for deprived populations	Reduced obesity; Reduced respiratory disease from vehicle emissions; Reduced child accident rates; Reduced social isolation

1. Choose a model for change

Different organizational models are available for bringing together people, ideas, and resources in order to achieve lasting improvement.

• in general, more collaborative approaches that involve members of the community take longer but achieve more lasting change, provided analytic and practical skills are 'cascaded' effectively

• communities may require different strategies at different times, depending on their confidence, experience, and available resources.

2. Prepare with data

(a) Identify the main problems

It usually helps to structure each problem in terms of which population is affected by which exposure; what intervention(s) is needed;

the level at which to act; what outcomes would be achieved, and what time period the intervention is needed for what follow-up period.

(b) Assess the size and scope of each problem

It is important to know its likely contributing factors and the context in which it manifests.

Different data collection methods include direct observation, interviews with key stakeholders, rapid appraisal mechanisms, focus groups, 'town hall' meetings, formal needs assessment, routine data (statistics or qualitative surveys), and specialist surveys (see chapters 1.1 and 1.4). Methods should be ethical and chosen to optimize scientific reliability and feasibility.

Information can be compiled to develop a 'health profile' of the community. These commonly include: socio-economic data (age, sex, income/expenditure, area), health status (morbidity and mortality from different conditions), functional status, quality of life, specific health risks, distribution of health care resources, and use of health care (see chapters 1.1 and 1.4). Triangulation (data from several sources) can improve estimates from imperfect sources.

(c) Assess costs and available resources

Resources may include money, skills and experience, time, organizational capacity, partners, and political influence. Costs may be assessed with cost–benefit analysis or simple budgeting. Assessment should include evaluation of the likely effectiveness of each intervention; opportunity costs of doing one thing rather than another; and non-monetary costs of interventions, including distress, dislocation, or reduced productivity resulting from changes to the social environment. (Such non-monetary costs are known as 'negative externalities' in economics.)

3. Prioritize options

It is rarely possible to address all issues at once. Problems can be prioritized in terms of how much disease and economic or social burden they place on society and how feasible they are to address. A problem may also be a priority for symbolic reasons rather than for immediate health gain. Depending on the nature of the problem, decision-tree analysis may help to separate options with uncertain outcomes.[12]

4. Plan each strategy: describe tasks and barriers

Describe systematically how to achieve different objectives as well as analysing possible barriers. A simple grid of four overlapping realms—psychological, political, professional, and technical—can help to prompt and classify tasks and potential pitfalls (Table 4.1.3).

Table 4.1.3 Examples of tasks and barriers affecting most change programmes.

Realm	Examples of tasks involved	Examples of potential barriers
Psychological	Engage people in ways that matter to them; Identify and support people who are effective community change agents (sometimes called 'product champions'); Use language that empowers, not excludes	Resistance of all kinds arising from key stakeholders' fear of loss of role, power, identity, social networks
Political	Ensure key stakeholder support; Phrase policies in language of current discourse	Failure to engage popular change agents; Poor timing, given political agenda
Professional	Identify and plan to meet professional and legal requirements, if any, for proposed changes; Identify and secure resources; set budgets	Regulations obstructing proposed changes
Technical	Secure equipment and map out process for data collection; Secure equipment and map out process for each change needed; Ensure requisite technical skills are available	Insufficient local skills or equipment to collect information

5. Evaluate

Programmes almost always require evaluation to improve future cycles of the programme; to close down ineffective or harmful programmes; and to empower participants. Although psychologically demanding of programme leaders, openness about negative feedback usually inspires more confidence in the long run than no evaluation efforts. Like initial data collection, evaluation methods can be relatively informal and inexpensive or highly structured. They include surveys of key stakeholders, routinely collected and specially collected data or formal epidemiological trials (including randomized controlled trials), ecological trials, and before-and-after trials.

Evaluation (including action research) should be planned from the beginning of the project and should include some kind of control group for comparison.

6. Build loyalty and trust

Efforts are usually wasted if change agents do not obtain the loyalty and trust of community members. Different strategies and lots of time are usually needed to build loyalty and trust, or 'social capital';[13] staff levels and time-frames for projects need to be set accordingly.

Further resources

Benzeval M, Judge K, and Whitehead M (ed.) (1995). *Tackling inequalities in health: an agenda for action*. King's Fund, London.

Durch JS, Bailey LA, and Stoto MA (ed.) (1997). *Improving health in the community: a role for performance monitoring*. National Academy Press, Washington DC.

Jacobson B, Smith A, and Whitehead M (1988). *The nation's health: a strategy for the 1990s*. King's Fund, London.

Kuh D and Ben-Shlomo Y (1997). *A life course approach to chronic disease epidemiology*. Oxford University Press, Oxford.

Wilkinson R (1997). *Unhealthy societies: the afflictions of inequality*. Routledge, London.

Wilkinson R and Marmot M (ed.) (1998). *Social determinants of health: the solid facts*. World Health Organization, Geneva.

Wilkinson R and Marmot M (ed.) (1999). *Social determinants of health*. Oxford University Press, Oxford.

References

1. Blane D, Brunner E, and Wilkinson R (1996). The evolution of public health policy: an anglocentric view of the last fifty years. In *Health and social organization*, (ed. D Blane, E Brunner, and R Wilkinson). Routledge, London.

2. Rose G (1985). Sick individuals and sick populations. *Int J of Epidemiology*, **14**, 32–8.

3. Marmot MG, Davey Smith G, Stansfeld S, Patel C, North F, and Head J (1991). Health inequalities among British civil servants: the Whitehall II study. *Lancet*, **337**, 1387–93.

4. Stansfeld S and Marmot MG (ed.) (2000). *Stress and heart disease*. BMJ Publications, London.

5. Hemingway H and Marmot MG (1999). Evidence based cardiology: psychosocial factors in the aetiology and prognosis of coronary heart disease: systematic review of prospective cohort studies. *BMJ*, **318**, 1460–7.

6. Lloyd EL (1999). The role of cold in ischaemic heart disease: a review. *Public Health*, **105**, 205–15.

7. Walberg P, McKee M, Shkolnikov V, Chenet L, and Leon DA (1998). Economic change, crime, and mortality crisis in Russia: regional analysis. *BMJ*, **317**, 312–8.

8. Department of Trade and Industry (1991). *Home and leisure accident research: twelfth annual report, 1988 data*. Department of Trade and Industry, Consumer Safety Unit, London.

9. Bartley M, Blane D, and Montgomery S (1997). Education and debate. Socio-economic determinants of health: health and the life course: why safety nets matter. *BMJ*, **314**, 1194.

10. Drever F and Whitehead M (ed.) (1997). *Health Inequalities*, decennial supplement, series DS No. 15. HMSO, London.
11. Acheson D (1998). *Report on the inquiry into health inequalities*. The Stationery Office, London.
12. Lilford RJ, Pauker SG, Braunholtz DA, and Chard J (1998). Getting research findings into practice: decision analysis and the implementation of research findings. *BMJ*, **317**, 405–9.
13. Pratt J, Plamping D, and Gordon P (1999). *Working whole systems*. King's Fund, London.

The quest for better health is the quest for social justice.

Kenneth Calman

4.2 **Effective health promotion programmes**

Don Nutbeam

Objectives

This chapter presents the different steps which need to be taken to plan, develop, test, and evaluate a health promotion intervention. Each stage provides different prompts for practitioners, which are intended to help systematically link relevant research, theory, and programme evaluation to 'real-life' experience and the practicalities of implementation.

Definition

Health promotion is defined by WHO as follows:

'Health promotion is the process of enabling people to exert control over, and to improve their health'.[1]

Thus, health promotion is described as a *process*, an activity directed towards *enabling people* to take action. Correspondingly, health promotion is not something that is done *on* or *to* people, it is done *with* people either as individuals or as groups. The purpose of this activity is to strengthen the skills and capabilities of individuals to take action, and the capacity of groups or communities to act collectively *to exert control over* the determinants of their health.

In tackling the determinants of health, health promotion will include actions directed towards changing both the determinants within the more immediate control of individuals, such as individual health behaviours, and those outside the immediate control of individuals, such as social, economic, and environmental conditions which influence health.

Basic assumptions concerning effective health promotion

The chapter is based on four basic assumptions concerning effective interventions:

1. Effective interventions are planned on the basis of a thorough analysis of the problem that indicates reasonable linkages between the short-term impact of interventions and subsequent changes in the determinants of health and in health outcomes. Such an analysis will usually indicate the scope and feasibility of successful intervention.

2. Effective interventions are informed by established theory, relevant to the type of intervention planned.

3. Effective interventions create the necessary conditions for successful implementation. This includes ensuring that there is sufficient public and political awareness of the issue and the need for action; developing capacity for programme delivery, and securing the resources required to implement and sustain a programme.

4. Effective interventions are of sufficient size, duration, and sophistication to be detectable above the 'background noise' of more general changes in society. Programmes which combine different intervention methods rather than relying on a single methodology are most likely to be successful.[2]

The stages and tasks of developing a health promotion intervention

Figure 4.2.1 provides a summary of the linkages between the different stages of planning, implementation, and evaluation of health promotion interventions. It indicates five distinct phases in the process, namely:

(a) problem definition

(b) solution generation

(c) capacity building

(d) implementation

(e) process, impact, and outcome evaluation.

Each of these stages is considered in turn.

(a) Problem definition—starting at the end

From the outset it is essential to be clear about the long-term goals and the short-term targets and priorities for an intervention by identifying priority health and social outcomes for a defined population, and the modifiable determinants of those priorities. This requires definition of outcomes to be achieved at the bottom part of the model in Figure 4.2.1 as a means to clarifying *what* and *who* might be the target of a programme intervention.

Many of the factors which might be considered important in deciding on these priorities have been examined in previous chapters and include, for example, what is known about:

• the size and distribution of a health problem in a population

• the determinants of the different health problems (behavioural, social, environmental, economic, genetic)

• the possibility and feasibility of changing these determinants

• community and political priorities (interests and motivation which may affect the opportunity to take action).

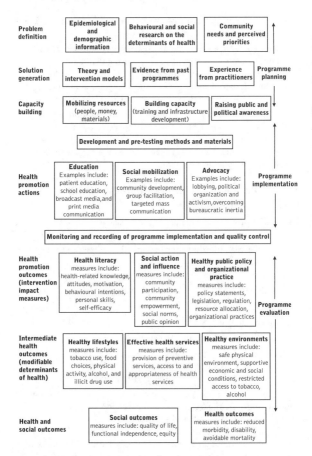

Figure 4.2.1 A planning model for health promotion.

Returning to the top of the model it should be possible to use local epidemiological and demographic information, together with available behavioural and social research to define measurable *programme goals*, and *programme objectives* as the basis for a structured *programme plan*.

- *programme goals* will usually be directed at changes to behaviours, or to social, economic, and environmental conditions which are the major determinants of the *health and social outcomes* being targeted. These programme goals will relate to the *intermediate health outcomes* in the model

◆ *programme objectives* will usually be directed at those personal, social, and organizational factors which are modifiable as a means to changing the determinants of health. These are the *health promotion outcomes* in the model.

In this way the beginning of the planning process is firmly fixed on the end of the evaluation process through a thorough and logical analysis of the linkages between intervention and outcome.

Unravelling complexities in causality

Figure 4.2.1 can be used not only to illustrate the vertical linkages between the different levels of input, process, and outcomes, but also the lateral relationships. For example at this stage of problem definition, analysis of epidemiological data may reveal excess coronary heart disease in a population, but it is only through analysis of the behavioural risks, social norms, and community preferences that this finding can be related to a comprehensive intervention programme—*what* modifiable factors and *who* might be the target of a programme.

What should also be obvious from the model in Figure 4.2.1 is that it is hard to identify a simple causal chain which links a health promotion action to changes in health status. Such a simplistic *reductionist* model for health promotion and disease prevention has long been discredited.[3] The link between health promotion action and eventual health outcomes is usually complex and difficult to trace. What the model can do is highlight these complexities, and at the same time offer an *expanded* model of health promotion which more adequately acknowledges the central place of social and environmental influences on health and quality of life, and the combination of interventions to achieve more substantial effects.

(b) Solution generation—what combination of actions is required?

The next task requires the use of a range of information and research evidence to determine the best solution to identified problems. This stage focuses on *how* and *when* change might be achieved in a target population. Decisions on the optimal *timing* and *sequencing* of interventions will also be made at this stage.

Figure 4.2.1 can again provide a useful guide to the issues which need to be considered. Health promotion action can be directed to achieve different health promotion outcomes by shifting the focus or emphasis to an intervention. Deciding on what represents the best starting point and how to combine the different actions to achieve desired health promotion outcomes is essential to effective practice in health promotion. Decisions at this stage will be guided by consideration of established health promotion theory and intervention models, alongside research evidence from past programmes, tempered by local knowledge of the context in which the programme is to be implemented.[4]

A typical health promotion programme might consist of interventions targeted at all three of the factors identified as health promotion outcomes in the model. For example a programme to reduce teenage smoking might consist of:

- *education* of young people concerning the negative consequences of smoking

- *social mobilization* of parents and other social role models to make smoking less socially attractive/acceptable to young people, and

- *advocacy* for legislative action to reduce access to tobacco and exposure to tobacco advertising.

Assessing the right combination of actions in the right sequence to achieve the programme goals and objectives decided earlier completes the process of developing a programme plan through the development of programme strategies.

Programme strategies will almost always involve combinations of action at multiple levels (individual, social, organizational) to achieve the programme objectives, and generally conform to the *health promotion actions* in the model.

(c) Capacity building: creating the optimal conditions for success

Once a programme plan has been developed the first phase in the implementation process is referred to as *capacity building* in the framework. This stage is not only concerned with obtaining the resources (such as money and materials) required for the successful implementation of a programme. It also refers to the need to build capacity in a community or organization so that a programme can be introduced and sustained, and to generate and maintain the community and political support necessary for successful implementation. This stage is concerned with *creating the optimal conditions for a successful intervention.*

A resource assessment will include:

- assessment of financial needs

- determination of the availability of human resources

- analysis of how to generate such resources.

Where the available resources, or community or political support, do not match that which is needed, it will be necessary to reformulate the programme objectives to better fit available resources, and/or to clarify the types of action which may be required to secure the greater community and political support that will generate the resources and opportunities for action which are required.

Failure to give sufficient time and attention to this capacity-building phase in the implementation of a programme is the commonest reason for programme failure. This is especially the case when programme implementation may involve working with other sectors, such as schools, work sites, and different agencies of government.

Engaging others in solving a public health problem

Building and sustaining relationships between sectors towards common goals is a difficult task. Many of the conditions for success (or failure) are in place long before any specific action is taken and it is important not only to plan the details of the project, but also to account for the context in which it is being undertaken, and the ability of the infrastructure of the organizations to deliver. Several issues are important in the implementation of a project that requires co-operation between different agencies:

- clear recognition of *why it is important for the organizations to work together*, including agreement on the role for different organizations in the implementation process
- acknowledgement that *the process is emergent and changing*; the need for flexibility in negotiation over roles and responsibilities
- definition of a *clearly articulated and achievable goal* that is understood and valued by the different organizations involved in a project
- *agreement on a way of working*; this may mean working on small, well-defined tasks initially to build trust and confidence in a working relationship before seeking to implement more significant changes
- *opportunities for renegotiation* including identification of the length of time to which organizations are committed, and allowing for redefinition of tasks, roles, and relationships
- *commitment to joint ownership*; any sense that one partner is imposing on another invariably leads to resistance and damage to the relationship
- *allocation of resources*; staff, space, money, information, and administrative support.

At the end of this stage the conditions for successful intervention need to be in place. This will have required close attention to:

- the *negotiations* required to secure political support and the co-operation of partner agencies
- *training* to motivate and improve the skills of the 'agents' for the intervention (for example, school-teachers, community health workers, administrators, general practitioners)
- *communication* to influence community awareness or to secure political support may be required before an intervention is commenced.

(d) Implementing the plan

The development and pre-testing of materials (such as pamphlets and other media) is an essential first step in the implementation of a programme. Testing materials on population segments, or in limited geographical areas, will provide vital information to allow fine-tuning of implementation strategies.

Combining interventions to achieve greatest effect

The implementation of a programme will often involve multiple *programme strategies* to achieve the *programme objectives and goals* emerging from initial analysis of the problem and its determinants. Traditionally, health promotion interventions have relied heavily on public *information, education, or communication* as a primary method for improving knowledge and changing attitudes and behaviours. Increasingly, health promotion programmes involve other forms of intervention designed to influence the social, environmental, and economic factors which determine health. This requires working with communities in different ways to *mobilize social action*, as well as *advocacy* for political and organizational change.

There is a dynamic interrelationship between these different health promotion actions. The implementation of any health promotion intervention will usually require a combination of actions, and as indicated above, the timing and sequence of these components is critical to success. These different health promotion actions can be directed to achieve different programme objectives by shifting the focus or balance of actions. For example, efforts to promote healthy nutrition can be directed at the consumer as an individual using traditional educational communication, or at food manufacturers and retailers to improve the supply and promotion of nutritious food, or at catering outlets (canteens, restaurants) to influence food preparation and supply.

Deciding on what represents the best starting point, how to combine the different actions and in what sequence, and managing people and resources to achieve the desired health promotion outcomes is at the core of 'best practice' in health promotion.

Managing people and resources

Good management of people and resources will make a major contribution to successful programme implementation. Increasing attention is being given to these management issues and to the development of *performance indicators* which can be used to assist this management process. Performance indicators are the measures which can be used to assess practitioner performance against stated criteria necessary to create conditions for successful programme implementation.

(e) Evaluation: how will you know when you have been successful?

Multiple intervention strategies lead to multiple outcomes and different levels of outcome which provide a basis for the evaluation of health promotion interventions, and there are many ways of determining success or failure in health promotion.

Although the measurement of these *outcomes* is important at this stage, understanding the *processes* which have occurred within programmes is also an essential part of evaluation. By systematic study and record keeping of the processes of implementation we are able to unravel the reasons for success and failure rather than just observe outcomes. This dimension to the evaluation task may include investigation of the organizational, practitioner, and community characteristics which underpin successful implementation, and define conditions for best practice.

Impact evaluation

This represents the first level of evaluation of a programme. Such impact measures would normally have been defined as *programme objectives* in the planning phase. These *health promotion outcomes* represent those personal, social, and environmental factors which are modifiable as a means to changing the determinants of health (intermediate health outcomes)—the starting point for the planning of the intervention. These outcomes also represent the most immediate impact of planned health promotion activities. *Health literacy* refers to the knowledge and skills which determine the ability of individuals to gain access to, understand, and use information to promote and maintain good health—typically the outcome of health education activities. *Social action and influence* describes the results of efforts to enhance the actions and control of social groups over the determinants of health—for example, efforts to mobilize older people towards the achievement of common health goals. *Healthy public policy and organizational practices* are the result of efforts to overcome structural barriers to health—typically the outcome of internal government policy development processes, and/or external advocacy and lobbying which may lead to legislative change. Examples of measures/indicators that can be used for this purpose are given in Figure 4.2.1.

Outcome evaluation

Changing the intermediate health outcomes (health determinants) is a fundamental goal in health promotion. Personal behaviours, such as smoking or physical activity, may increase or decrease the risk of ill health, and are summarized as *healthy lifestyles*. *Healthy environments* consist of the physical, economic, and social conditions that can both impact directly on health, as well as support healthy lifestyles—for example by making it more or less easy for an individual to smoke, or adopt a healthy diet. Access to, appropriate provision of, and appropriate use of health services are acknowledged as important determinants of health status, and are represented as *effective health services* in this model.

At this stage, feedback on success or failure in relation to programme objectives can already be used to redefine the problem (stage (a)), or to re-examine potential solutions (stage (b)).

Programme failure can almost always be traced to problems at stage (c) in the model—*capacity building.*

At the end of these stages it should be possible to:

• assess whether or not a programme can achieve predetermined programme goals and objectives

• understand the essential organizational, practitioner, and community characteristics which underpin successful implementation, and define conditions for best practice

• determine whether or not these conditions for success can be reproduced in different circumstances.

Strengths and weaknesses of planning models

The planning model summarized in Figure 4.2.1 will not answer all questions likely to arise in the planning, evaluation, and maintenance of a health promotion programme. Decision making never follows such a smooth pathway as that described above. Most people engaged in health promotion, whether as paid health workers or as volunteers, will not start with a blank piece of paper on which they are asked to plot out their perfect programme for a perfect world. Most people who are engaged in 'doing' health promotion will be working in established settings such as schools and work sites, or in a defined geographical area. Often people are working on solving predetermined problems such as drug and alcohol misuse, road traffic injury, or cardiovascular disease—representing defined directions and priorities over which they will have had only minimal influence.

Adapting not adopting

This model is provided as a guide to action, intended to be *adapted* to prevailing circumstances, rather than *adopted* wholesale without critical examination of its usefulness. In such circumstances, what models of this kind can do is highlight the need for an expanded view of a problem and how to solve it. Because few of us engaged in practical programme development will have the resources, opportunities, and skills to apply this model in the systematic way described in this section of the book, it is important to be able to:

• identify what *is* possible

• clarify and make explicit the constraints on what is being attempted

• indicate what else might be done to strengthen and improve chances of success in solving the public health problem being addressed.

Knowing the limits

Knowing the limits to what can be achieved in different circumstances is not only important for planning a successful programme, but also important for framing community and political expectations of health promotion programmes. In this sense the framework in the model serves as a useful reference point in decision making.

More importantly, application of this model promotes recognition that health promotion is a complex and sophisticated activity, which requires careful planning and skilful execution if success is to be achieved.

Further resources

Downie RS, Tannahill C, and Tannahill A (1996). *Health promotion—models and values*, (2nd edn). Oxford University Press, Oxford.

Thorogood M and Coombes Y (1999). *Evaluating health promotion: practice and methods*. Oxford University Press, Oxford.

References

1. World Health Organization (1986). *Ottawa Charter for Health Promotion*. WHO, Geneva.
2. Nutbeam D (1999). Making the case for health promotion: the questions to be answered. In *The evidence of health promotion effectiveness: shaping public health in a new Europe*, (ed. D Boddy). European Union, Brussels.
3. Chapman S (1993). Unravelling gossamer with boxing gloves: problems in explaining the decline in smoking. *BMJ*, **307**, 429–32.
4. Nutbeam D and Harris E (1999). *Theory in a nutshell: a guide to health promotion theory*. McGraw-Hill, Sydney.

4.3 Protecting and promoting health—behavioural approaches

Jeff French

Objectives

This chapter poses a number of questions about the use of behavioural change approaches to protecting and promoting health. Each question is followed by a brief review of key issues of relevance to practitioners as they contemplate the use of behavioural change interventions.

What is the contribution of behavioural approaches to protecting and promoting health?

Interventions directed at changing behaviour have been a mainstay of most national public health programmes. Behavioural change approaches to promoting health are broad in scope and operate at a number of levels. Lalonde[1] in his description of the 'Health Field concept' clearly identified health behaviour as one of the key determinants of health and disease. He also made a powerful argument for recognition of the interconnection between lifestyle and behaviour and the other major determinants of ill-health. Public health action directed at behaviour change related to lifestyle should be integrated with and complementary to action directed at the other elements, determinants, and influences on health (see chapter 4.2).

Box 4.3.1 **Elements of the Health Field concept**

1. Lifestyle and behaviour
2. Health, social, and other service provision
3. Socio-economic and physical environment
4. Biological processes

(from Lalonde[1])

Behavioural change approaches are used with individuals in relation to personal health behaviour and in relation to compliance with health care interventions. Individual health behaviour change approaches can also make a contribution towards promoting personal and family health protection, for example through encouraging mothers to lay infants on their backs in order to reduce the incidence of cot death. At a group level, behavioural approaches can be used to engage communities in identifying health concerns and developing community solutions. The contribution of behavioural change interventions directed at the uptake of services such as screening and immunization programmes is also significant.

Individual and group behaviour can clearly promote, maintain, or damage health. Health-related behaviour is best understood as a dynamic phenomenon that is influenced by individual attitudes, beliefs, and motivations, societal norms, socio-economic factors, and physiological genetic, and neural hormonal effects.

Should we attempt to change health behaviour?

This question relates to the value systems that individual health practitioners, organizations, government, and society at large hold. In a democratic system individuals have the right to behave in any way they choose providing it does not have negative consequences for others. However individual choices often have negative effects on people other than the individual making them.

Practitioners should be aware of two key concepts in relation to this issue:

+ victim blaming
+ voluntarism.[†]

The concept of victim blaming has been used to describe a process in which individuals who adopt health-damaging behaviours such as smoking are blamed for their decisions when in fact they are victims of a coalition of societal pressures that to a large extent force them into a position of adopting such behaviours. Rather than addressing the determinants of health-damaging behaviour, health campaigns that focus on individual responsibility for behavioural change have often been criticized for adopting such a victim-blaming approach.

The concept of voluntarism is one that is often used to guide practice. In essence voluntarism is concerned with ensuring that individuals, groups, or communities are willing and active parties in any attempt to change behaviour and that there is no covert manipulation of behaviour even if it is deemed by a health professional to be 'for the best'. Voluntarism implies a partnership between a health professional and client in relation to any attempt to change behaviour. Voluntarism is a concept rooted in an educational model of practice that stresses the importance of freedom to choose among alternative health-related activities.

....

† The principle of relying on voluntary action. *New Oxford dictionary of English*, (1998). Oxford University Press, Oxford.

Does behavioural change work?

This question needs to be asked more specifically of particular interventions within specific situations dealing with specific population groups. There is however a great deal of evidence of the effectiveness of behavioural approaches to health protection and promotion. This evidence is available from:

- macro epidemiological and behavioural evidence
- meta studies
- specific studies in particular areas of practice.

At the level of population change there is good evidence of significant and sustained changes in behaviour resulting from sustained health education and health promotion interventions. A good example of such a change is the fall in smoking rates amongst advantaged groups in developed countries. Meta studies of interventions have also demonstrated the positive and significant contribution of behavioural change approaches.[2]

What are the characteristics of successful behavioural change interventions?

Successful health promotion initiatives tend to have a number of common characteristics (see chapter 4.2). When establishing or reviewing behavioural change programmes, practitioners should assure themselves that interventions are:

- systematically planned and informed by relevant theory; programmes need clear aims and objectives, which are measurable
- achievable; the behavioural change should be possible for people to achieve within the circumstances of their lives
- sufficiently focused on an assessment of structures and systems in society and how these may facilitate or act as barriers to change
- sufficiently resourced, allowing for both delivery and evaluation of the intervention.

What insights can practitioners gain from the theoretical and research base about behavioural change?

What has more than sixty years of research shown us about the relationship between knowledge, attitude, and behaviour? The simple answer is that these relationships are positive but very small. Attitudes and behaviour do not seem to be closely related. This conclusion gives little comfort to those health practitioners who advocate a traditional belief that if people can be given accurate information they will change their attitudes and stop behaving in unhealthy ways and start behaving in a more healthy way.

Jackson[3] has set out eight principles that can be used to guide the use of behavioural approaches to health promotion. These principles are drawn from the evidence of effectiveness:

- acquiring new behaviours is a process, not an event, and often entails learning by performing successive approximations of the behaviour
- psychological factors, notably beliefs and values, influence how people behave
- the more beneficial or rewarding an experience, the more likely it is to be repeated: the more punishing or unpleasant an experience the less likely it is to be repeated
- behavioural experience can influence individuals' experience and values
- individuals are not passive responders, but have a proactive role in the behaviour change process
- social relationships and social norms have a substantial and persistent influence on how people behave
- behaviour is not independent of the context in which it occurs; people influence and are influenced by their physical and social environments
- the process of applying behavioural science theories in practical situations should be guided by research and evaluation methods.

Choosing your approach

A number of theories of behaviour change in the health field have been developed. All of these theoretical models provide insights into how and why people change their behaviour or do not. Practitioners should be aware of the key components of these models and their implications for planned interventions.

Based on the work of Bandura[4] and colleagues, *social learning theory* asserts that modelling is a key influence on learning. In simple terms, people watch others' behaviour, and then adopt similar behaviours. Practitioners should note that the important elements in the learning process are the credibility of the role model observed and reinforcement of learned behaviour. Positive reinforcement leads to a greater likelihood of the behaviour being retained or repeated.

Developed by Becker,[5] the *health belief model* suggests that when faced with the possibility of changing health behaviour individuals consider the advantages and disadvantages of change and then take a rational decision. Their behaviour will depend on their view of their susceptibility to the illness or danger, the perceived seriousness of the illness, and the relative costs and benefits of the possible change. Practitioners will need to address these issues when developing interventions.

Devised by Tones,[6] the *health action model* builds on the health belief model by incorporating the additional element of 'self-esteem', which is concerned with our beliefs about our appearance, intelligence, skills, and how we believe others perceive us. People with high self-esteem are likely, the model argues, to be more receptive to health messages. The model also identifies a number of factors, such as knowledge, and supportive environment, which can influence health decision making. Within the model individuals are considered to have the potential to take charge of their own health if complementary health promotion work is directed towards making the environment within which health choices are made conducive and supportive. The key factors here for practitioners are the need to build esteem-raising initiatives into intervention programmes and to simultaneously address factors in the environment that may help or hinder an individual's attempts at change.

A great deal of current health behaviour change interventions use the *stages of change model* developed by Prochaska and DiClemente.[7] This model attempts to describe how change happens at an individual level. It suggests that change moves from a stage of contemplation through to preparation for change and finally maintenance or relapse from a change. This is a useful model for practitioners in that it can be used to focus efforts on the particular stage of change that individuals are at, with the intention of helping them to move through the cycle towards making a positive change and maintaining it, rather than attempting to move from a contemplation of change stage to a maintenance stage in one jump. Further insights are provided by Ajensen and Fishbein's theory of reasoned action,[8] which suggests that people's behaviour can best be predicted by an assessment of their intentions. Intentions flow from attitudes that are in turn based on beliefs about what will be the consequences of behaviour. In addition to beliefs about the consequences of behaviour, intentions are also influenced by beliefs about what 'significant others' expect individuals to do. This theory emphasizes the need for practitioners to develop a clear understanding of the attitudes and belief systems that underpin individuals' or groups' behaviour if successful interventions and helping strategies are to be developed.

Maximizing the impact

Health promotion focused on behavioural change can be effective. A greater effect is possible when behavioural change approaches are considered as part of a wider strategy to improve health. Approaches to health promotion which emphasize general empowerment through health education, community development, and organizational development and change, together with health promotion efforts aimed at social, administrative, and political change, have been shown to be most effective. Within this context, behavioural change has a significant and complementary role.

Further resources

International Union for Health Promotion and Education (2000). *Evidence of health promotion effectiveness: shaping public health in a new Europe. A* report for the European Commission. IUHPE, Vanes.

Tones K and Tilford S (1994). *Health education effectiveness efficiency and equality*, (2nd edn). Chapman Hall, London.

References

1. Lalonde M (1974). *A new perspective on the health of Canadians*. Government of Canada, Ottawa.
2. Liedekerken P, Jonkers R, Haes W, Kok G, and Saan J (1990). *Effectiveness of health education. Review and analysis*. Dutch Health Education Centre, Van Gorcum/Uitgeverij voor Gezondheidsbevordering bv Assen, The Netherlands.
3. Jackson C (1997). Behavioural science and principles for practice in health education. *Health Education Research*, **12(1)**, 143–50.
4. Bandura A (1977). *Social learning theory*. Prentice Hall, Engelwood Cliffs.
5. Becker M (ed.) (1974). *The health belief model and personal health behaviour*. Slack, Thorofare, New Jersey.
6. Tones K (1991). *Health promotion, self empowerment and the concept of control*. Leeds Polytechnic, Leeds.
7. Prochaska JO, DiClemente CC (1983). Stages and processes of self change of smoking: toward an integrative model of change. *Journal of Consulting and Clinical Psychology*, 51(3), 390–5.
8. Ajenzen J and Fishbein M (1980). *Understanding attitudes and predicting social behaviour*. Prentice Hall, New Jersey.

4.4 **Protecting health, sustaining the environment**

Roscoe Taylor and Charles Guest

Introduction

By reading this chapter you will be better able to understand the nature of environmental health and the process of identifying, evaluating, and planning a response to an environmental health threat.

Why is this an important public health issue?

Threats to public health from environmental hazards are continually emerging. Impacts range from relatively small-scale and local, to widespread exposures affecting whole populations. It is now clear that ecosystem degradation threatens health at the global level.[1] Although environmental health protection and sustainability are effectively the same thing, the practice usually fails this rhetoric.

Social and economic factors are powerful determinants of the health of the environment, and hence the health of the public. A new public health has emerged in which healthy environments that include a healthy social and economic milieu are seen as the way forward to improve population health. However, differing beliefs about what constitutes a 'healthy economic milieu' underlie community debate about 'development' vs. 'growth'.

Public health has its developmental roots in the identification and control of environmental health threats. For example poor sanitation, food, or water supply contamination leading to outbreaks of communicable disease, or air pollution episodes causing increased respiratory morbidity and mortality, were triggers for major advances in health protection.[2] It remains a basic function of environmental health practitioners to understand, predict, prevent, monitor, and respond to such threats. But while enforcement of statutory provisions was the mainstay of practice in the past, the emphasis now is more on prevention—calling into play a broad range of strategies including advocacy, intersectoral collaboration, and community development models in addition to development of policy, standards, and guidelines. An ongoing capacity for monitoring and surveillance is also necessary for early identification of environmental hazards.

Definitions

Environmental health encompasses those aspects of human health, including quality of life, determined by physical, chemical, biological, social, and psycho-social factors in the environment. The discipline involves the theory and practice of assessing, correcting, controlling, and preventing those factors in the environment that can potentially affect adversely the health of present and future generations.[3]

Environmental health practitioners may operate at a local (municipal), regional, or national and international level, and be involved in a vast range of issues (see Box 4.4.1).

Box 4.4.1 The wide range of issues and exposures that environmental health practitioners may encounter includes:

Household exposures
Indoor air quality
Sanitation and clean drinking water
Communicable diseases
Housing quality
Soil and dust contamination
Noise

The occupational environment
Agriculture
Mining and extraction
Construction
Manufacturing
Service occupations

Community-level exposures
Outdoor air quality
Traffic and transport
Industry and manufacturing
Waste management
Microbiological contamination of water and food
Chemical contamination of water and food
Urbanization

Regional exposures
Atmospheric dispersion of contaminants
Land use and water engineering

Global environmental change

Hazard* is the intrinsic capacity of an agent, a condition, or a situation to produce an adverse health or environmental effect.

Whilst information about a source of emissions and environmental concentrations of contaminants is essential to environmental health protection, it does not indicate how much toxin actually reaches the individual. An agent may be hazardous but not necessarily result in a risk until exposure occurs and a dose is delivered to target organs. Compare exposure and dose, as follows:

Exposure* refers to actual contact with an agent (usually chemical, physical, or biological).

Dose* is the stated quantity of a substance to which an organism is exposed. The *applied* dose is the amount of the substance in contact with the primary absorption sites (e.g. skin, lungs, gut) and available for absorption. The *absorbed* dose is the amount crossing a specific absorption site, and the amount actually available for interaction with any particular organ or cell is the *delivered* dose. The latter may be particularly difficult or impossible to measure.

Dose–response assessment is the determination of the relationship between the magnitude of the dose or level of exposure to an agent or hazard, and the incidence or severity of the associated effect.

Exposure assessment is the estimation of the magnitude, frequency, duration, and pathway of contact of an agent encountered by humans in the course of their activities e.g. via inhalation, ingestion, or dermal contact. In contrast to dose, exposure does not indicate absorption, metabolism, excretion, or storage of a toxin.[4]
   Different types of exposure indices include:

- ambient environmental exposure (e.g. average air pollution in a city)
- individualized measures (e.g. hours per week over known periods in an occupational environment)
- total exposure assessment (integration of various exposure pathways affecting a community or individual, e.g. from a soil contaminant).[5]

Risk assessment is the process of estimating the potential impact of a chemical, physical, microbiological, or psycho-social hazard on a specified human population or ecological system under a specific set of conditions and for a certain timeframe.[6,7]
   Where good dose–response relationship and other information is available, risks may be quantifiable. However risk assessments must also take into account qualitative information about the nature of health effects in the context of particular communities.

Environmental health indicators are environmental or health indicators, chosen because they are both measurable and associated either with a known environmental exposure or a health-effect relationship. These indicators should be directed at an issue of specific policy or management concern, presented in a form to improve the evidence base for decision making.[8]

Protecting against an environmental health threat

In order to protect against a perceived environmental health threat, a framework for assessing health risk should be used. The steps involved typically include:[9]

- identifying the hazard
- determining the relationship between the hazard and the effect (dose–response assessment)
- exposure assessment
- risk characterization.

Identifying the hazard

Before embarking on a formal risk assessment the specific issues should be identified with key stakeholders. Specific concerns and their context should be identified. It is most important to establish if the issue is actually amenable to risk assessment. Successful management requires transparency and a strong involvement of the affected communities as far as possible in every aspect of the process. Hazard identification generally relies on prior knowledge and published literature, including animal toxicology and epidemiological studies.

Dose–response information

Dose–response information is also derived from prior knowledge and the literature. However, there are often gaps in such data. This is partly due to difficulties in measuring exposure and dose in human studies (which tend to be opportunistic and retrospective), but also because methodological weaknesses are common. Even when human data are available, it may be difficult to extrapolate dose–response relationships from high-exposure studies to situations involving low exposures.

Perspective and priority

Commonly, environmental exposures (e.g. via soil, water, or ambient air) present lower dose rates and total doses than those experienced through personal ('lifestyle') behaviours or occupational sources. Such exposures may incur relatively small increases in risk. However, because they are perceived as being outside the control of individuals, there is often a large 'outrage' factor; this may require attention that seems out of proportion to their impact if they are involuntary (see chapter 7.5).

Environmental factors with only a small additional risk for individuals can still have a major impact on populations if many people are exposed—for example, low-level childhood lead exposure.

Some environmental hazards are also amenable to control more readily than lifestyle exposure factors and therefore present opportunities for efficient and effective public health interventions. This is analogous to 'engineered' injury prevention measures that separate the person from the hazard.

In establishing priorities when there are multiple environmental health problems, consider:

- the urgency of the threat (see chapter 4.9)
- the number of people affected, and their experience of the impacts
- whether the exposure is increasing (amount / numbers of sources)
- the consequences of 'doing nothing'
- vulnerability / identifiability of population subgroups
- amenability of issues to investigation
- availability of interventions or remedies.

Proactive versus reactive approaches

Periodic, systematic review is important to ensure that priorities are not only reactive. For example, there is an urgent need to address long-term environmental issues (including the abatement of greenhouse gas emissions) by considering the health perspective, as well as the health impacts of immediate problems related to the environment. Our preoccupations include food, water, fuel, waste disposal (particularly in developing countries), together with unemployment, violence, drugs, and debt (everywhere). Ecosystem disruption remains the looming but neglected threat whilst these more immediate issues demand attention.

Maintaining the environment and mitigating risk

Maintenance of a healthy environment requires:

- legislation and other regulation, with enforcement
- healthy public policy
- appropriate guidelines and standards
- economic incentives
- demonstration projects
- attitudinal change
- community involvement
- accurate information.

Although legislative controls and regulatory mechanisms may be available to deal with an environmental health threat (and are sometimes essential as a back-up measure), this is not usually the first course of action. It is preferable to establish collaborative approaches.

Options for risk mitigation

Depending on the situation a wide range of potential strategies may be available to control or prevent risks, including:

(i) Reduction in hazard at point of generation

- alteration of systems and human behaviours that underlie the production of a hazard (e.g. increased use of public transport)
- enforced shutdown of activity
- cleaner processing systems
- improved emission controls.

(ii) Reduction in exposure to hazard

- removal of contaminant from medium (e.g. drinking water treatment)
- physical separation of exposed community from source
  - relocation of activity
  - buffer zones between emission source and community
  - barriers (e.g. noise barriers, clean topsoil cover, shade creation)
- altered personal behaviour to reduce exposure
  - dietary consumption (e.g. reduced intake of mercury-contaminated fish)
  - avoidance (e.g. recreational water contact during blue-green algal blooms).

(iii) Protection at the individual level

- biological measures (e.g. Hepatitis A vaccination to reduce risk of this disease from an unclean water supply).

Note that options higher up in this list are in general preferable as (unlike the later options) they address the root causes. Neglect of root causes world-wide reflects the difficulties we face in promoting 'ecologically sustainable development' (ESD)(Box 4.4.2).

Uncertainty and the precautionary principle

Whilst an evidence-based approach should underpin environmental health action, there are many instances where information is lacking. In such circumstances, a precautionary approach should apply, recognizing the existence of uncertainty and ignorance and accepting that lack of full scientific certainty should not be used as a reason to postpone preventative measures. Proponents of environmental modification need to be able to demonstrate that, to a very high degree of probability, a project will not cause significant harm to the environment.

Health risk assessments need to be explicit about uncertainties. Look for bias and identify what further information could reduce the uncertainty. This also assists in setting priorities in research and monitoring.

Box 4.4.2 **Ecologically sustainable development (ESD) and human health**

Principles for ecologically sustainable development:

- live off 'interest'(renewable resources) rather than (non-renewable)'capital'
- aim for diversity and variety
- 'closed cycle' system designs (e.g. waste water recycling)
- population levels should be in balance with available resources
- work with rather than against natural topography and biological systems.

It is essential that ecologically sustainable development is linked to investment. Projects—in public health and other sectors—should aim to:

- focus on what is possible
- solve small problems to influence larger ones
- involve people's creativity and energy
- foster responsibility of those who pollute or degrade.

Some projects that have aimed to promote sustainability and health have had low participation rates. New projects that bring the questions of sustainability in the indefinite future into focus in the present are required. These may be developed by:

- identifying the critical quality-of-life issues in a region
- establishing how these issues relate to longer-term sustainability issues
- identifying simultaneous solutions for sustainability and quality-of-life issues
- obtaining resources to make solutions happen.

Sustainable health projects should simultaneously promote:

- economic efficiency
- social equity
- environmental responsibility
- human livability.

What are the competencies needed to achieve these tasks?

The domain of environmental health interest is very broad, potentially requiring practical knowledge of principles underlying food, water, air and soil quality, waste disposal, drugs and poisons, vector control, communicable diseases, health promotion, healthy cities and municipal health planning, disaster planning, preparedness and response, and (increasingly) ecosystem health.

Necessary competencies may include communication, advocacy, policy, and planning together with an understanding of epidemiology, toxicology, microbiology, and a range of other biological, physical, and social sciences—or at least an ability to recognize when additional specialist input is needed.

Who are the other people that might need to be involved?

In conjunction with the breadth of inputs mentioned above, efforts to protect public health from environmental threats require engagement with community groups and many government and non-government sectors other than health. Development of a shared understanding with such partners is a key strategy—for example in injury prevention by altering the physical environment through town planning measures, or in minimizing exposure to air pollutants from vehicle emissions.

Potential pitfalls

Epidemiological studies of adverse health outcomes from environmental exposures can be a weak link in health risk assessments, with inadequate measures of exposure a common failing. Other problems may include lag times between exposures and potential health effects. In addition, health effects may be poorly defined, and low-level effects may be very difficult to distinguish from 'background' incidences of common health problems. There may be groups within a population that are more susceptible to certain hazards, or more highly exposed (e.g. children), and to whom risk assessment assumptions do not apply. Compounding of risk by other exposures or possible synergism between co-pollutants may also lead to underestimates of risk.

Communities often call for a 'study' of their own health status when concerned about impacts from an existing exposure. However, epidemiological investigations in relation to environmental exposures should not be undertaken lightly. Many factors need to be considered in examining their feasibility.[10] Such studies are often inconclusive (particularly in small populations) and may even serve to delay implementation of satisfactory exposure reduction measures.

It is often more appropriate to carry out thorough exposure assessment and rely on pre-existing information (e.g. dose–response data of a known toxicant, environmental guidelines) to help interpret the exposure data.

Lessons from success and failure

Successful public health practice is usually invisible, while failures often attract attention.

(a) Successes

Globally there are many examples of benefit from activities under the auspices of the World Health Organization's Healthy Cities programme, and Local Agenda 21. Consider the local action to create shade protection against UV light exposure (Box 4.4.3).

Another success involved the management of contamination of a dietary supplement. The powerful linkage of epidemiology with

---

Box 4.4.3 **Creating shade: a case study**

A high mortality rate from skin cancer (particularly malignant melanoma), arising from excessive exposure to sunlight and UV radiation, is a major public health issue in Australia. Extensive promotional efforts have led to high public awareness but have not been sufficiently effective in encouraging people to adopt 'sunsmart' behaviours.

More sustainable approaches combine individual and community responsibility through interventions such as the creation of shade—however there is no legislative mandate regarding provision of shade.

Local governments are very well placed to implement shade creation policies, but at this stage only some have adopted such policies. Research into barriers and facilitative factors combined with shade audits in local government areas demonstrated the following 'critical success' factors:

- support from elected council members

- quarantined funding for provision of natural and manufactured shade

- appointment of an officer to facilitate actions emanating from the shade creation policy whilst maintaining links with staff in all local government departments (including planning, engineering, parks and gardens, finance, executive officers, and environmental health)

- transferring responsibility for shade creation to other parties, for example by including shade provision as a condition of approval of development applications for facilities to be used by the public

- active inclusion of community members and groups in development, adoption, and implementation phases of the policy.

(Adapted from The National Environmental Health Strategy, enHealth Council of Australia, 1999.
www.health.gov.au/pubhlth/publicat/document/metadata/envstrat.htm
(accessed 14 September 2000).)

laboratory, surveillance, and communications systems rapidly identified the cause of a food-borne disease and then achieved its removal.[11]

(b) Failures

Construction of dams to increase certainty of water supply for irrigation-based agriculture has been a widespread practice resulting in short-term economic gain but sometimes highly adverse long-term social and ecological consequences.[12]

Industrial accidents such as the disastrous methyl isocyanate leak at Bhopal in 1984 highlight the potential for risks to be compounded in many developing countries, with fewer environmental controls, planning, and safety measures.

Human conflicts continue to occur with the potential to create major environmental health threats for populations through dislocation, loss of basic public health infrastructure, bioterrorism activities, and ecosystem destruction.

Failure to consider the principles of ESD remains common in public health practice, as well as in health care itself. The Australian Hospital Association and Environment Protection Agency, for example, developed a green health care project—but were unable to achieve satisfactory levels of participation.[13] The Centre for Greening the National Health Service has been more successful, playing a central part in the development of guidelines about sustainability for health care organizations.[14] Nevertheless, the rising costs of waste disposal have probably been more important than the action of a pressure group in alerting managers to the need to consider the challenges of sustainability more actively.

Key determinants of success

In acute situations where environmental exposures clearly threaten health, adequate legislation and emergency powers to support public health interventions may be essential to ensure that exposures are abated as soon as possible.

Risk assessment and management practices need to be sound and accountable.

Empowerment of local authorities and communities to integrate environment, health,and sustainable development in local strategies is fundamental to the creation of healthy environments.[15]

How will you know if you have been successful?

+ reduced exposure to a hazard (usually easier to measure than health outcomes)

+ 'process' measures such as improvements in policy or community satisfaction with the process of risk assessment and management

• reduced morbidity or mortality associated with the exposure, when health surveillance/epidemiological methods allow.

Further resources

Bassett WH (1992). *Clay's handbook of environmental health*, (16th edn.). Chapman and Hall, London.

Beck U (1992). *Risk society*. Sage, London.

Harr J (1996). *A civil action*. Vintage Press, New York. (A courtroom drama that shows the difficulties of establishing environmental causation of disease—and of obtaining justice. For related materials, see cyber.law. harvard.edu/acivilaction/ (accessed 25 August 2000).)

Jackson MH (1989). *Environmental health reference book*. Butterworth, London.

The President's Council on Sustainable Development (1999). *Towards a sustainable America: advancing prosperity, opportunity, and a healthy environment for the 21st century*. PCSD, Washington DC.

References

1. McMichael AJ (1993). *Planetary overload: global environmental change and the health of the human species*. Cambridge University Press, Cambridge.

2. Moeller DW (1992). *Environmental health*. Harvard University Press, Cambridge MA.

3. World Health Organization (1993). *Health, environment and development: approaches to drafting country-level strategies for human well-being under Agenda 21*. World Health Organization, Geneva.

4. Armstrong BK, White E, and Saracci R (1994). *Exposure assessment in epidemiology*. Oxford University Press, Oxford.

5. McMichael AJ, Kjellstrom T, and Smith KR (2000). Environment and health. In *International Public Health*, (ed. M Merson, R Black, and A Mills). Aspen Press, Gaithersburg MD.

6. Aldrich T and Griffith J (1993). *Environmental epidemiology and risk assessment*. Van Nostrand Reinhold, New York.

7. enHealth Council. *Environmental health risk assessment*. Department of Health and Aged Care, Australia. www.health.gov.au/pubhlth/strateg/envhlth/risk/ (accessed 25 August 2000).

8. Briggs D, Corvalan C, and Nurminen M (ed.) (1996). *Linkage methods for environment and health analysis*. WHO; Office of Global and Integrated Environmental Health, Geneva.

9. National Research Council (1983). *Risk assessment in the Federal Government: managing the process*. National Academy Press, Washington DC.

10. Agency for Toxic Substances and Disease Registry (April 1996). *Guidance for ATSDR Health Studies*. US Department of Health and Human Services. www.atsdr.cdc.gov/HS/gd1.html (accessed 25 August 2000).

11. Taylor R and McNeil J (1993). Eosinophilia-myalgia syndrome: lessons for public health researchers. *Med J Aust*, **158**, 51–5

12. Brewster D (1999). Environmental management for vector control. Is it worth a dam if it worsens malaria? *BMJ*, **319**, 651–2.

13. Australian Hospital Association (1996). *Green health care. Environmental assessment manual*. AHA, Canberra.

14. Gray M and Keeble B (1989). Greening the NHS. *BMJ*, **299**, 4–5.

15. Environmental Health Commission (1997). *Agendas for change*. Chadwick House Group. Chartered Institute of Environmental Health, London.

We do not inherit the earth from our ancestors, we borrow it from our children.

4.5 **Protecting and promoting health in the workplace**

TC Aw, Malcolm Harrington, and
Stuart Whitaker

Objectives

By reading this chapter you will:

- become familiar with the major causes of occupational ill-health
- develop a systematic approach for dealing with occupational and environmental health concerns in the workplace
- know who to approach for further assistance, information, and guidance on occupational health and safety issues.

Definition

Occupational health is about managing the health of people at work.
This process encompasses four dimensions:

- exposures in the workplace that cause or contribute to occupational disease and workplace injury
- chronic illness, disability, or predisposing factors that may be exacerbated by workplace exposures
- protection from risks to health for the local community, or those who may be adversely affected by the company's processes or operations
- the promotion of safe systems of work, and the promotion of healthy lifestyles through campaigns at the workplace.

Why is this an important public health issue?

The maintenance of optimum health for the economically active section of the population is an important public health issue, because ill health and injury in the working population reduces the effective contribution of the individual to his welfare, the family, the community, and the nation. Managing the health of the working population with a wide age range from 16 to 65 years or more will reduce the overall burden on the national health care system. The main health issues facing workforces today (following the effective control of exposures to many recognized occupational chemical hazards) are occupational musculo-skeletal disorders and psychosocial health problems in the workplace.

Subdividing this issue into defined tasks

There are three main ways in which health in the workplace can be approached:

(a) occupationally-related illness or injury

(b) workers with pre-existing illnesses or disability

(c) promoting general health in the workplace.

Taking each of these three methods in turn:

(a) Occupationally-related illness or injury

For occupationally-related illness or injury, there are six main tasks:

1. Identifying hazards at the work setting (hazard identification)

2. Determining the population exposed to such hazards

3. Assessing the risks from exposure to the hazards (risk assessment)

4. Taking appropriate preventive action by one or more of the following actions to reduce those risks:

   • elimination, substitution, or containment of the hazards

   • limiting numbers of workers exposed

   • reducing the time each person is required at specific areas where hazards are not easily eliminated.

   • providing personal protective equipment, as a last resort

5. Audit and reassess the efficacy of the preventive measures

6. Consider the need for a suitable health surveillance programme or periodic monitoring system for the workforce.

(b) Workers with pre-existing illnesses or disability

For workers with pre-existing illnesses or disability, the four main tasks involved are:

1. Identification of relevant risk factors e.g. atopy, previous asthma, or previous history of several episodes of low back pain, so that suitable advice, job placement, and work modification can be considered.

2. Assessment of job duties.

3. Pre-placement assessment and advice.

4. Health surveillance, including periodic review of health status and sickness absence record.

For some occupational groups e.g. health care workers, specific tasks include checking the immune status and providing immunization as required. An example of this is the Hepatitis B immune status for health care workers.

Furthermore, the quality of working life, which is the subject of national government and European Union attention, is partly determined by the degree to which workplace risks are controlled, how well the workforce perceive themselves to be valued, and how healthy their workplace is. Other factors such as job security, opportunities for advancement, and social contact are also important.

(c) Promoting general health in the workplace

There two main tasks involved in health promotion at the workplace.

1. *Specific*: suitable and sufficient information, instruction, and training in working safely should be provided where there are recognized hazards at the workplace.

2. *General*: issues should be identified that relate to healthy lifestyles. Workplace advice and information should be actively provided on alcohol intake, smoking, diet, exercise, safe driving, and precautions in the course of working elsewhere e.g. travelling abroad on work duties.

The workplace, along with other settings such as the school, the home, and the local community, is an important setting in which to deliver health education and promotion. The workplace has a number of unique features which can be used to support health promotion activities. Health promotion initiatives in the workplace can be underpinned by organizational change, such as changing the food provided in the works canteen, establishing a no-smoking policy or by providing subsidized membership of sports facilities. The workplace also offers good opportunities for establishing peer support; such initiatives can be targeted towards those who are most at risk.

The workplace offers a good setting in which to carry out health promotion, as it affords ready access to a population which is often difficult to reach by other means. The workplace can provide an opportunity for long-term involvement with a well-defined population and can be used as a venue to offer support during periods of change. Employers are generally supportive of initiatives, which the staff perceive to be in their best interests; some employers may believe that health promotion may help them to reduce economic losses through the reduction of sickness absence or increased productivity.

There can be potential disadvantages to workplace health promotion. The main problem to be aware of is the risk that attention and resources may be diverted away from ensuring that potentially more serious occupational health and safety risks are properly assessed and controlled.

What are the tasks needed to achieve effective change?

In order to minimize the risk to health at work from particular hazards, ensure the following steps are addressed:

- identify the (potential) problem (adverse health outcome or excessive exposure to a hazard)
- communicate these concerns to management and workforce representatives

- get commitment at the highest level to rectify the problem
- identify skills needed to undertake the tasks
- ensure that individuals involved are clear about what needs to be done, and their role in the process
- undertake the appropriate tasks outlined above
- review and evaluate success or failure. '

Who are the other people that might need to be involved?

While the occupational physician or public health physician may have a major interest and be given a lead role in promoting health in the workplace, other groups of professionals will often need to be involved:

- management at all levels, as they ultimately have the responsibility for managing occupational health issues and, in practical terms, control the access to resources. Occupational health professionals are their advisers
- the workforce and their representatives, as the measures proposed will affect them. Worker co-operation and participation is essential for the measures to succeed
- occupational hygienists—experts in assessment of exposure to workplace hazards
- occupational psychologists and sociologists
- occupational health nurses
- health promotion personnel
- toxicologists
- epidemiologists.

In order to engage the workforce with the actions being taken to protect and promote their health, it is important to understand that genuine teamwork is crucial. Publicity through in-house newsletters, seminars, and even effective use of media are crucial elements of creating effective change. Above all, the workforce must be not only informed but actively engaged in the whole process where appropriate.

Potential pitfalls

The four key areas where occupational health analysis and action can founder are:

1. Misinterpretation of motives for action by either management or workforce.
2. Misguided and ill-informed media coverage.
3. Inappropriate risk perception.
4. Inappropriate or inaccurate health belief models.

Guard against all of these at the earliest opportunity.

Fallacies in occupational health

Fallacy 1: The data are abundant

Due to lack of awareness and access to reliable data, public health practitioners may not appreciate the extent to which the health of the working population may be adversely affected by occupational hazards.

Fallacy 2: If there are no data, exhortation will be sufficient

Until accurate data on the incidence and prevalence of work-related conditions become available, it may be difficult to impress upon the public, employers, and government the extent of any problem.

Fallacy 3: Most clinicians are well trained in occupational health

Training in occupational medicine and occupational health in medical and nursing schools is limited. Consequently, medical and nursing professionals often have only a very general understanding of what can be done to prevent ill-health and injury at the workplace.

Examples of occupational health incidents

Bhopal disaster—where workplace problem caused acute and chronic health effects among the workforce and surrounding community. Chemical agent involved: methyl isocyanate.

Chernobyl —where effects from an out-of-control 'industrial process'—partly related to operator fatigue, became a major public health problem (occupational and environmental). Agent involved: radioactive materials.

Dibromochloropropane (DBCP) problem —questions on male infertility and inability to start a family amongst workforce led to occupational and industry-wide epidemiological investigation that resulted in cessation of manufacture of DBCP for use as a pesticide.

Gynaecomastia in pharmaceutical company —led to investigations showing that for some potent biologically-active workplace materials, the level of containment to prevent health effects may need to be greatly increased. Agent involved: estrogenic compounds.

Asbestos —pulmonary fibrosis, bronchogenic carcinoma, and pleural and peritoneal mesothelioma in those exposed to asbestos fibres. The risk of lung cancer for asbestos exposure was noted to be multiplied where there was concomitant cigarette smoking. Similar health effects occurred from secondary exposure of wives who had to clean the asbestos-contaminated overalls of these workers.

Vinyl chloride —four cases of a very rare malignancy—angiosarcoma of the liver—were described at a tyre factory amongst workers responsible for cleaning polymerization chambers for PVC manufacture. Prompt preventive action led to rapid reduction in worker exposure to the chemical agent—vinyl chloride monomer. This is a gas which is polymerized to form the relatively inert and non-toxic polyvinyl chloride (PVC). Corroborative animal evidence of similar tumours in rodents came to light at about the same time.

Four important lessons

1. Prompt public health action may be needed even if not all of the desired information is available. Don't let the desire for perfection hinder the need for pragmatism.

2. Clusters of a *rare* illness (mesothelioma, angiosarcoma) are often easier to identify as resulting from an occupational exposure than more common diseases such as lung cancer.

3. Effects on workforce, wider community, and the environment can result from workplace hazards.

4. Public health vigilance and clinical case reports can both lead to identification of health hazards at the workplace.

Predictors of success and failure

Success

- a good quality team of occupational and public health professionals can identify problems early in order to initiate preventive action

- a sympathetic and supportive management and workforce aids this process.

Failure

- ensure that health promotion in the workplace is not done at the expense of control of workplace hazards

- a multi-disciplinary approach will not work if co-ordination of activities is poor and there is a lack of understanding of the roles of each team member

- an over-reliance on the medical model may prove to be ineffective in addressing the problems encountered at the workplace. Identification of cases, correct diagnosis, treatment, and reporting procedures, important though those activities are, will do little to prevent further cases from occurring unless risks to health can be communicated effectively to the public, politicians, decision-makers, employers, and employees. All of these groups have a part to play in ensuring that effective action is taken to prevent exposure to hazardous working conditions.

How will you know if you have been successful?

To check how successful you are being, assess the following five criteria:

1. Reduction in the incidence and prevalence of occupational ill-health and injury.

2. Reduction of risk or frequency of hazardous exposures.

3. Improved knowledge of risks and awareness by the working population.

4. Positive changes in behaviour and attitudes towards occupational risks by the working population.

5. No inappropriately adverse publicity by the media.

Further resources

Adams P, Baxter PA, Aw TC, Cockcroft A, and Harrington JM (ed.) (2000). *Hunter's diseases of occupations*, (9th edn). Edward Arnold, London.

American Conference of Governmental Industrial Hygienists, Inc. www.acgih.org/ (accessed 10 September 2000).

American Journal of Industrial Medicine.

Cox RAF, Edwards FC, and McCallum RJ (ed.) (1995). *Fitness for work: the medical aspects*, (2nd edn). Oxford Medical Publications, Oxford.

Databases (available on CD-ROM):
  TOMES (Toxicology, Occupational Medicine and Environmental Science).
  HSELINE (Health and Safety Executive, UK).
  NIOSHTIC (National Institute for Occupational Safety and Health, USA).
  CISDOC (International Labour Office, Geneva).

Faculty of Occupational Medicine, UK, www.facoccmed.ac.uk/ (accessed 10 September 2000).

Finnish Institute of Occupational Health, www.occuphealth.fi/e/ (accessed 10 September 2000).

Hansson SO (1998). *Setting the limit: occupational health standards and the limits of science*. Oxford University Press, Oxford.

Harrington JM, Gill FS, Aw TC, and Gardiner K (1998). *Pocket consultant on occupational health*, (4th edn). Blackwell Science, Oxford.

Health and Safety Executive, UK. www.open.gov.uk/hse/hsehome.htm (accessed 10 September 2000).

Institute of Occupational Health, Birmingham, UK. www.bham.ac.uk/ioh (accessed 10 September 2000).

Occupational and Environmental Medicine.

Sadhra SS and Rampal KG (ed.) (1999). *Occupational health: risk assessment and management*. Blackwell Science, Oxford.

Scandinavian Journal of Work, Environment and Health.

University of Edinburgh. www.med.ed.ac.uk/hew (accessed 10 September 2000).

4.6 'Hard to reach' populations

Julia Carr, Don Matheson, and
David Tipene-Leach

Objectives

After reading this chapter you will:

- think carefully before using the term 'hard to reach'
- understand the relevance of the structural determinants of personal and public health
- be sensitive to the gap between the rhetoric about the charters relating to health promotion and the reality of day-to-day public health practice
- understand the difference between health promotion and health education
- understand which responses are likely to be effective in improving the health status of marginalized populations and which approaches are likely to perpetuate inequalities in health status.

Definition

When the health status of populations most affected by inequity and alienation fails to improve despite the efforts of conventional public health approaches, these groups are deemed 'hard to reach'. The term is generally applied to those marginalized by poverty, ethnicity, geography, and different cultural or behavioural norms (like IV drug use or sexual orientation).

Why is this issue important?

By using terms such as 'hard to reach', dominant groups subtly reinforce a political system that denies certain groups or individuals access to wealth, opportunities, health care, and knowledge.[1] While the term 'hard to reach' reflects historical reality (that many public health programmes have had little impact on the populations with the lowest health status), there is a strong sense that their poor health outcomes are somehow a problem of their own making, a result of barriers erected between themselves and the expertise that could 'deliver' better health. It is important to use language consistent with public health's commitment to social justice; language that speaks of the reciprocity and interdependence which characterize community;[2] to replace terms that reflect a 'deficit' model with terms that reflect health as a right.

The framework in which health is understood influences the actions taken. If we focus on the context of people's lives, on issues such as power, dominance, dispossession, paternalism, racism, and their implication for how diseases are created, distributed, and treated, this leads to a different approach than a framework that perceives health as a privilege or as an individual responsibility.[3]

The idea that poor health is generally the result of 'unhealthy' choices leads to the 'educational' approaches seen so commonly. The belief behind the activity is that you can improve health by marketing a certain way of living. Extra attention and innovative methods are 'targeted' at certain social groups and, while social determinants of health are acknowledged, the focus is on lifestyle 'choices'—diet, smoking, and exercise.

Conceptualizing health as a right and 'Health for All' as a collective responsibility leads to a different set of responses. The WHO model of health promotion of the early 1980s emerged from increasing recognition that health education in isolation from other measures would not result in the radical changes necessary to achieve improvements in health.

The Ottawa Charter for Health Promotion[4] is perhaps the best known expression of this broader approach and it is a much-quoted document. Unfortunately the gap between the rhetoric and everyday health sector activity is a reality that remains a challenge for all public health practitioners.

What's the difference?

The Ottawa Charter emphasizes that health promotion works through concrete and effective community action in setting priorities, making decisions, planning strategies and implementing them in order to achieve better health. At the heart of this process is the empowerment of communities, their ownership and control of their own destinies.

Endorsing this implies at the very least:

- acknowledging inequalities in power, ownership, and control and vested interests in maintaining inequalities
- challenging professional control of health promotion
- validating and supporting community health initiatives that are seeking to transform the distribution of power, ownership, and control.[5]

What are the approaches to a programme of work and the tasks involved?

While there is no single method for putting the Ottawa Charter into action, the community development approach is consistent with the principles and has been tested in many environments. Community development as a public health practice has been defined as 'the process of organising and/or supporting community groups in identifying their health issues, planning and acting upon their strategies for social action/change and gaining increased self-reliance and decision making power as a result of their activities'.[6]

There are many examples of such community development projects. See chapter 4.1 on community action or, for a detailed theoretical discussion and practical list of recommended procedures, using a New Zealand example, see Voyle and Simmons.[7]

What are the pitfalls of a community development approach?

Community empowerment challenges the concepts of expertise and professionalism that are now dominant. It also runs counter to the structures and time-frames for decision making of most public bureaucracies. It takes a long-term view of health gain and does not fit neatly with single-issue programmes. Nor does it sit well with contracts that tightly specify service outputs.

Given the difficulty of addressing disparities in health status between privileged and deprived groups, many public health practitioners retreat to a reductionist, problem-based approach. However, this limited view of the possibilities for practice is not ethically sound. Health improvement comes from addressing structural root causes of ill health, rather than a targeted, narrowly-defined intervention.[3] In tackling single issues by interventions that will give a desirable short-term outcome, it is important to be aware that there may be longer-term adverse outcomes, such as increased dependency on public services. For example, a study in 1991 revealed that only 33% of poor children surveyed in an area were fully immunized and another study reported that, by linking immunization with a Federal food subsidy programme (offering free vaccinations at the welfare offices and giving only one month of food vouchers instead of three), immunization rates rose from 56% to 89%. Because of this it was suggested that 'Now all we have to do is replicate this program across the US and we can raise immunisation rates among the vast majority of poor US children'. However, the longer-term effects of such a policy might be to further stigmatize and isolate this group.[8]

On the other hand, there is evidence that certain interventions, such as providing smoking cessation programmes to pregnant women or promoting the use of fluoride, can indeed reduce inequalities in particular health outcomes.[10] Such improvements, however, are unlikely to be sustained, unless the intervention has been developed in partnership with the community, with shared decision making and the potential to follow local rather than imposed priorities.

Examples of success and failure

Two striking examples of the effectiveness of different approaches are provided by steps taken to address sudden infant death syndrome

(SIDS) in New Zealand and the approach adopted to control the spread of HIV/AIDS.

SIDS in New Zealand

In the early 1980s, New Zealand had a higher rate of SIDS (Sudden Infant Death Syndrome) than comparable countries, with a particularly high rate among the indigenous Maori population. SIDS, by its tragically and uniquely quantifiable outcome, has provided an unprecedented opportunity to observe how Maori health outcomes are influenced by the strategic approach taken. By 1991, there was published evidence that SIDS was a multiple risk factor syndrome with three significant 'modifiable' risk factors—prone sleeping position, lack of breast-feeding, and maternal cigarette smoking. Other significant risk factors, like low socio-economic status, young motherhood, young maternal school leaving age, low birth weight, prematurity, and admission to neonatal intensive care, were not postulated to be modifiable.[11]

This conceptual dichotomy led to the development in 1991 of a national SIDS prevention campaign, comprised of intensive publicity about the three risk factors. Subsequent SIDS prevention activities were based around a minimal intervention, risk reduction approach that provided simple health information, relying on individual change of behaviour without any form of personal or community support.

Between 1988 and 1992, national SIDS mortality fell by 48% (from 4.4/1000 live births to 2.3/1000). Maori SIDS rates were twice as high and, during the same period, a more modest fall of 24% was observed (from 9.1/1000 to 6.9/1000).[12]

Although Maori mothers readily adopted the 'easy to do' prone-sleeping position for their babies, the impersonal 'educational' approach did not foster a commitment among Maori women or communities to deal with the 'difficult' risk factor: cigarette smoking. There was no Maori strategy and no specific funding to address Maori health needs.

In 1994, after considerable advocacy by Maori public health professionals, the Maori SIDS prevention programme was launched, based on:

- information sharing and consultation in Maori communities, particularly with influential women elders
- consistently utilizing Maori protocols
- promotional messages couched within a Maori world view
- development of resources for smoking cessation and breast-feeding promotion that Maori women 'owned'
- identification of disempowering factors in the lives of Maori mothers and work with communities for change
- attempts to induce structural change within maternal and child health care to provide accessible and acceptable services.

Although it has taken five years to achieve, this broad-based community development approach to health promotion has seen the Maori SIDS rate fall to half the 1994 rate.[13]

Example of a community development approach: HIV/AIDS in New Zealand

The response of the gay community to HIV/AIDS and the AIDS campaign in New Zealand illustrates many aspects of the Ottawa Charter in action. The AIDS campaign has been effective in limiting the spread of HIV/AIDS in gay men, and extensive spread into other groups has not occurred.

The initial response to news of the AIDS epidemic was through informal networking, information, and counselling service provision within the gay community itself. It is not possible to detail the complexity of the developments over the early 1980s, but key points are:

- recognition of the potential health problem came from within the group most 'at risk' and leadership came from within that community
- capacity-building started early, with significant mobilization of the gay community and organization-building
- partnerships with key people in the health sector and influential people outside the gay community were developed to assist in meeting the demands of the corporate health sector and political environment
- affected communities gained representation at government advisory level—the original Council included two people with HIV infection and representatives of gay, sex worker, intravenous drug user, Maori, and Pacific communities
- a multi-level approach was adopted.

In addition to publicity and promotion of safe sex practices, the AIDS prevention campaign included actions as diverse as:

- establishment of a needle-exchange scheme
- a human rights campaign to include sexual orientation and HIV status in the Human Rights Commission Act
- the HERO project, a direct attempt (beginning with a dance party) to strengthen the gay community's identification with and involvement in the epidemic, and raise the profile of the issues in the wider community.[14]

This multi-faceted, participatory strategy has been effective in limiting the spread of HIV in New Zealand.

Alternative approaches

Some of the most effective interventions may be at a structural or environmental level. For example, adolescent smoking may be decreased by mechanisms such as legislation limiting retail practices, taxation policy, and advertising bans. Fluoridation of water supplies to improve dental health is a classic 'environmental' approach; road engineering changes in response to accidents, another. With 'upstream' interventions, input from affected communities is still valuable in providing opportunity for insights that might otherwise be missed.

What are the competencies needed to achieve health gains in marginalized groups?

This chapter has attempted to illustrate that 'hard to reach' groups are a construct of a 'top-down' public health perspective that fails to acknowledge the historical, social, and economic forces that have denied certain sectors of society the choices available to others.

As public health workers, we can be part of the problem or part of the solution. Taking an issue-by-issue approach to population health without addressing disparities between population groups, and supporting 'quick-fix' solutions without questioning the context in which health problems are generated contributes to the perpetuation of inequality.

We can contribute by:

- legitimizing and promoting approaches that are rooted in community health action
- stimulating debate about the structural barriers to achieving health for all
- monitoring the gap between rhetoric and reality
- challenging the monopolization of health promotion by health professionals
- constantly raising and setting up mechanisms for participation by marginalized people in decision making.

A key role for public health professionals is to influence the distribution of health resources. There is a variety of mechanisms for matching resources to need both at a population level (through population-based funding formulae that include variables such as deprivation indices, ethnicity, etc.) and at provider level (see chapter 6.7).

Organizational development to achieve health gains in marginalized groups

How do decisions about existing or new resources (including funding, personnel, 'pilots', research grants) reflect the needs of 'hard to reach' groups within your agency? Marginalized communities often express amusement at being labelled 'hard to reach' when, in their experience, they are 'locked out' (either in the literal sense or by the barriers created by corporate culture) of meaningful participation in these kinds of decisions. The 'micro-equity' decisions about resource allocation within agencies (and who makes them) can be as influential as the macro-equity resource allocation policies. It is essential to review the way in which the public health agency works—its culture and systems—as well as developing the competencies of individual practitioners.

Developing partnerships

Day-to-day public health activity with communities usually involves some form of partnership. Partnerships inevitably raise issues of power and control.[15] It is helpful to be clear about the type of partnership you are intending. Shared expectations are a constructive starting point.

Three important types of community partnerships:

◆ *community action partnerships* in which the partnership forms to address a specific issue or pursue a specific opportunity

◆ *community organization partnerships* in which a set of organizations in a similar service sector agree to collaborate for mutually agreed goals

◆ *community development partnerships,* in which a partnership attempts to increase participation by people and organizations in collaborative activities on multiple fronts or contribute to community assets and services in multiple areas.[16]

What are the key determinants of success in working with marginalized communities?

There are some important features that are associated with success in working with marginalized groups of people:

◆ good analysis of the 'problem' and whose problem it is—this means having time to think about and debate the issues both before and whilst working with the community

◆ open-ended meetings with communities to determine what their priorities are and how the public health perspective fits or does not fit with these

◆ development of partnership and sharing of knowledge and research

◆ participation and ownership by the community

◆ capacity-building within the community and support for locally-generated solutions—information, funding, training, people resources, evaluation tools

◆ ongoing communication in an atmosphere that supports critical analysis, honesty, and flexibility.

Although these points look self-evident, in practice it takes patience and a high level of commitment. The temptation is to submit to pressures to adopt faster methods.

Many communities have a legacy of mistrust based on historical experience of health agencies or state institutions and this has to be overcome. Failure of the contemporary health system to meet immediate curative needs may lead to scepticism about initiatives in other areas or a lack of willingness to engage.

Lay knowledge is often not valued by health professionals. These attitudes are readily internalized by communities themselves so that they may appear reluctant to make suggestions or take leadership roles initially. Such challenges are common and it is wise to identify mentors or experienced people from the communities involved to provide supervision and support.

How will you know when/if you are successful?

The community will be owning and driving a strategy and will have the information, confidence, and resources to implement it. The institutions of power will feel challenged and those within them may be making themselves hard to reach.

Further resources

Carr-Hill R, Sheldon T, Smith P, *et al.* (1994). Allocating resources to health authorities: development of method for small area analysis of use of inpatient services. *BMJ*, **309**, 1046–9.

Sanders D and Carver R (1985). *The struggle for health. Medicine and politics of underdevelopment*. Macmillan, London.

Smith P, Sheldon TA, Carr Hill RA, Hardman G, Martin S, and Peacock S (1994). Allocating resources to health authorities: results and policy implications of small area analysis of use of inpatient services. *BMJ*, **309**, 1050–4.

References

1. LeBlanc R (1997). Definitions of oppression. *Nurs Inq*, **4**, 257–61.
2. Robertson A (1998). Critical reflections on the politics of need: implications for public health. *Soc Sci Med*, **47**, 1419–30.
3. Adams L and Pintus S (1994). A challenge to prevailing theory and practice. *Critical Public Health*, **5**, 17–29.
4. World Health Organization (1986). Ottawa Charter for Health Promotion. WHO, Geneva.
5. Farrant W (1994). Addressing the contradictions: health promotion and community health action in the United Kingdom. *Critical Public Health*, **5**, 5–17.
6. Labonte R (1993). Community development and partnerships. *Canadian J Public Health*, **84**, 237–40.
7. Voyle J and Simmons D (1999). Community development through partnership: promoting health in an urban indigenous community in New Zealand. *Soc Sci Med*, **49**, 1035–50.

8. Wood D (1999). *Evidence-based Healthcare*, 3, 93–4. Commentary on: Hoekstra E, LeBaron CW, Megaloeconomou Y, Guerrero H, Byers C, Johnson-Partlow T, Lyons B, Mihalek E, *et al.* (1998). Impact of large-scale immunisation initiative in the special supplemental nutrition program for women, infants and children. *JAMA*, **280**, 1143–7.

9. Mayer ML, Clark SJ, Konrad TR, Freeman, VA, and Slifkin RT (1999). The role of state policies and programs in buffering the effects of poverty on children's immunization receipt. *Am J Public Health*, **89**, 164–70.

10. Arblaster L, Lambert M, Entwistle V, Foster M, Fullerton D, *et al.* (1996). A systematic review of the effectiveness of health service interventions aimed at reducing inequalities in health. *J Health Serv Res Policy*, **1**, 93–103.

11. Mitchell E, Scragg R, Stewart A, Becroft D, Hassal I, *et al.* (1991). Results from the first year of the New Zealand Cot Death Study. *NZ Med J*, **104**, 71–6.

12. New Zealand Health Information Service (1993). Ministry of Health, Wellington.

13. Te Puni Kokiri (2000). Progress towards closing social and economic gaps between Maori and non-Maori. Te Puni Kokiri, Wellington.

14. Lindberg W and McMorland J (1996). From grassroots to business suits: the gay community response to AIDS. In *Intimate details and vital statistics. Aids, sexuality and the social order in New Zealand*, (ed. Peter Davis). Auckland University Press, Auckland.

15. Popay J and Williams G (1998). Partnership in health: beyond the rhetoric. *J Epidemiol Community Health*, **52**, 410–1.

16. Gamm L (1998). Advancing community health through community health partnerships. *J Healthcare Management*, **43**, 51–67.

4.7 Screening

Alexandra Barratt, Les Irwig, Paul Glasziou,
Robert Cumming, Angela Raffle, Nicholas Hicks,
and Gordon Guyatt

Objectives

After reading this chapter you should be better able to:

- review evidence about a screening programme
- apply criteria about when screening is worthwhile.

Introduction

Early detection and intervention is an instinctively attractive idea. Consequently many screening tests have been developed. These include Pap tests (for cervical cancer), mammography (for breast cancer), faecal occult blood tests (for colorectal cancer), Guthrie test (for phenylketonuria in neonates), blood tests (for high cholesterol), and blood pressure checks, to list only a few.[1,2]

Screening has the potential to provide important and long-lasting benefits. However there is also potential for harm and therefore a thorough understanding of the issues involved in screening is important for good public health practice.

'Some screening programmes can help; all screening programmes can harm.'

Box 4.7.1 gives one definition of screening. There are many others.[3,4,5]

Box 4.7.1

Screening is the systematic application of a test or inquiry, to identify individuals at sufficient risk of a specific disorder to benefit from further investigation or direct preventive action, among persons who have not sought medical attention on account of symptoms of that disorder.[6]

- Screening is undergone by well people, without symptoms of the target disorder

  Because people who are screened are, by definition, free of symptoms, there is the possibility that screening may, inadvertently, reduce the health of participants. It is important to have good quality evidence about the benefits of screening and to make sure that participants understand the possible consequences of being screened.

• Screening tests generally do not provide a definitive diagnosis

Also by definition, screening tests just indicate a high or low probability of the target disorder. Subsequent tests are used to establish or rule out the disorder. Inevitably, some people will be misclassified by the screening test. People with positive screening tests but normal subsequent tests are described as having false positive screening test results. People with negative (normal) screening tests but who do have the target disorder are described as having false negative screening test results (see Table 4.7.1). The column headed 'Disease or risk factor present' is subdivided. This is because some screening programmes identify diseases or risk factors in some people, only a proportion of whom go on to develop clinically important disease. An example is screening for cervical cancer, which involves detection of thousands of women with low grade cervical changes in order to avert one death from cervical cancer.

Table 4.7.1 Summary of benefits and harms of screening by underlying disease state.

	Reference standard results	
	Disease or risk factor present	**Disease or risk factor absent**
Screening test positive	a^0 True positives (significant disease) a^1 'True' positives (inconsequential disease)	b False positives
Screening test negative	c^0 False negatives (significant disease) c^1 'False' negatives (inconsequential disease)	d True negatives

Key:
a^0 disease or risk factor which will cause symptoms in the future (significant disease)
a^1 disease or risk factor asymptomatic until death (inconsequential disease)
b   false positives
c^0 missed disease which will be significant in the future
c^1 missed disease which will be inconsequential in the future
d   true negatives
Note: sensitivity = a/(a+c) and specificity = d/(b+d)
$a = a^0 + a^1$
$c = c^0 + c^1$

Deciding whether screening is worthwhile

Wilson and Jungner developed a set of criteria for deciding when screening is worthwhile in 1968.[3] Their careful consideration of the issues served public health well in the following decades. New criteria (shown in Box 4.7.2) update the Wilson and Jungner approach to assist policy makers to decide whether screening is worth offering as part of health care, and to aid individuals to make their own judgements about whether to participate in screening.

Box 4.7.2 **New criteria for deciding whether screening is worthwhile**

1. Is there randomized trial evidence that earlier intervention works?
2. Were the data identified, selected, and combined in an unbiased fashion?
3. What are the benefits?
4. What are the harms?
5. How do these compare in different people and with different screening strategies?
6. What is the impact of people's values and preferences?
7. What is the impact of uncertainty?
8. What is the cost-effectiveness?

(Reproduced with permission[7])

---

1. Is there randomized controlled trial evidence that earlier intervention works?

Unless the benefit is very large (as in, for example, screening for phenylketonuria), randomized controlled trials are needed to evaluate whether early detection and treatment is better than treatment given later (when the disease becomes symptomatic). Two designs can be used for this (see Figure 4.7.1). The trial may assess the entire screening process (early detection and early intervention, Figure 4.7.1(a)). Trials of mammography screening use this approach.[8,9] Alternatively the trial may assess only the effect of treatment in those who screen positive (Figure 4.7.1(b)). Trials of screening for high blood pressure and high cholesterol have used this design.[10,11] Both designs can provide valid information.

Randomized controlled trials are needed because observational studies may be affected by biases, such as lead time and length time bias, which can make early detection and intervention appear beneficial even if it is not. For example, if survival is measured from the date of diagnosis, disease that is detected earlier will appear to have better survival when in reality the earlier detection may only mean that people live with the diagnosis for longer (lead time bias). Slowly progressing disease is also more likely to be detected by screening than rapidly progressing disease (length time bias). Furthermore, people who volunteer to be screened are known to be

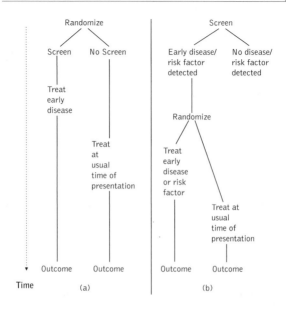

Figure 4.7.1 Designs for randomized trials of screening.
(Adapted with permission from Barratt *et al.* 1999.[7])

healthier and have better survival prospects than those who do not.
For a fuller discussion of these issues, see chapter 5 of *Clinical epidemiology: a basic science for clinical medicine.*[5]

2. Were the data identified, selected, and combined in an unbiased fashion?

The data from trials (if there is more than one trial) should be combined in a systematic review. Guidance is available on how to decide whether the systematic review is valid and useful.[12]

3. What are the benefits?

Ideally a point estimate of the benefit should be given. Benefits should be expressed as absolute risk reductions, as well as relative risk reductions, because the latter always appear more impressive and may be misleading.[13]

4. What are the harms?

Next you need some information about harms. These may be physical (such as the risk of bleeding, bowel perforation, or death from colonoscopy[14]) or psychological (such as the anxiety associated with

Table 4.7.2 Anticipated outcomes of ten years of biennial screening offered to 10,000 Australian women from 40 years of age.

	Total attributable to ten years of screening
No. of screens	50,000
No. of assessments (further imaging tests)	2,820
No. of biopsies	300
No. of invasive cancers	129
No. of DCIS[†]	28
No. of deaths prevented after 13 years	8.8 (95% CL -1.84, 19.3)

[†] Ductal carcinoma *in situ*
(Adapted from Irwig, *et al.*[17])

having an abnormal mammogram[15]). Benefits can be presented along with the harms in a 'balance sheet'[16] as in Table 4.7.2. It is clear from Table 4.7.2 that while many women undergoing screening mammography will 'test positive' (that is, will be given an abnormal screening report and recalled for more tests), few of these women actually have cancer. In the example shown in Table 4.7.2, 4.6% of women recalled for assessment because of an abnormal mammogram have invasive cancer. Harms will be greater if many people are found to have 'inconsequential' disease (see Table 4.7.1).

5. How do benefits and harms compare in different people and with different screening strategies?

Benefits of screening will be greater among people at higher risk of the target disorder. For example, people with existing heart disease will experience greater benefits from cholesterol screening than people at low risk of heart disease[18,19] and people aged 60–69 years are more likely to benefit from colorectal cancer screening than those aged 40–49 years.[20]

Benefits and harms will also vary according to the tests available and the cut-off points used. For example, a test which is more sensitive will pick up a greater proportion of the target disorder. This is a benefit if most of the additional cases detected are important; if the new test just picks up more cases of inconsequential disease then there will be little (if any) marginal benefit of the new test.[21] If a new test is more specific (results in fewer false positive results) then the harm of screening will be reduced.

6. What is the impact of people's values and preferences?

The benefits and harms of screening may be finely balanced so that whether there is a net benefit will depend on how the individual values the possible consequences of screening. For example, consider couples contemplating antenatal screening for Down syndrome.

Those who screen 'positive' may have an amniocentesis to provide a definitive result and there is about a 1% risk of miscarriage with amniocentesis. Some couples will want to be screened and will have a termination if the baby is affected. Some would like the advance warning of having a Down Syndrome child, even though they would not terminate the pregnancy. Others will refuse screening because they do not wish to know early, and they would not have a termination even if the baby is affected. Others will not want to be screened because of the risk that the follow-up tests might cause miscarriage. Clearly the value people place on the pregnancy, an unaffected child, and an affected child all influence whether couples will decide there is benefit for them in being screened.[22]

7. What is the impact of uncertainty?

There is much uncertainty in screening. Estimates of benefit have wide confidence intervals, because there are usually only a few trials, if any. Precise data on the frequency and severity of harms (especially psychological harms) may be difficult to find. It is important to acknowledge the uncertainty in the estimates when providing information to potential users of screening services.

8. What is the cost-effectiveness?

Generally screening is expensive because large numbers of people are involved and the costs can quickly mount up. Even if the initial screening test is cheap, the follow-up investigations are often relatively expensive. In order to achieve the same benefits as demonstrated in randomized trials, the screening programme must have similarly good facilities and services, which may be expensive to set up and maintain. Screening programmes may be highly cost-effective (for example screening young women for chlamydia trachomatis[23]) or may be very expensive (for example, the incremental cost of expanding mammographic screening to include women aged 40–49 years has been estimated at US$105,000 per life-year saved[24]). The society considering the screening programme must therefore consider the cost-effectiveness of screening relative to other health interventions which could be offered instead.[25]

Conclusion

High quality screening programmes have the potential to provide substantial health benefits to populations and individuals. However, because of the potential for harm as well as benefit, a decision to implement a screening programme needs to be based on strong evidence of benefit, usually from randomized trials.

Benefits and harms of screening programmes may be finely balanced so that individuals considering whether to be screened may make different, yet rational, choices depending on their own values and preferences. People are more likely to benefit from screening if they are at high risk of the target disorder, if they value the future highly, and if they are not bothered by the anxiety, discomfort, and costs associated with screening and follow-up tests. To make informed choices about screening programmes, people need evidence-based, balanced, and up-to-date information.

Further resources

Austoker J (1999). Gaining informed consent for screening. *BMJ*, **319**, 722–3.

Holland WW (1993). Screening: reasons to be cautious. *BMJ*, **306**, 1222–3.

Raffle AE (1997). Informed participation in screening is essential. *BMJ*, **314**, 1762–3.

UK National Screening Committee. www.doh.gov.uk/nsc/index.htm (accessed 5 February 2001).

References

1. US Preventive Services Task Force (1996). *Guide to clinical preventive services*, (2nd edn). Williams and Wilkins, Baltimore.

2. Canadian Task Force on the Periodic Health Examination. (1994). *Canadian guide to clinical preventive health care*. Canada Communication Group, Ottawa.

3. Wilson JMG and Jungner G (1968). *Principles and practice of screening for disease*. World Health Organization, Geneva.

4. Muir Gray JA (1997). *Evidence-based healthcare*. Churchill Livingstone, New York.

5. Sackett DL, Haynes RB, and Tugwell P (1991). *Clinical epidemiology: a basic science for clinical medicine*, (2nd edn). Little Brown and Co., Boston MA.

6. Wald NJ (1994). Guidance on terminology. *J Medical Screening*, **1**, 76.

7. Barratt A, Irwig L, Glasziou P, *et al.* (1999). Users' guides to the medical literature XVII: how to use guidelines and recommendations about screening. *JAMA*, **281**, 2029–34.

8. Andersson I, Aspegren K, Janzon L, *et al.* (1988). Mammographic screening and mortality from breast cancer: the Malmo mammographic screening trial. *BMJ*, **297**, 943–8.

9. Tabar L, Fagerberg G, Duffy S, *et al.* (1989). The Swedish two county trial of mammographic screening for breast cancer: recent results and calculation of benefit. *J Epidemiol Commun Health*, **43**, 107–14.

10. Multiple Risk Factor Intervention Trial Research Group (1982). Multiple Risk Factor Intervention Trial: risk factor changes and mortality results. *JAMA*, **248**, 1465–77.

11. Frick MH, Elo E, Haapa K, *et al.* (1987). Helsinki Heart Study: primary prevention trial with gemfibrizil in middle-aged men with dyslipidemia. *N Engl J Med*, **317**, 1237–45.

12. Oxman AD, Cook DJ, and Guyatt GH (1994). Users' guides to the medical literature VI: how to use an overview. *JAMA*, **272**, 1367–71.

13. Fahey T, Griffiths S, and Peters TJ (1995). Evidence based purchasing: understanding results of clinical trials and systematic reviews. *BMJ*, **311**, 1056–9.

14. Winawer SJ, Fletcher RH, Millar L, *et al.* (1997). Colorectal cancer screening: clinical guidelines and rationale. *Gastroenterology*, **112**, 594–642.

15. Lerman C, Trock B, Rimer BK, *et al.* (1991). Psychological side effects of breast cancer screening. *Health Psychology*, **10**, 259–67.

16. Eddy D (1996). Comparing benefits and harms: the balance sheet. In *Clinical decision making: from theory to practice: a collection of essays from the Journal of the American Medical Association*. Jones and Bartlett Publishers, Sudbury MA.

17. Irwig L, Glasziou P, Barratt A, and Salkeld G (1997). *Review of the evidence about the value of mammographic screening in 40–49 year old women*. NHMRC National Breast Cancer Centre, Sydney.

18. Khaw KT and Rose G (1989). Cholesterol screening programmes: how much potential benefit? *BMJ*, **299**, 606–7.

19. Davey Smith G, Song F, and Sheldon TA (1993). Cholesterol lowering and mortality: the importance of considering initial level of risk. *BMJ*, **306**, 1367–73.

20. Towler B, Irwig L, Glasziou P, *et al.* (1998). A systematic review of the effects of screening for colorectal cancer using the faecal occult blood test Hemoccult. *BMJ*, **317**, 559–65.

21. Raffle AE (1998). New tests in cervical screening. *Lancet*, **351**, 297.

22. Fletcher J, Hicks NR, Kay JDS, and Boyd PA (1995). Using decision analysis to compare policies for antenatal screening for Down's syndrome. *BMJ*, **311**, 351–6.

23. Howell MR, Quinn TC, and Gaydos CA (1998). Screening for chlamydia trachomatis in asymptomatic women attending family planning clinics. A cost-effectiveness analysis of three strategies. *Annals of Internal Medicine*, **128**, 277–84.

24. Salzmann P, Kerlikowske K, and Phillips K (1997). Cost-effectiveness of extending screening mammography guidelines to include women 40–49 years of age. *Annals of Internal Medicine*, **127**, 955–65.

25. Baum M (1995). Screening for breast cancer, time to think—and stop? *Lancet*, **346**, 436.

4.8 **Managing a communicable disease outbreak**

Fraser Hadden and Sarah O'Brien

Objectives

After reading this chapter you will:

* understand the principle of outbreak management
* be able to develop a framework for your own practice and that of your department.

What is an outbreak?

An outbreak is two or more cases of illness thought to be linked in time and place. This contrasts with an epidemic, where disease incidence exceeds that expected for the time and place—a single case of, say, malaria originating in the UK would thus represent an epidemic but not an outbreak.

Last defines an outbreak as 'an epidemic limited to localised increase in the incidence of a disease'.[1]

Outbreaks may be acute e.g. where many cases of food poisoning arise a day or two after a major gathering, or chronic e.g. detailed laboratory reports revealing escalating numbers of an unusual organism. Although the former appears more dramatic, the latter poses the greater threat to public health, as awareness has dawned late; there is no immediate indication as to the source of the problem and many more cases may be in the pipeline.

The acute outbreak

This must be managed systematically and rapidly. Much prior preparation is possible.

The management of an acute outbreak is divided into stages, though in practice some stages will run in parallel. The stages are:

(a) the preliminary enquiry

(b) ascertainment of *all* those exposed—those unaffected are as important to the investigation as the affected

(c) collection of data—including microbiological sampling and choice of study

(d) analysis of data

(e) implementation of control measures and legal issues.

(a) The preliminary enquiry

This is to:

- establish that an outbreak has truly occurred
- confirm the diagnosis
- establish a case-definition
- suggest a hypothesis as to cause
- immediate control measures.

Establishing that an outbreak has truly occurred

An apparent outbreak may be spurious—cases of pneumonia in an air-conditioned hotel may present as an outbreak of legionnaires' disease yet on investigation turn out to be neither legionnaires' disease nor related in any other way. Similarly, laboratory contamination incidents, though uncommon, can generate apparently robust evidence of an outbreak.

Confirming the diagnosis

Arrange for appropriate specimens to be obtained and examined. Since laboratory diagnosis takes time and should not delay the investigation, look for a degree of commonality of symptoms which can then form the case-definition.

Establishing a case-definition

The case-definition is a list of symptoms and their time of onset which, taken together, suggest that a person's illness forms part of the outbreak. A case-definition for a foodborne outbreak takes the form 'any person attending <establishment> between <date> and <date> who develops within <hours> of the attendance any of all or vomiting, diarrhoea, and fever'.

When constructing a case-definition, it is advisable to use the range of incubation periods associated with a particular infection, rather than just the median incubation period. This means that cases presenting late will be included. It is helpful to consider classical as well as common symptoms.

Forming a hypothesis

In a point-source outbreak—one where all the primary cases have an exposure common in place and have arisen over a short period—formation of a hypothesis is not absolutely critical. For instance, in a food-poisoning outbreak centred upon a gathering, the approach is to examine all the exposures and test how they relate to the illness.

Where the exposure is not plain, the investigator must arrive at a likely diagnosis from the symptoms of the cases and the apparent incubation period of the illness. This diagnosis will suggest aetiological agents for the outbreak and an investigation can then proceed on this basis.

Where the focus of the outbreak is not clear, the cases should be plotted on a map to give an indication of possible sources of exposure e.g. in a community outbreak of Legionnaires' Disease.

Immediate control measures

There are two purposes to instituting immediate control measures:

1. Preventing new primary cases arising, which may be by:
   - destroying all the foods left over from a gathering
   - destroying all foods from the same batch, and maybe the same production or distribution source, but not yet distributed.

2. Preventing secondary cases. This may involve:
   - instituting personal hygiene and/or isolation measures
   - treatment of the primary cases
   - use of vaccine in contacts of cases
   - selectively limiting the return to work of cases.

(b) Ascertainment of cases

It is important to describe completely the total number of cases and thus be able to calculate the attack-rate—the number ill divided by the number exposed. Epidemiological investigation relies on comparing cases and non-cases and needs adequate numbers of each. Very low and very high attack-rates both militate against reliable analytical results.

Where an outbreak is centred upon an event or a place of accommodation, try to obtain the contact details of all those exposed, using, for instance, guest lists. Where the outbreak is less well-defined, it may be necessary to trawl through laboratory returns or approach GPs concerning cases they may have seen but not recognised as part of a larger picture.

(c) Collection of data

Choice of study

This is between a cohort study and a case-control study and the choice is straightforward. If the event is so well delineated that all those at risk, both ill and well, can be identified, then a cohort study is appropriate.

If all those at risk cannot be delineated e.g. where a general excess of disease is apparent in the community but its origin is not, a case-control study is appropriate.

Controls should be matched, but not over-matched, to the cases, being:

- within 10% of age—saying within five years of age is a nonsense if the outbreak involves many children
- resident within, say, the ring of cases when the cases are plotted on a map.

Foods are not gender-sensitive, by and large, and so there is no value in matching for sex in a food-borne outbreak.

Controls must have had the opportunity of exposure to the hypothesized source. In a community outbreak, the controls must be drawn from that community.

Controls can be nominated by the cases but cases are often unwilling to admit their illness to others in their community. Other possible sources of controls include staff at local workplaces. Be sure that the chosen staff actually *live* within the ring of the cases.

The case-control questionnaire must garner information about shopping habits and must enquire about a wide range of foods.

Microbiological data

Specimens of suspect materials and of faeces are obtained by environmental health officers who, in the event of a food-borne outbreak, will also collect important details such as food preparation and storage practices and carry out an inspection of the premises. Discarded foods can yield useful microbiological data, as identification of toxins and recovery of organisms from deep within the food are still likely to be significant.

In large outbreaks, it is a kindness to the laboratory to forewarn of a large influx of specimens so that workload can be planned.

Factual data

Typically this is obtained by questionnaire. Many questions are common to all types of investigation, enabling preparation of large elements of the questionnaires in advance, taking pressure off the investigator when the outbreak occurs.

Core data elements:

- personal demographic data: name; address; date of birth; sex and occupation
- clinical details: date of onset of illness; a listing of symptoms from which the case can select those affecting them; duration of illness; days off work and need for admission to hospital; outcome of illness
- variably: travel history; immunization history.

Context-specific data elements:

- in food-borne outbreaks: complete food histories
- in outbreaks due to spread between persons: a complete list of possible sources and their contacts.

(d) Analysis of data

To establish whether the source is on-going

Dates of onsets of cases should be plotted. A point-source outbreak yields the pattern shown in Figure 4.8.1.

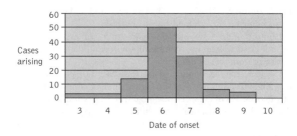

Figure 4.8.1 The profile of a point-source outbreak.

A continuing source or an outbreak with person-to-person transmission produces a flattened curve over a longer period of time.

To find the root cause

The purpose of this analysis is to detect whether there is a significant difference between the attack-rate in those who consumed a given food and the attack-rate in those who didn't. If there is, then the food consumed is significantly associated with the subsequent development of illness.

From the questionnaire answers, a sheet should be constructed as in Table 4.8.1.

Table 4.8.1 Form for analysing questionnaire answers.

	Consumed			Not consumed			
Food	Ill	Not Ill	Attack-rate	Ill	Not Ill	Attack-rate	Statistic e.g.:
A	a	u	a/(a+u)	d	x	d/(d+x)	0.002
B	b	v	b/(b+v)	e	y	e/(e+y)	0.05
C	c	w	c/(c+w)	f	z	f/(f+z)	0.0003

The statistic needs interpretation. If many foods are examined, there will be chance associations between consumption and illness and these must be weeded out. For example, if the analysis of a campylobacter-mediated outbreak yields significant associations with chicken and fried fish, the investigator must use their knowledge of the epidemiology of campylobacter infection to identify the likelier cause.

The statistics can be generated by a conventional spreadsheet or a dedicated computer program such as *Epi-Info*. *Epi-Info* is constantly refined and is increasingly user-friendly—an essential in a program which may only be used infrequently. *Epi-Info 2000*, and its predecessor *Epi-Info 6*, are free and can be downloaded from the CDC website.[2]

Combining information from the epidemiological, environmental, and microbiological investigations allows the investigating team to develop a picture of what went wrong and why, and helps them formulate both immediate control measures and measures to prevent a recurrence in the longer term.

(e) Implementation of control measures and legal issues

Immediate control measures have been discussed earlier in this chapter. It may be worth seeking expert advice, as control measures do evolve. For example, it is now clear that vaccine has a role in the limitation of spread of hepatitis A, whereas up to now, normal immunoglobulin has been the therapeutic mainstay.

Control measures in foodborne outbreaks

Control measures to prevent recurrent episodes of food-borne illness are almost always governed by national legislation. For instance, in the UK, the principal legislation, in date order:

- Milk and Dairies Regulations 1959
- Public Health (Control of Disease) Act 1984
- Food Safety Act 1990
- Food Safety (General Food Hygiene) Regulations 1995.

Broadly they empower local government officials to:

- require examination of a person suspected of harbouring one of a range of illnesses
- require people to stop work
- enter premises 'at all reasonable hours'
- inspect, detain, and seize food
- require that milk be heat-treated
- serve improvement notices and prohibition orders
- prosecute food producers and handlers
- compensate food providers in selected instances of loss consequent upon outbreak investigations.

Standards of evidence

Outbreak investigation is not just a matter of elucidating the cause, but also of establishing why the causal circumstance(s) arose. Information seeking, to meet the first purpose, conflicts with evidence gathering to meet the second. The standards of evidence have to be preserved throughout the investigation—allowing for, for instance, the passage of a laboratory specimen through several laboratories for precise identification, typing, etc.

Spoken evidence, as from the caterer, has to comply with the Police and Criminal Evidence Act (PACE) 1984 and with the Criminal Procedures and Investigations Act 1996. Under PACE, a caution must be issued before seeking to acquire information that might subsequently be used in a criminal prosecution.

Section 20 of the Health and Safety at Work Act can be used to require a person to answer questions to aid an investigation—they sign a declaration to this effect—but the replies cannot be used in a criminal prosecution.

Section 33 of the Food Safety Act defines the offence of failing to give information but does not require a person to answer questions that might incriminate them. Again, any answers cannot be used in a criminal prosecution.

There is also the consideration of the confidentiality of information gained in an investigation, though such information can be divulged if the Proper Officer thinks it necessary.

Working with the media

Outbreaks may attract media attention or, much less commonly, media attention may be sought by outbreak investigators to aid tracking down of people to participate in the investigation. The cardinal rule of investigations, as with all other media contact, is to stick to the established facts of the case and not to extrapolate unreasonably from the modest information available at the start of an outbreak investigation (see chapter 7.4).

Summary

Above all, remember these four things:

- be sure that an outbreak has occurred before embarking upon an extensive investigation
- act quickly—memories of exposures are short-lived
- to obtain the best response-rates, keep questionnaires brief. Only seek the data you really need—you can always go back for greater detail of, for instance, demographic information
- remember that, in all studies, the exposures of the non-cases contribute as much to the analysis as the histories of the cases.

Further resources

Centers for Disease Control and Prevention (CDC), Atlanta. www.cdc.gov/ (accessed 14 September 2000).

Chin J (2000). *Control of communicable diseases manual*. American Public Health Association, Washington DC. (Previously edited by Benenson.)

Communicable Disease Surveillance Centre (CDSC). www.phls.co.uk/ (accessed 14 September 2000).

Donaldson LJ and Donaldson RJ (2000). *Essential public health*, (2nd edn). Petroc Press, Newbury.

World Health Organization. www.who.ch/ (accessed 14 September 2000).

References

1. Last JM (ed.) (2001). *A dictionary of epidemiology*. Oxford University Press, Oxford.
2. *Epi-Info 2000*. www.cdc.gov/epiinfo (accessed 5 February 2001).

Yet the captain of all these men of death that came against him to take him away was the consumption, for it was that that brought him down to the grave.

John Bunyan, 1680;
The life and death of Mr. Badman

4.9 Managing disasters and other public health crises

Paul Bolton

Objective

After reading this chapter you should be familiar with a basic public health approach to disasters and other crises.

Classification and definition

The term 'disaster' is used in many different ways. To get an overview of all the ways in which the word is used, see Box 4.9.1:

Box 4.9.1 **Natural and Human Disasters**

I. Disasters of *natural* origin
   (a) sudden onset (earthquakes, landslides, floods, etc.)
   (b) slower onset (drought, famine, etc.)
II. Disasters of *human* origin
   (a) industrial (e.g. Chernobyl)
   (b) transportation (e.g. train crash)
   (c) complex emergencies (e.g. wars, civil strife, and other disasters causing displaced persons and refugees.)

(Adapted from Noji[1])

This chapter focuses on the more complex disasters, with the understanding that many of the issues and approaches described apply equally to other types of disasters and lesser crises.

In a descriptive sense, a public health crisis is an event(s) that overwhelms the capacity of local systems to maintain a community's health. Therefore, outside resources are temporarily required. Crises can range from specific health issues—such as a disease outbreak in an otherwise unaffected community—to a full-scale disaster with property destruction and/or population displacement and multiple public health issues.

Principles of response

The public health response to any disaster or crisis is based on these principles:

1. securing the basics that all humans require to maintain health

2. determining the current and likely health threats to the affected community, given the local environment and the community's resources, knowledge, and behaviour

3. finding and providing the resources required to address (1) and (2).

The first action is a rapid assessment of (1) and (2) in order to initiate (3) as soon as possible. Too often assessment is delayed due to a misguided fear of delaying assistance. Instead organizations may rush to supply materials and personnel without checking what is actually needed. After a major disaster these supplies can choke the transport system with unneeded goods while needed goods cannot get through. Even in a limited crisis, time and money may be wasted sorting through, storing, and/or destroying useless donated supplies.[†] Remember to quickly assess first, by the aphorism 'don't just do something, stand there (and assess)'. If conducting an assessment for a particular agency, then any assessments should include co-ordination with local government, community leaders, and other assisting and co-ordinating organizations (such as the UN or non-governmental organizations (NGOs)). This is necessary to determine their capacities and intentions and to avoid duplication of efforts.

This chapter concentrates on the initial rapid assessment as the basis for response. More detailed assessments and response should be done after the practitioner has been joined by persons skilled in the necessary techniques.

The initial rapid assessment

Assessment involves determining what is needed, and how much. What is needed is decided by considering the principles mentioned above:

(a) Consider the basics required for health

Clean water and sanitation

Each person requires a minimum of 15 litres/day; three for drinking (more in hot weather or with exertion), two for food preparation, five for personal hygiene, and four for cleaning clothes and food utensils. Drinking water need not be pure, as long as it is reasonably clear, free of toxic substances and faecal contamination, and has acceptable taste. Simple testing kits of water quality are widely available. Where water is compromised, you should consult with a water and sanitation engineer to reconstruct damaged systems or set up temporary new ones.

[†] WHO have issued guidelines on drug donations during disasters that have helped improve this situation. These guidelines are available from WHO or from various sites on the internet, including www.who.int/repo/eha/TG/DON/ddon.htm (accessed 30 August 2000).

Food

Food aid is most often required after man-made disasters and when people have been displaced from their usual food sources. After natural disasters, crops usually remain intact and people usually do not leave the area, so that large supplies of food are not required. An exception to this can be in cases of flooding.

When outside supplies of food are required the major considerations are adequate calories, adequate micronutrients, acceptability to the local population, and ease of preparation. To survive, a population requires an average of at least 2100 Kcal/person/day. If a population is already malnourished, or the emergency lasts months, they will require more. Acceptability to the population refers to supplying foods that people are familiar with and will eat. Ease of preparation is an important factor: if foods require cooking then supplies of fuel (such as piped gas or firewood) must be available. Alternatively, cooked meals may be provided directly in the short term.

When food must be supplied a nutritional survey conducted by nutritional experts should be done as soon as possible to determine the correct food needs. Securing and transporting adequate supplies of food will require the expertise of a food logistician.

Shelter and clothing

People are best housed in their own homes, except if a disaster has rendered these structures unsafe. They should never be moved from their homes just to ease provision of assistance. If shelter must be provided, people should be housed in small groups, such as families or groups of families, to reduce general crowding and exposure to disease. In cold weather, attention to insulation and heating is necessary.

Additional clothing is rarely required as people already have clothes appropriate to their environment and manage to retain sufficient supplies. Exceptions may occur where a population is displaced from a hot to a cold area. However, facilities for washing clothes are more frequently required. Estimating and supplying shelter and clothing material needs fall under general logistics.

Health services

Adequate health care provides treatment for illness, reassurance to the population who will feel unsafe without it, and forms the basis of the Health Information System (see below). 'Adequate' means reasonable access to drugs, equipment, and infrastructure necessary to treat likely problems, as well as trained staff skilled in treating those problems with those facilities. This is important to remember in considering what type (if any) of outside medical staff are required. For example, an internist accustomed to Western illnesses and advanced diagnostic facilities is not considered adequate staff for a crisis in a tropical area with limited resources; a skilled local nurse is likely to be more useful. Good 'access' means that people know about the services, know they are eligible for them, and do not have to travel so far, wait so long, or pay so much as to make them disinclined to use them. Setting up these services requires clinical, pharmaceutical, and medical supply personnel with emergency experience.

Medical personnel will also need to assess the potential for epidemics, and assess the need for vaccination. Keep in mind that epidemics cannot occur unless the causative organism is present. For example, cholera cannot occur in a community, not matter how crowded or how poor the sanitation, without the presence of *vibrio cholerae*. Therefore epidemic risk assessment includes finding out about the previous disease patterns of both the area of the disaster and the affected population. Among disaster-affected populations exposed to exhaustion, malnutrition, and crowding, measles vaccination assumes prime importance, due to increased susceptibility, morbidity, and mortality under these conditions. Measles vaccination is recommended for children aged six months to 12 years. This is particularly important among populations for which measles vaccine coverage prior to the disaster was low. Coverage of other routine child vaccinations should be maintained, although not as urgently as the provision of measles vaccination.

For large scale emergencies WHO provides a recommended list of drugs and materials (including quantities) to serve 10,000 people for three months. These materials are available in kit forms.[2]

Information

This is often neglected but is nevertheless a fundamental requirement of the disaster response. In unaccustomed circumstances people require new information on how to maintain their health. They also require information on what is happening and is likely to happen. In the absence of information rumour will take over, causing insecurity and mistrust of those handling the emergency. Rumours may even force inappropriate diversion of resources to minor or non-existent problems, to appease the population. Therefore, a system of good communication between those assessing the situation and in charge, and the affected population, is vital. Any accessible means of transmitting information is appropriate, as long as it communicates directly with the population and not through a third party (to avoid distortion). Collaboration with local persons in designing the messages is important to ensure a style and approach which is understandable to the population. Methods can include radio and TV, pamphlets, posters, advice by health workers in the clinics, and even megaphones.

(b) Consider the current and likely health threats, given local conditions

Current health problems

Describing population health should include measurement of crude mortality rates, causes of mortality, and the nature of health problems—their current incidence and severity (including case fatality rates) and potential for change. Rates are important to determining disease trends in the face of varying population size. Measuring rates requires both numerators (the frequency of events, such as illness or death) and denominators (an estimate of population size).

For the initial assessment, numerator information can be gathered by visiting the available treatment centres, talking with staff, and reviewing daily records of diagnoses and treatment. These records form the basis of the Health Information System (HIS), which should be established as part of the initial assessment. In most cases setting up the HIS requires developing case-definitions for the important health problems and establishing treatment protocols to ensure sufficient medical supplies for treatment and prevention. Case-definitions are required because laboratory facilities are usually not adequate to test all suspected cases of illness. Rather, the (usually limited) testing facilities are used to confirm the presence of specific illnesses among the population (particularly those with epidemic potential such as meningitis) by testing the first suspect cases, and to develop case-definitions for these diseases once confirmed. These case-definitions are then used to diagnose subsequent suspected cases.

If the affected population is spread over a wide area and transport is poor, an effort should also be made to visit areas far from the treatment centres, to ask people about the problems affecting them. In these situations, rates calculated on the basis of the HIS are likely to be underestimates, since many people will not attend the health centres. However, by visiting outlying areas you should still be able to form a general idea of the main problems and trends.

Denominators can be difficult to calculate (see below). Although much less useful, proportional mortality ratios can be used if the denominator cannot be determined with any confidence.

All efforts should be made to identify the leader(s) among the population, to meet them early on, get their impressions of the main problems, and enlist their support for your efforts.

Another important aspect of current health and disease threat is the health knowledge and behaviour of the population. Failure to take precautions, such as washing hands, can render populations more susceptible to illness. Such behaviours are relatively more important when one is dealing with overcrowding, or with a specific health crisis like a single transmissible disease. Local knowledge and behaviour can be assessed by direct observation, and by interviews in which local people are asked how they prevent particular illnesses of concern, such as diarrhoea. Gaps in knowledge and behaviour form part of the information needs discussed previously.

General condition of the population
Talk with health workers and walk through the community. Observe and talk with people. The aim is to form an overall impression of the state of nutrition and available supplies, including clean

water and food, cooking supplies and fuel, shelter and clothing (particularly in a cold environment). Assess whether people appear to be getting enough supplies. Observe how people get water, to estimate the risk and potential for contamination. Ask how people are disposing of their faeces. Estimate adequacy of access to medical treatment, given the distance, available transport, cost, and degree of crowding of the clinics.

Condition of the environment

Assess the need for shelter in terms of the weather. Get a weather report. Observe the water sources and whether the water from these sources looks clean or turbid. Observe where people are defecating, the adequacy of available latrines, water drainage, and the likelihood that the water supply and faeces will come in contact. If there is a sewerage system, investigate whether the system has been damaged, whether it is being attended to, and whether water treatment supplies are adequate.

If the area is known to harbour transmissible disease, then monitor for those diseases as part of the disease surveillance system (see below). Supplies needed to address these illnesses must be investigated and prepared by the health team and logisticians. As previously noted, remember that transmissible agents can only occur if the agent is present in the environment. Information on disease endemicity is usually available from local authorities, and from regional health organizations like WHO or the Pan-American Health Organization (PAHO).

Injuries and diseases augmented by crowding—such as any respiratory or gastrointestinal infections—will be more likely where populations have left their homes and are crowded into an unfamiliar environment.

Security issues

These may be both health problems in their own right—such as violence—or threats which preclude access to resources and affect behaviour. For example, people may be unable to go to a clinic or collect supplies if this exposes them to danger. Similarly health personnel may be unwilling to work or unable to do their jobs. Even limited health emergencies may engender violence, often through ill-feeling and rumour due to lack of information. Security can be assessed by talking with local people about how secure they feel. Addressing these issues requires close co-operation with the police or even the military.

Having assessed what is needed, assess how much must be provided. This depends on how much is required less how much is available, which comes down to the size of the population and local capacity.

Size of the affected or vulnerable population

This is one of the most important pieces of information about the population. Without this 'denominator' the amounts of resources required cannot be assessed. Moreover, rates cannot be calculated, making it impossible—in public health terms—to determine the size of a problem or trends by prevalence or incidence.

Early in an emergency, rough estimates are acceptable, and can be based on pre-existing information, estimates of knowledgeable persons, or even (in the case of a mass displacement of people to an open area) 'eyeballing' from a high piece of ground. Later more sophisticated sampling and survey methods should be used (by a demographer or epidemiologist), or even a count if possible.

Demography of the affected population

Usually some groups are more vulnerable to problems than others. In a limited crisis, such as a disease outbreak, this may be because of disease susceptibility; for example children are more susceptible to measles. In a full-scale disaster with crowding and limited resources, some groups are at a disadvantage in securing their needs. This is particularly true in developing countries and can include women (particularly if pregnant or lactating), children (especially those without adult protectors), the elderly, and the handicapped. The size and location of these groups should be determined and particular attention given to meeting their needs.

Assessing capacity

In meeting needs the emphasis should be on reconstructing or supporting the system that met those needs before the emergency, rather than on creating a parallel system. Determine what that system was/is and who is in charge. Work with that person to identify what they need to meet the current crisis, and try to provide it. This is particularly true after a disaster, yet this simple principle is often ignored. Where a system has been damaged rather than simply overwhelmed, this does not mean reconstituting it the way it was, but rather providing those elements required to meet demand. For example, during an emergency you may not rebuild a destroyed hospital but instead provide tents, supplies, etc.

Compared with the creation of new system, reconstruction:

- requires fewer outside resources
- uses locally appropriate resources, and so will be sustainable
- builds local capacity to address this emergency, other problems, and future emergencies
- provides employment
- uses people who know the local population best
- restores a sense of self-reliance.

Assessing local systems in detail requires persons skilled in that field, for example a sanitation engineer to assess sewerage, or a health information specialist/epidemiologist to assess a health information system. As always, suitable local people with these skills are preferable to outsiders, as these will be the people who will maintain these systems in the long term.

Surveillance

After the initial assessment, a surveillance system must be created to monitor health trends and detect incipient epidemics. In any displaced and crowded population, surveillance should include measles and the common serious diseases known to occur among the population and in the geographical area. These may include important epidemic diseases like cholera and other diarrhoeal diseases, dysentery, malaria, dengue fever, meningitis, hepatitis, typhoid and paratyphoid, typhus, and viral encephalitis.

Surveillance information must be provided to all involved, including the affected population and those in charge politically. It will provide the information to determine whether the response to the crisis is effective. The surveillance system must be capable of rapidly investigating and either confirming or debunking rumours.

Setting up surveillance will require consultation with the other organizations providing health assistance; to agree on standard case-definitions and reporting formats. Access to a laboratory will be required to confirm diagnoses, particularly in the early phases of an epidemic. The system should be under the direction of an epidemiologist.

Logistics

For all external supplies, consider:

- where to get them in sufficient quality and quantity
- how to pay for them
- how quickly they are needed
- available transportation methods for these requirements
- how the situation is likely to change.

All these considerations will require co-operation between an experienced logistician and local people familiar with local suppliers and markets.

Skills and knowledge

After a disaster, the following skills and knowledge are required:

- rapid assessment and survey skills
- clinical

- water and sanitation
- food and nutrition
- logistics
- familiarity with local language, culture, environment, and the affected population
- relationships with important local persons whose assistance and support will be needed
- sensitivity in dealing with the affected population
- ability to communicate ideas and problems well, and to write coherent and clear reports
- ability to deal with the media.

Personnel

These skills and knowledge translate into the following personnel:

- project director
- epidemiologist
- logistician
- local people (familiar with local culture and language)
- water and sanitation expert
- nutritionist
- clinical staff (familiar with likely problems and resources).

Fallacies

In his book *The public health consequences of disasters*[1], Eric Noji describes some of the important myths and realities about disasters collected by The Pan American Health Organization. Awareness of these myths is useful in approaching emergency response:

1. Foreign medical volunteers are always needed.
2. Any kind of international assistance is urgently required.
3. Epidemics are inevitable after disasters.
4. Disasters bring out the worst in people.
5. Affected populations are too shocked and helpless to help themselves.
6. Disasters kill randomly.
7. Locating disaster victims in temporary settlements is the best shelter solution.
8. Food aid is always required after natural disasters.
9. Clothing is always needed.
10. Conditions return to normal after a few weeks.

All of these myths (except (4) and (10)) have been dealt with previously in this chapter. Most workers would agree that disasters overwhelmingly bring out the positive side of human nature, and that community spirit is usually enhanced. Far from resolving quickly, the effects of most disasters last for years, or even decades. This is true even in developed countries, where increased debt and interruption in economic activity can create long-term financial burdens.

Conclusion

As a public health professional/team, there is much you can do to help in a disaster. Effective disaster and crisis response is predicated on rapid assessment of the situation prior to initiating a response, and on focusing on the public health principles outlined in this chapter.

Further resources

Chin J (ed.) (2000). *Control of communicable diseases manual.* American Public Health Association, Washington DC. (Previously edited by Benenson.)

Hanquet G (ed.) (1997). *Refugee health. An approach to emergency situations.* Macmillan/Medecins Sans Frontieres, London.

Office for Foreign Disaster Assistance. *Field operations guide.* www.info.usaid. gov/hum_response/ofda/fog/foghme.htm (accessed 14 September 2000).

Perrin P (1996). *War and public health.* International Committee of the Red Cross, Geneva.

References

1. Noji E (ed.) (1997). *The public health consequences of disasters.* Oxford University Press, New York.
2. World Health Organization (1990). *The new emergency health kit.* World Health Organization, Geneva. (Document WHO/DAP/90.1.)

4.10 The public health professional as political activist

J.A. Muir Gray

'One person is a crank, two people are a pressure group, three people are public opinion.'

Objectives

By reading this chapter, you should be more clear as to how action can be initiated by raising the profile of a public health issue through lobbying and direct action.

Case study

The first report of The Royal Commission on Environmental Pollution was published in 1971 in the UK. It had highlighted the problems of the illicit dumping of toxic waste—known as 'fly tipping'—at sites, such as waste ground, not registered to receive it. Although the problem had first been identified in 1963, the government had not acted. Throughout 1971, the Royal Commission lobbied the government to act on this matter, because of the potential danger to water supplies and the risk to public health, but to no avail. Until one day a Midlands lorry driver called Lonnie Downes took the matter into his own hands. He had discovered that fellow drivers were being given a bonus of £20 a week to dump toxic waste (which was described as 'suds oil'). After complaining to the management, he was threatened with dismissal. Several weeks later, he was offered a promotion; Lonnie declined. Lastly, he was offered £300 to leave the firm; again Lonnie declined. Instead, he went to the local branch of the Conservation Society, which then sent a detailed report to the Secretary of State for the Environment. Despite this, the Government still decided not to act.

The Conservation Society then sent its findings to the press. The story was published in the Birmingham *Sunday Mercury* on 10 January 1972. On 24 February that same year, 36 drums of sodium cyanide were found on a derelict piece of ground near Nuneaton where children were known to play. The government finally acted. A Bill was drafted and passed into law by 30 March 1972.

On this occasion, the evidence alone, even that from a scientifically respectable government report, was not enough to determine policy. Decisions taken by policy makers and managers can be made either in response to public pressure or from an ideological position in which the scientific evidence may play only a negligible part.

Making and amending laws

The process by which law is made or amended is sometimes weird and wonderful, but the public health professional can make an impact by doing one or more of the following:

- raising the public awareness of an issue
- lobbying politicians personally
- lobbying politicians through pressure groups
- becoming a politician
- breaking the law.

Political action can be very exciting and seductive, so it is wise to pause before suddenly embarking on the campaign, and reflect on the following questions.

Box 4.10.1 Five points to ponder before getting politically active:

- could present legislation be enforced more effectively?
- what do the public think about this problem and the proposed legislation?
- what is the current best evidence about the need for, and benefits of, legislative change?
- what else should I stop doing to create time for political action?
- what will my boss and my employer think about my getting involved?

Raising the issue with the public

This is the first step. The fact that some change is required, and the reason for that change, needs to be raised within the consciousness of the electorate, either as a new idea or as an issue that is more important than they previously considered. It may be sufficient to say something must be done but it is more effective to describe what should be done.

Issues can be raised by press releases and other means of getting coverage in the media (see chapters 3.5 and 7.4). However, as in so many aspects of life, it is insufficient by itself and other steps must be taken to change the law.

Lobbying politicians personally

A lobby is an open space in a house of legislature, open in architecture and open in style, for politicians and the public to meet. Lobbying is the process of influencing the members of a legislature and it is the right of every citizen to influence their representative. Lobbying is an art, not a science, and there is no evidence on which to base guidelines other than experience, but it is possible to identify ways of lobbying that appear to be more effective

---

Box 4.10.2 **Guidelines for effective lobbying**

- focus: don't lobby politicians on everything but let them know you are willing to give information on any public health issue
- aim at the right level—start locally and work up
- don't rely on letters alone—make an appointment for an interview
- in an interview, listen, and leave a note of your main points
- don't embarrass your employer—keep people informed about your political activities.

It is essential to lobby the representative of the population concerned even though they appear to be powerless or even though they are known to be opposed to the desired course of action. Even if lobbying does not change the politician's mind, it has an impact on the vehemence of their feelings and this may be very important.

Lobbying politicians through pressure groups

In the United States the word 'lobby' has come to mean the pressure group itself. For example, the gun lobby works with highly paid consultants running sophisticated campaigns to influence politicians by a wide variety of methods, usually stopping just short of corruption by money.

Corruption need not be money alone, for it is defined as 'the perversion of integrity by money or favours', and in many countries favours are used by those promoting goods or services hostile to the public health.

There have been pressure groups for health for many years but it was in the sixties that consumer pressure groups blossomed, as attitudes changed and leaders emerged. Ralph Nader, who took on the American car industry on the issue of safety, became an icon of this activity in this period.

There are now hosts of health pressure groups. Public health professionals who wish to influence policy should ask the questions presented in Figure 4.10.1.

ASH (Action on Smoking and Health), Greenpeace, Amnesty International are all examples of pressure groups who are powerful forces for health improvement. They usually have highly skilled and committed staff who may have some reservations concerning the public health professional who wants to get involved. Pressure

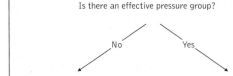

Is there an effective pressure group?

No   Yes

- What would be the risks, costs and benefits of starting one?
- Who could help?
- What should be its constitution? Informal or formal, charity or company?
- Could any resources from my organization be used or should it be entirely within my free time and resources?
- Would the pressure group put me in conflict with my employer?

- What would be the risks, costs and benefits of getting involved?
- Should I get close or use it as an external agency for change?
- If I get close, should I join or have observer status?
- Would it be better to put my energies into a national or local pressure group?
- What would my employer think?

Figure 4.10.1 Pressure groups.

group workers are usually on low pay and shorter contracts, so it is wise to approach with humility and an eagerness to learn from very effective operators.

Becoming a politician

If many of the causes of ill-health can be tackled effectively by political action, it could be argued that every public health professional should become a politician; if some do, then why not all?

There is no formal study of this issue with a single conclusion, but possible reasons why not all public health practitioners are politicians are set out below:

- a politician has to sign up to a broad range of party policies, some of which require the individual to compromise
- policies are often based on ideology not evidence, because politics is based on values: the person who likes evidence-based decision making may find this unsatisfactory
- politicians in power have power; those who are not may have less power than the public health professional managing a budget
- the politician has to cover many issues other than those which directly affect health; the public health professional can focus on health issues.

Even the public health professional who becomes a successful politician may find that they are steered away from health jobs for fear they will go native and fail to do what politicians are there to do: bring values to decision making and challenge the professionals. The politician's role has been most eloquently described by Enoch Powell in his book *A new look at medicine and politics*[1], in which he argued not only that doctors were not necessarily better Ministers of Health than generalists (and could be less effective) but also that any politician in a post for more than two years started using the jargon of their officials and had lost the edge they contributed to a department before they became institutionalized.

Breaking the law

Most public health professionals break the law frequently, but usually in a way that endangers the public health rather than protecting it. Speeding is one of the most common offences and has a significant effect on mortality. However, the type of law-breaking that might protect the public health—an environmental protest that triggers police action, for example—is less commonly committed by a public health professional, particularly if they are employed, directly or indirectly, by a government. Law-breaking may be necessary to improve the public health, but law-making and enforcement has had an even greater impact and the skills of the public health professional are best used in this activity.

Personal survival amongst organizational change

Structural change in government and health care organizations is frequent. In times of structural change in an organization, the job of the orthopaedic surgeon is relatively secure. The public health practitioner, however, is more exposed, often because of our inability to describe what we do quickly and clearly and concisely.

The following experience-based survival skills tips I pass on, gleaned from those people who have survived a series of organizational changes:

- never try to guess the future; always do the job you are currently paid to do to the best of your ability
- never put your faith in institutions, only in individuals
- make sure you can describe public health and your own contribution to the service in one minute if someone asks you to do so
- keep fit, constantly attend training courses, and keep a good record of the training and the professional development that you have done, and plan to do.

Further resources

Machiavelli N (1998). *The Prince*. Penguin, Harmondsworth.
Chapter 3.5, this handbook: Using media advocacy to shape policy.
Chapter 7.4, this handbook: Working with the media.

References

1. Powell JE (1976). *Medicine and politics; 1975 and after*. Pitman Medical, London. (The best guide to how to work with full-time politicians and senior civil servants.)

To help people change, try the following, in order: 1) make it understandable and relevant (education); 2) make it easy (training); 3) make it desirable (incentives); 4) make it obligatory (regulation).

Part 5
Health care assessment

Introduction

Advances in clinical practice dominated the debate about health in the second half of the twentieth century. Astonishing progress has been made that has contributed to an increase in life expectancy. We are, however, coming to the end of an era of exuberant growth and development. In almost every country there is now major concern about health care costs. The pressures of population ageing, rising public and professional expectations, and the continuing development of new knowledge and technology, mean that in almost every country there is a growing gap between what can be done and what can be afforded. This is a tension between needs and demands on the one hand and the ability of health services, and those who pay for them, to respond on the other. These issues and their consequences, such as commissioning and rationing care, have made debates about clinical care important debates on the public health agenda.

Most health is won or lost through the big four determinants of health: genes, environment and behaviour, and health care.[1] It is mainly through the development and modification of 'systems' that public health endeavours improve health. A health system, in its broadest sense, is composed of 'personal health care, public health services and other inter-sectoral initiatives'.[2]

The role of public health is to contribute 'to the health of the public through assessment of health and health needs, policy formulation, and assurance of the availability of services'.[3] Assessment of health and health needs was addressed in part 1, policy was dealt with in part 3, with assessment and assurance of health care being dealt with in parts 5 and 6.

These next two parts highlight the specific contributions that public health practitioners, if appropriately skilled, can make to assessing and assuring the quality and accountability of health care. In addition, they present the mechanisms by which people and organizations can be held accountable for this quality as part of a process of continuous improvement.

Many public health practitioners have been taught that personal health services are almost completely irrelevant in the determination of health. The radical critiques of McKeown, in his 1979 book *The role of medicine*[4] and Illich, in his book *Medical nemesis*[5] have become powerful, but not wholly valid, orthodoxies, with significant effects upon movements such as Health for All 2000. A comprehensive understanding of these issues is vital for effective public health practice.

McKeown argued that much of the reduction in standardized mortality in England and Wales between 1841 and 1971 was due to nutritional, environmental, and behaviour changes and was little influenced by medical interventions. The key points are summarized below:

- age/sex standardized (1901 population standard) mortality in England and Wales fell from 22 to 6 per 1000 per year between 1841 and 1971; 75% of this due to a fall in infectious disease deaths

- for tuberculosis, measles, pertussis, and tetanus only a very modest part (10–15%) of the decline in mortality from these conditions since 1841 occurred *after* the introduction of specific medical interventions (immunization and/or treatment)

- in the cases of polio, smallpox, and diphtheria, a larger proportion of the decline (at least 30%) occurred after medical interventions were introduced

- improved nutrition (due to increased food production and more efficient food distribution) coupled with improved sanitation, and housing are held to be mainly responsible; medical care was relatively unimportant.

Illich strongly asserted that medical care is not only generally ineffective but also inflicts clinical and social iatrogenesis. His key arguments are:

- environmental factors are the key determinants of health

- clinical iatrogenesis manifests itself as antibiotic resistance, drug interactions, unnecessary surgery, and the hazards of diagnostic procedures; 20% of hospital patients experience an iatrogenic problem, causing death in 3%

- social iatrogenesis increases individuals' dependency on health professionals and reduces both their autonomy and their ability to cope with illness

- within health care there is excess expenditure on treatment of the sick rather than on public health services, especially in developing countries

- consumer empowerment and increased public control of doctors are inadequate approaches to the problem. Instead a radical rejection of the 'scientism in health care' is needed.

The British physician and epidemiologist, Archie Cochrane, focused attention upon the uncertain effectiveness of many medical interventions rather than fundamentally questioning the important underlying role of medicine. In *Effectiveness and efficiency*[6] he demonstrated that, within the UK National Health Service, the relationship between increased inputs (staff, drugs, and procedures) and increased health outcomes (increased longevity and quality of life) was not clearly present. He advocated the wider application of the randomized controlled trial both to individual therapies and to issues of health care organization, such as length of hospital stay. In this way, he argued, clinical effectiveness and efficiency could be enhanced: 'It is surely a great criticism of our profession that we have not organised a critical summary, by specialty or subspecialty, updated periodically, of all randomised controlled trials'.[7]

Cochrane made his initial influential observations in 1972. To what extent has the situation improved? The number and size of published trials has increased enormously, and the International Cochrane Collaboration[8]* has developed to summarize randomized trial evidence in the form of systematic reviews.

Recent empirical findings are mixed. The National Institutes of Health in the USA found in 1990 that only 21% of 126 therapeutic and diagnostic technologies were soundly evidence-based.[9] This may be a biased estimate, however, as it focused on expensive and sometimes rarely-used technologies. Conversely, two UK studies, based in routine medical and surgical practice, suggest a more favourable picture:

• 53% of 109 consecutive medical patients received treatment supported by RCT evidence. Only 18% were treated in a non-evidence-based fashion[10]

• 95% of 100 consecutive surgical patients received evidence-based treatment (24% supported by RCTs[11]).

It seems likely that, while the evidential base for health care is improving, clear difficulties in translating research evidence into routine practice persist (see chapters 6.9 and 6.10).

McKeown's and Illich's analyses of the unimportance or even malign influence of health care have been criticized:

• McKeown's evidence is relatively weak that improved nutrition was the key factor in declining mortality in the nineteenth century

• other historical analyses suggest that specific public and personal health measures (such as sanitation, food hygiene, eradication of bovine TB, and segregation of TB patients) were of major importance[12]

• though falls in mortality rates had tended to level off by the 1960s (despite expanding health care expenditure), since 1970 there has been an accelerating decline (3–6% per annum) in mortality in many age groups in developed countries from conditions judged amenable to modern medical intervention (so-called 'avoidable deaths').

Overall it seems possible that medical care, though not the dominant factor it was once believed to be, may not be as impotent as has been alleged. But what is the evidence?

• a detailed econometric analysis of 1970 data from groups of counties in the USA[13] indicated that more medical care use was associated with lower mortality rates, after controlling for a wide range of confounding variables (income, education, marital status, tobacco consumption, and disability prevalence). A 10% increase in medical care spend was associated with a reduction of between 0.8% and 3.2% in mortality rates, depending on age and ethnic group

- the strongest beneficial relationship was between medical care spend and deaths from ischaemic heart disease and cerebrovascular disease. Cancer death rates were little influenced

- increased medical care cost $85,000 per death averted (compared with $300,000 per death averted for income redistribution policies).

John Bunker[14] has used clinical trial evidence to assess the likely impact of modern medical interventions on common causes of death. He suggests that medical care can be credited with only two years of the 23-year increase in longevity between 1900 and 1950, but with three of the seven years' improvement in mean life expectancy seen since 1950.

To detect a disease early (secondary prevention) or, better still, to prevent it developing in the first place (primary prevention), has an immediate intuitive appeal, compared with the alternative of allowing the disease to develop to a point at which it causes symptoms. By using preventive strategies, suffering of patients and their carers is apparently avoided and less costly procedures (if any are needed at all) suffice. This view is simplistic. Each preventive programme (whether primary or secondary) needs to be argued on its merits, based on demonstrable benefit (preferably derived from randomized experiments) for defined population groups, offset against direct, indirect, and intangible costs. The biggest challenge is to demonstrate that early detection and treatment of disease gains significant survival and/or quality-of-life advantage for those screened (rather than merely causing prolonged anxiety and post-treatment side-effects). Screening for prostatic cancer, cervical cancer, and raised serum cholesterol in low-risk subjects remains unsupported by randomized trial evidence of net benefit.[15] Even immunization programmes—which have generally been shining examples of successful primary prevention—need to be kept under review to consider whether the threat from the disease has declined to a point at which rare vaccine side-effects outweigh their advantages.[16] Smallpox vaccination and BCG against tuberculosis (in some locations) provide examples (see chapter 4.7).

Summary

- McKeown and Illich usefully remind us that personal medical care contributed relatively little to overall mortality improvements since the beginning of the nineteenth century

- developments in health technology and closer attention to the evaluation of effectiveness of interventions appears to be producing improvements in longevity in developed countries over the last 40 years that are modest but nonetheless important

- societies may, at a certain level of prosperity, reach an epidemiological transition point[17] when the absolute standard of living ceases to be the main influence on population health. Instead other factors—including income distribution and medical care—may become proportionately more influential

- public health contributes through assessment of health and health needs, through policy formulation, and by assuring the quality of the health system

- a health system is a combination and interaction of personal health care services, public health services, and other inter-sectoral initiatives.

To understand how health care quality can be improved, it is essential to have a framework of the dimensions of health care around which quality can be assessed and improved. Models of quality vary around the world, but they all contain similar basic concepts. It is imperative that public health practitioners, and teams in which they work, have a specific, shared model of quality and how they hope to influence it, before they make a significant contribution. An overview of how the dimension of quality can be framed and perceived is offered in the introduction to chapter 5.1.

Once an appreciation of the dimensions (and how they relate and compete) is established, the next step is an appreciation of the different ways in which health care quality can be assessed. First, Newton (chapter 5.2) demonstrates the need to understand the strengths and weaknesses of routine data when used for evaluation, and how you can develop your ability to design, conduct and interpret such evaluations.

The health technologies (processes, systems, devices, interventions...) have a significant influence on the quality of health care. Stevens and Milne, in chapter 5.3, explain what health technology assessment is, how it is done and how it relates to public health.

It is important to understand the assessment of the quality of health care in terms of both process and outcome. Each perspective offers particular advantages. Jessop and Fitzpatrick address these dimensions in chapters 5.4 and 5.5 respectively.

The ability to assess health care quality from different perspectives enables a more complete and systematic picture of a complex area. Assessing health care technologies is an increasingly important public health skill world-wide as more critical and cost-conscious health systems develop.

IH,DP

Further resources

Haynes B (1999). Can it work? Does it work? Is it worth it? *BMJ*, **319**(7211), 652–3.

References

1. Lalonde M (1974). *A new perspective on the health of Canadians: a working document*. Department of National Health and Welfare, Ottawa.
2. World Health Organization (2000). *World health report 2000. Health systems: improving performance*. World Health Organization, Geneva. www.who.int/whr (accessed 6 February 2001).
3. Institute of Medicine (1988). *The future of public health*, and Stoto M, Abel C, Dievler A (ed.) (1996). *Healthy communities—new partnerships for the future of public health*. Institute of Medicine. Both available from www.nap.edu (accessed 17 August 2000).
4. McKeown T (1979). *The role of medicine*. Basil Blackwell, Oxford.
5. Illich I (1976). *Medical nemesis: the expropriation of health*. Marion Boyars, London.
6. Cochrane AL (1972). *Effectiveness and efficiency*. Nuffield Provincial Hospitals Trust, London.
7. Cochrane AL (1979). A critical review with particular reference to the medical profession. In *Medicines for the year 2000*. Office of Health Economics, London.
8. International Cochrane Collaboration (2000). *Cochrane Library*, Issue 3. Update Software, Oxford.
9. Dubinsky M and Ferguson JH (1990). Analysis of the National Institutes of Health Medicare coverage assessment. *Int J Technol Assess Health Care*, **6**, 480–8.
10. Ellis J, Mulligan I, Rowe J, and Sackett DL (1995). Inpatient general medicine is evidence based. *Lancet*, **346**, 407–10.
11. Howes N, Chagla L, Thorpe M, and McCulloch P (1997). Surgical practice is evidence based. *Br J Surg*, **84**, 1220–3.
12. Fairchild AL and Oppenheimer GM (1998). Public health nihilism vs. pragmatism: history, politics and the control of tuberculosis. *Am J Public Health*, **88**, 1105–17.
13. Hadley J (1982). *More medical care, better health?* Urban Institute Press, Washington DC.
14. Bunker J (1995). Medicine matters after all. *J Roy Coll Phys Lond*, **29**, 105–12.
15. Russell LB (1994). *Educated guesses: making policy about medical screening tests*. University of California Press, Berkeley.
16. Russell LB (1986). *Is prevention better than cure?* The Brookings Institution, Washington DC.
17. Wilkinson R (1996). How can secular improvements in life expectancy be explained? In *Health and social organisation*, (ed. D Blane, E Brunner, R Wilkinson). Routledge, London.

> Doctors are people who give treatments about which they know little, for diseases about which they know less, to people about whom they know nothing.
>
> *Voltaire*

5.1 The meaning of quality in health care

Nick Wareham, David Pencheon, and David Melzer

Scoping quality in health care

Lack of quality in health care can be easy to recognize, when for example the wrong kidney is removed, the wrong drug prescribed, or where communication between different professionals breaks down. Being systematic about what quality is, how its presence or absence can be measured, and how to improve quality is far more challenging. This introductory chapter will concentrate on the dimensions of quality, with emphasis on approaches to measuring quality. Other chapters in this part will address other mechanisms for assessing quality. The next part of the handbook (part 6) addresses the methods of improving quality.

Defining and measuring the quality of health care

It is not simple to measure quality. As Donabedian said:

> 'There was a time, not too long ago when this question could not have been asked. The quality of care was considered to be something of a mystery: real, capable of being perceived and appreciated, but not subject to measurement. The very attempt to define and measure quality seemed, then, to denature and belittle it'.[1]

However, times have changed. The issue of quality is now paramount. The Institute of Medicine in the United States offers the following definition:

> 'Quality of Care is the degree to which health services for individuals and populations increase the likelihood of desired health outcomes and are consistent with current professional knowledge'.[2]

This definition explicitly acknowledges that:

- quality is measured as a scale or *degree* rather than as a binary phenomenon
- quality encompasses all aspects of care by referring to *health services*
- quality of health care provision can be observed from an *individual* as well as a *population* perspective
- quality outcomes are *desired* without specifying for whom, thus allowing the possibility of differing perspectives on which aspects

of quality are most important (professional, patient, public, political . . .)

- the link between the quality of care and outcomes is rarely causal (what is measured is a *likelihood* or probability)
- the phrase: 'consistency *with current professional knowledge*' indicates that quality of care can only be judged relative to what is known at that moment in time.

Another definition, more prevalent after the election of a new Labour government in the UK in the 1990s, states that quality care consisted of:

- doing the *right* things (*what*)
- to the *right* people (*to whom*)
- at the *right* time (*when*)
- and doing things *right* first time.

However, despite quality often being perceived as difficult to define, Donabedian constantly stresses that the quality of a service is the degree to which it conforms to pre-set *standards* of good care.

An important dimension of measuring (and thus defining) quality is to make the standards against which one is assessing quality explicit and pre-set. The importance of the words 'standards' and 'right' in the definition above is that they emphasize and make explicit the *subjective nature of quality* (i.e. 'quality is in the eye of the beholder or begetter').

Defining or measuring?

One method of defining quality is not to ask which words should be used to define it but to ask which approaches, methods, or measures could be used to describe (and sometimes quantify) it.

While many definitions of quality have been offered, they are only usually helpful in that they make explicit the dimensions being considered and assumptions being made. The great challenge in health care quality is to systematically assess or measure it. *Attempting to measure quality will immediately clarify what you mean by 'quality' in any particular context.*

Dimensions of quality

The first step toward assessing or measuring quality is to deconstruct it into its core dimensions.

Six dimensions of quality

Maxwell suggested six dimensions which form the basis of quality of care.[3,4] This classification has the advantage of making it easier to operationalize the definition: i.e. to measure these dimensions individually.

Box 5.1.1 **Maxwell's original dimensions of quality**

Effectiveness: Does the intervention in question produce the desired effect? Is the treatment given the best available in a technical sense, according to those best equipped to judge? What is their evidence? What is the overall result of the treatment? To what degree are achievable health benefits actually achieved?

Efficiency: Is the output (e.g. health) maximized for a given input or (conversely) is the input minimized for a given level of output? How does the unit cost compare with the unit cost elsewhere for the same treatment/service?

Acceptability: How humanely and considerately is this treatment/service delivered? What does the patient think of it? What would/does an observant third party think of it? (How would I feel if it were my nearest and dearest?) What is the setting like? Are privacy and confidentiality safeguarded? i.e. to what extent does the service conform to patient/public expectations?

Access: Can people get this treatment/service when they need it? Are there identifiable barriers to service—for example, lack of information, large distances to travel, inability to pay, and waiting times—or straightforward breakdowns in supply?

Equity: Is this patient or group of patients being fairly treated relative to others? Are there any identifiable failings in equity—for example, are some people (perceived as) being dealt with less favourably than others?

Relevance: Is the overall pattern and balance of services the best that could be achieved, taking account of needs and wants of the population as a whole?

(Adapted from Maxwell[4])

Access, efficiency, and equity

There are many variants, acronyms of the six dimensions mentioned in Box 5.1.1. They all have in common three broad areas, shown in Table 5.1.1.

Whose quality is it?

Clinicians and others directly involved in the provision of care frequently have a deeply-held belief that maximizing the effectiveness

Table 5.1.1 Three areas of quality.

1. Effectiveness/efficacy/ appropriateness[†]/safety	Appropriate[†] and safe
Whether the service actually delivers in the way it is claimed (either under ideal conditions (efficacy) or in practice (effectiveness))	Can it work? (efficacy) Does it work? Does it do more good than harm? (effectiveness)
2. Cost/efficiency	**Cost**
Are there more efficient ways to deliver this service or are there other services that would be a better use of the resources? (eliminating waste and improving efficiency are integral to quality)	Is it worth it? (efficiency e.g. cost–benefit) Is it wasteful?
3. Equity/acceptability/access/ ownership/ relevance/legitimacy/ responsiveness	**Ownership**
How is the service received by those who (might) receive it? Is it relevant, fair, flexible, responsive to demand? Is it what patients want? Is it what professionals judge what the public 'need'?	Is the system fair? (equity) Can people use it? (accessible) Is it what individuals/society wants, and if not, can the system be changed accordingly? (acceptability, legitimacy, and responsiveness)

[†]Some definitions of appropriateness will include the issue of resources (see below: 'Appropriateness').

of their treatment for a given patient is the most important aspect of the care that they are providing. The Institute of Medicine definition of quality acknowledges that this may not necessarily be the case by including the phrase 'increasing the likelihood of desired health outcomes'.

The definition recognizes that the link between care and outcomes is rarely deterministic, and also qualifies outcomes as having to be desirable. But for whom should they be desirable? The perspective on quality, and the priority given to particular aspects of quality, can depend on who the interested party is.

Table 5.1.2 gives a summary of the different perspectives of quality depending on who is considering it.

Structure, process, or outcomes?

For each of Maxwell's dimension of quality, measures of quality can usually be derived based on assessment of system structure, processes, or outcomes of care (or resources, actions, and results).[5] The structures of care include people, buildings, and facilities, whereas the processes characterize what care is actually delivered.

Measuring the outcome of care would intuitively appear to be the final arbiter, but outcomes are not necessarily the best measures of

Table 5.1.2 Differing perspectives of quality.

Interested party	High priority elements of quality
Consumers/patients/public (i.e. those who demand and receive the care)	Responsiveness to perceived care needs; Level of communication, concern and courtesy; Degree of symptom relief; Level of functional improvement
Practitioners/clinicians (i.e. those who actually deliver the care)	Degree to which care meets the current technical state of the art; Freedom to act in the full interest of the patient; Accountability to 'professional standards'
Commissioners/ funders/ purchasers (i.e. those who actually sanction and pay for the health care)	Efficient use of funds available for health care; Appropriate use of health care resources; Maximum possible contribution of health care to reduction in lost productivity; Accountability to politically set philosophy, objectives, targets, goals

quality. Take the example of foot care for people with diabetes: should you try to measure quality by assessing the clinics and chiropodists (structure), or alternatively should you measure quality by the number of patients seen in specialized foot clinics or the proportion of all patients with diabetes who have a routine foot examination (process)? Perhaps it is preferable to compare amputation rates (outcomes)?

It is often tempting to measure outcomes, which are ultimately what you are trying to achieve (or avoid, if the potential outcomes in question are undesirable). There are, however, important limitations in measuring quality through outcomes.

Using 'outcomes' as indicators of quality

(See chapter 5.5.)

There are six important questions (modified from Donabedian[6]) to ask yourself if you intend to use *outcomes* as your predominant measurement of quality:

(a) How strong is the link between the care provided to the patients, and outcome?

Outcomes do not directly assess the quality of performance. They only permit an inference about the quality of the processes and structures of care. The degree of confidence in that inference depends upon the strength of the predetermined causal relationship.

(b) Am I sure that my assumptions about the relationship between outcome and quality will be statistically sound?

Because that causal relationship is modified by factors other than health care, corrections must be made for the effects of these factors, by casemix standardization or other means so that like can be compared to like.

Because the relationship between process and outcome is a probability, it is necessary to collect an appropriately large number of cases before one can infer if care is better or worse or meets specific standards. Often the numbers required are larger than are seen by individual clinicians and units over relatively long periods of time.

(c) Is it fair to assume that poor outcomes imply poor quality care?

Poor outcomes can identify a set of cases that merit analysis of the processes and structures of care in search of possible causes for the poor outcomes.

Outcomes have the important advantage of being 'integrative' (i.e. many different factors are 'integrated' into the end result or outcome). For instance, outcomes often reflect the contributions of patients to their own care. Outcomes also reflect skill in execution as well as appropriateness of choice of a strategy of care. (It may not be the wrong thing being done, but the right thing being done wrongly.)

(d) Am I clear *whose* outcomes I am measuring?

There are many outcomes that can be measured: some patient-focused and some system-focused. All can be legitimate. However, it is important to ask which aspect of quality (and specifically whose values and perspectives) is being addressed, and for what purpose of likely improvement.

(e) Does measuring outcomes help *identify* the problem?

The integrative property of outcomes is necessarily accompanied by an inability to isolate with certainty the specific errors that have contributed to bad or good outcomes. Work backwards from the outcome: analyse the process ((1.) things done right? and then (2.) right things done?), and then the structure.

Outcomes measurement requires specification of the appropriate 'time window'. This is the time period when outcome differences caused by degrees of quality in health care are most manifest. (For instance, poor quality outcome may be due to a factor that has subsequently been improved—conversely, although the outcome today may be optimal, processes and structures may be slipping which will result in predictable poor quality in outcomes in the future.)

The varying time windows of specific outcomes determine the manner and degree of their usefulness in assessments. Immediate outcomes can be used for concurrent monitoring of care so that modifications in care can be made accordingly. Delayed outcomes are useful for retrospective monitoring, leading to improvements in future care.

(f) Does measuring outcome itself have a cost?

Outcomes as indicators of quality are more comprehensible to patients and the public at large than are indicators of the process of technical (but not interpersonal) care. But outcomes are also open to misrepresentation and misunderstanding by the public if the problem of multiple causation is not understood.

As in all evaluation activities, the availability of information, its completeness, its accuracy, its susceptibility to manipulation, and the cost of acquisition are important considerations.

Consideration of these attributes of outcomes as indicators of quality is sobering, and may suppress some of the over-enthusiastic inferences that might otherwise be made. The statistical problem of accumulating enough cases with a homogenous intervention providing a frequent and easily defined adverse endpoint, means that few examples outside coronary surgery have been investigated.[7]

Example

In the case of surgery for coronary artery disease, it may be appealing to measure quality by comparing outcome in coronary artery bypass graft operations. The outcome being considered could be post-operative mortality rates between institutions, departments, or even between individual physicians. This would seem to be closer to the issue of quality than simply counting the number of surgeons or operations undertaken (structure and process). However, unless you take into account other important determinants of outcome (e.g. casemix), outcomes may be not only misleading as indicators of quality, but can also be unhelpful and even damaging if not considered carefully.

Safety and process of care

As our environment generally, and health care in particular, becomes increasing complex, safety is an increasingly important dimension of quality. Although some domains of our existence have become both increasingly complex and relatively safer (e.g. air travel), there is little evidence that increasing safety is matching increasing complexity in health care. In the USA, where most analysis has been done '... more people die in a given year as a result of medical errors than from motor vehicle accidents (43,458), breast cancer (42,297), or AIDS (16,516)'.[8]

Analysing and addressing safety in health care

It is important to *define* (e.g. 'freedom from accidental injury') and *quantify* errors in the system. It is important to know *where* errors occur in a system. This needs a careful, explicit, and valid analysis, often along epidemiological lines. These analyses can be conducted by defining adverse incidents, measuring them, and comparing them across time and space. The assumptions made and the values implicit in this process should be made explicit wherever possible.

It is important to know *why* errors occur. The reason is often that the system unwittingly allows a person to make a mistake too easily.

It is important to know *how to address* errors. Attributing blame is rarely the first nor the most effective thing to do, however tempting or however much the pressure (e.g. from the public/politicians) is to do that: ' . . . fear, reprisal and punishment produce not safety, but rather defensiveness, secrecy, and enormous human anguish.' ' . . . safety depends not on exhortation, but rather on the proper design of equipment, jobs, support systems, and organisation. If we truly want safer care we will have to design safer care systems.'[9] Consider the role of reporting systems and the setting of standards (see above).

'Errors can be prevented by designing systems that make it hard for people to do the wrong thing and easy for people to do the right thing.'[10]

Appropriateness of clinical interventions

Bob Brooks, of the RAND Corporation Health group in the USA, defined appropriateness of health care interventions as the degree to which benefit of care exceeded the expected negative consequences.[11] Through this concept, it is possible to establish a set of rules or standards of care based on identifying appropriate interventions which should be used in specific clinical situations, either on the basis of trial evidence or on clinical judgement. Delphi group or other procedures can be used to systematically explore expert opinion on the precise types of clinical cases in which the intervention should be appropriately used. Having defined appropriate standards of clinical care, clinical cases can be reviewed (often through examination of case notes) to assess the degree to which appropriate or inappropriate care is being derived.

In the UK, appropriateness is related to the UK government definition of quality, namely 'is the treatment that has been shown to be effective in research studies actually being given to the right patients at the right time?' However, a working group on behalf of the UK NHS Research and Development Strategy[12] has (unsurprisingly in a more resource-limited health care system) chosen to include two other dimensions under the umbrella of 'appropriateness':

- the individuality of the patient
- the availability of health care resources.

Important dimensions of quality are the over-use or under-use of effective treatment. As the pressure on resources increases, it is common for people to press for the removal of ineffective therapies from a range of services offered. Even if this is done, however, there can still be major concerns about the appropriateness of use of effective therapies with either over-use or under-use being a matter of concern.

The RAND studies[11] have:

- developed a *robust methodology* for classifying health care interventions into groups such as necessary, appropriate, inappropriate, or equivocal
- examined why the level of procedures deemed inappropriate and equivocal varied so much
- demonstrated that cost containment procedures reduced the *overall* level of activity; levels of both appropriate *and* inappropriate interventions were reduced.

Setting quality standards

Most approaches to assessing quality require the setting of standards. Imagine, for example, that there are a hundred orthopaedic services in a country. The casemix-adjusted unplanned readmission rate after surgery (a measure of certain adverse short-term outcomes) across units varies from 1% to 5% and the range of readmission rates can be plotted as a distribution curve. What rate of unplanned readmission should we adopt as an indicator of high quality care? If we adopt the lowest standard, we may be ignoring avoidable problems even in the best units. On the other hand, the highest standard may set impossible targets that cannot be achieved. Similar questions arise in setting process or structure based standards.

Should the benchmark be the average or the best possible?

It is important to decide the principles underlying the standards adopted. For instance, there has been a long tradition of considering and adopting the status quo as the standard, rather than adapting the best known practice to local use.[13]

Different levels of standards are typically used. For instance, many people aspire to a mean (average standard) whereas others aspire to excellence.

- *excellent standards*: these are the standards which are used by the best services, and the top 10% can be taken as an example of excellence, although this is entirely arbitrary; the performance level of the best service, the only service that has a 1% readmission rate, could be taken as excellence. Highlighting the best that one team can achieve is often used as part of a process of encouraging others (or more likely, challenging the excuses used by others). Witness the 'Model Villages' displayed with pride in rural China in the 1970s, or the 'Beacon' sites used by the UK's Department of Health in the late 1990s.

- *minimal acceptable standards* are those below which no service should fall; again it could be deemed (arbitrarily because standard setting is always arbitrary) that the minimal acceptable readmission rate should be 6%, so that all the services were above the minimal acceptable standard. Alternatively those responsible for service quality could arbitrarily choose 4.5% as the readmission rate that indicates the minimal acceptable standard. With this definition a readmission rate higher than 4.5% would be below the minimal acceptable standard and action must be taken.

- *achievable standards*: it has been fashionable to preach the pursuit of excellence, and although excellence is a worthy target, for many services in the middle of a distribution curve the excellent services, the top 1 or 2%, are often perceived as unattainable. Sometimes, therefore, standard setters set a more modest, achievable standard. In the UK Breast Cancer Screening Programme, achievable standards were set arbitrarily by picking the cut-off point between the top quartile and the rest of the distribution curve as the achievable standard.

In practice standards must fulfil two criteria to be useful:[14]

- it must be clear what *individuals* need to do to achieve them (the link between individual activity and achievement is important)

- the standards must be attainable; i.e. a balance needs to be struck between standards of excellence (which may be desirable but not always attainable and thus leading to a feeling of failure and frustration) and achievable standards (which may not provide a sufficient incentive for those who have the opportunity to do even better).

Local or (inter)national standards?

Like guidelines, in order to get standards agreed to, implemented, and achieved, there has to be local ownership. However, it can be problematic and inconsistent if standards differ everywhere. National standards need to be examined and explicitly made relevant to the local situation. This principle of subsidiarity means that comparable and evidence-based standards can be owned and implemented locally. Moreover, the cost of establishing standards can be minimized by basing them, in the first instance, on internationally reliable evidence (e.g. an evidence, criteria and standards 'toolkit'), and then adapting them explicitly to local conditions.[14]

Trading off dimensions of quality

The reduction of the complex phenomenon of 'quality' to sub-dimensions may allow aspects of quality to be debated, analysed, and measured more easily. However, it quickly becomes obvious that these different dimensions, rather than being independent, may inter-relate and conflict with each other. It is often necessary to trade off one dimension of quality for another. For instance, it may be fair and accessible to have a Trauma Unit on the corner of every block, but it is clearly not the best overall use of resources. How much more do people value the *longer-term outcome* of the health care (e.g. functional improvement, symptom relief, readmission rate) over the *shorter-term infrastructure and process* of care (comfort, facilities, cleanliness, waiting time, courtesy, dignity . . .).

Not only do different people value different dimensions but the same individual may value different dimensions over time or depending on the condition that needs attention.

Costs

The perspective held by those who commission health care, for whom efficiency is a high priority element of quality, can create uneasy tensions.[15] The economic notion of an 'opportunity cost' can apply where improving, for example, access or responsiveness of services conflicts with improving efficiency. A high value placed on a particular dimension of 'quality' can result in benefits forsaken in other areas, or the cost of an alternative opportunity sacrificed (see chapter 2.6).

Including economic efficiency in the definition of quality is hotly debated. The Institute of Medicine definition does not include any mention of efficiency, in contrast to the Maxwell dimensions of quality. The real issue is whether including economic efficiency in the definition of quality has any effect on how we set about measuring and improving it.

The US health care system has been characterized as having two main problems: exclusion of large numbers of people from medical insurance and the need for cost containment. To some, efforts to improve quality are part of a wider attempt to limit the overall amount of money spent on health care. As a result, systems were developed to try to reduce inappropriate care (usually the product of supplier-induced demand, one of the side-effects of market-based health care).

In general, separating systems for measuring quality and cost is important because the issues and solutions to these two problems are different. A wide spectrum of systems and checks have been introduced to limit the cost of necessary care, and to reduce the provision of unnecessary 'harmless' care. These *efficiency* review systems may lead to a reduction in the total cost of care, but they can also have the undesirable consequence of making access to necessary care more difficult. Conversely, *effectiveness* monitoring may increase the provision of necessary care and reduce the unnecessary 'harmful' care, leading to a net improvement in health. The effect on cost here could actually be an increase.[16]

Separating systems aimed at improving value for money and quality avoids unrealistic expectations. In non-market-based health care systems, the problems are somewhat different. The NHS is not typically characterized by the provision of inappropriate care, and the control of global budgets tends to create a system characterized by a shortfall in necessary care. Whether we choose to meet that shortfall is a political decision and consequently, for many people, falls outside the definition of quality.

For more details about the use of resources (especially opportunity cost, ethics of choice, technical vs. allocative efficiency) in delivering services for health see chapter 2.6.

Perspectives on improving quality

No one would doubt that assessing quality through mechanisms such as monitoring, audit, and evaluation is essential. However, there are different philosophical and practical approaches to how a system's quality is maintained and improved. At their extremes, they are characterized by the 'bad apple approach' on the one hand, and continuous quality improvement on the other.

One approach is to identify the *individual* whose quality of care is unacceptable. Thus, performance tables comparing surgeons aim to identify the worst, and stop them from practising, at least until they are retrained. This approach has some superficial attraction politically in identifying 'the person responsible', but does little to drive up standards for the bulk of patients. In addition, punitive atmospheres will rapidly lead to secrecy and conflict.

In the alternative approach of 'continuous quality improvement', emphasis is placed on learning from mistakes, and modifying the *system* of care to make them less likely to happen again (see 'Safety' above). Doing more trials to identify the best way to treat a particular condition may be the best response to evidence of a wide variation in practice with little consensus over what's best. Doing more training, or developing a quality culture, may result in more improvement to the system of care than identifying the individual who happened to be there when a mistake was made by the system.

Both approaches require measuring quality, but in the first accountability, punishments, and awarding selective accreditation are emphasized. 'It is not possible to learn without measuring, but it is possible, and very wasteful, to measure without learning.'[13]

Summary: questions to ask when addressing 'quality'

Public health practitioners are often called on to either actively measure quality of health care, or more often, help others with the process. Consider the following check-list. It should help scope the issues (and possible ways forward) in your own head, and thus in the minds of the people with whom you are hoping to work.

(a) *Why* measure quality?

Ask people why they want to measure quality. (There may be tangentially-related issues at stake which may need addressing in completely different ways.)

(b) *What* do you actually plan to measure?

Discuss with them what they mean by quality of care and agree a common definition. (If this appears to be difficult as a textual definition, then enquire what would be considered good measures of quality of care. This may quickly give an indication of what sub-dimensions and approaches to quality are considered most important.

(c) *Who* are you planning to involve in this whole process?

Consult other people who might have a stake in this issue and consider their perspective on quality.

(d) *Which* aspect(s) of quality are you planning to address?

Break quality of care down into measurable sub-dimensions and then agree which ones will be measured.

(e) *Whose* perspectives are you going to consider most?

* are you going to concentrate on the professionals' approach to quality?
  * this is not likely to be perfect, as evidenced by large variations in practice unexplained by casemix*
  * methods for appraising, distilling, distributing, and using clinical evidence in practice are still imperfect (see chapters 5.3, 6.6, 6.9, and 6.10)
* are you going to concentrate on lay people's approach to quality?

Distinguish between:

* the views of patients
* the views of the public who may be well

(Pay special attention to the validity of the measurement of these views (e.g. combining a perception of effectiveness with individuals' values (see chapters 2.7 and 8.2)), and the paternalism with which they may be incorporated.)

◆ are you going to concentrate on the society's approach to quality?

Distinguish between:

- *population* appropriateness (effectiveness, modified by societal judgements and resources—a synthesis of a professional/ technical perspective with a societal/political perspective)

- *individual* appropriateness (effectiveness, modified by patient characteristics and preferences).[12]

(f) *Which* approach (or combination of approaches) are you planning to use?

◆ a management ethos that actively manages risk and learns from complaints—the genuinely learning organization

◆ a quantitative measurement ethos where quality is measured via audit, criteria, and standards and fed back to practitioners and managers

◆ a lean, simple system—making it more difficult to make errors and more difficult to be inefficient.

◆ an educational model of quality—promote an enquiring and open-minded workforce with respect to clinical practice—encourage practitioners to use the latest evidence in clinical practice— acknowledge that many quality issues cannot be addressed by changing the system but by changing the way individual professionals make decisions

◆ an evaluative and regulatory culture where all interventions are rigorously assessed and licensed, and all professionals are revalidated and reaccredited.

(g) *Which* dimension: structure, process, or outcome?

Under these headings of structure, process, and outcome, a great range of measures can be developed. The following questions might help to focus on the most important areas for each particular quality-monitoring 'case' or project.

◆ is the system/environment/organization right?

- is the service structured and resourced in such a way as to allow quality care to be delivered?

- how safe is the system/environment/organization? (is the system designed so that making errors is as difficult as possible?)

- how central is the active pursuit of quality to the organizational culture? (how difficult is it to admit sub-optimal quality in yourself or others (e.g. 'whistle-blowing')?)

- what are the mechanisms and incentives (financial, career progression . . .) that promote quality and minimize perverse incentives?

◆ are professionals competent?

- do good information systems exist (clinical decision support, making good evidence available...)
- are educational opportunities genuinely available? (to help professionals implement good evidence, and share and learn from best practice ...)
- what are the methods of improving professional practice? (regulation, continuing medical education (CME), continuing professional development (CPD), revalidation and re-licensing)

- are the interventions that are performed:
  - safe?
  - rigorously evaluated?
  - appropriate?
  - the best possible use of available resources?
  - fairly distributed and accessible?

- when such errors and lapses in quality *do* happen:
  - are they acknowledged?
  - are they investigated? (confidential enquiries, critical incident analysis)
  - is the learning fed back into the system? (is this a genuinely learning organization nurturing lifelong learners?)

Further resources

Deming WE (1993). *Out of the crisis*. Massachusetts Institute of Technology, Center for Advanced Engineering Study, Cambridge MA.

Enthoven AC (2000). In pursuit of an improving National Health Service. *Health Affairs*, **19**(3), 102–19.

Leape LL and Berwick DM (2000). Safe health care: are we up to it? *BMJ*, **320**, 725–6—and whole of same special Issue: (18 March 2000) *Errors in medicine*.

Øvretveit J (1992). *Health service quality*. Blackwell, Oxford.

Thomson R (1998). Quality to the fore in health policy—at last. *BMJ*, **317**, 95–6.

References

1. Donabedian A (1988). The quality of care: how can it be assessed? *JAMA*, **260**, 1743–8.
2. Lohr KN (1990). *Medicare: a strategy for quality assurance*. National Academy Press, Washington DC.
3. Maxwell RJ (1992). Dimensions of quality revisited: from thought to action. *Quality in Health Care*, **1**, 171–7.
4. Maxwell RJ (1984). Quality assessment in health. *BMJ*, **288**, 1470–2.
5. Donabedian A (1980). *The definition of quality and approaches to its assessment*. Health Administration Press, Ann Arbor, Michigan.
6. Donabedian A (1992). The role of outcomes in quality assessment and assurance. *QRB*, 356–60.
7. Luft HS and Hunt SS (1986). Evaluating individual hospital quality through outcome statistics. *JAMA*, **255**, 2780–4.

8. Centers for Disease Control and Prevention (National Center for Health Statistics) (1999). Births and deaths: preliminary data for 1998. *National Vital Statistics Reports*, **47**(25), 6. Quoted in: Kohn LT, Corrigan JM, and Donaldson MS (ed.) *To err is human: building a safer health system*. National Academy Press, Washington DC (available at books.nap.edu/catalog/9728.html accessed 24 August 2000).

9. Berwick DM and Leape LL (1999). Reducing errors in medicine. *BMJ*, **318**, 136–7, reproduced in *Quality in Health Care*, **8**, 145–6.

10. Kohn LT, Corrigan JM, and Donaldson MS (ed.) *To err is human: building a safer health system*. National Academy Press, Washington DC (available at books.nap.edu/catalog/9728.html accessed 24 August 2000).

11. McCormick KA, Moore SR, and Siegel RA (1994). The RAND/UCLA Appropriateness Model. In *Clinical practice guidelines development: methodology perspectives*. DHHS/PHS/AHCPR, AHCPR No. 95–0009, Rockville, MD *Assessing the appropriateness of care*, RAND www.rand.org/organization/health/healthpubnav.html (accessed 23 August 2000).

12. *What do we mean by appropriate health care?* Report of a working group prepared for the Director of Research and Development of the UK NHS Management Executive, pp. 117–23, 1993.

13. Berwick DM (1998). The NHS's 50th anniversary. Looking forward. The NHS: feeling well and thriving at 75. *BMJ*, **317**, 57–61.

14. Jewell D (1992). Setting standards: from passing fashion to essential clinical activity. *Qual Health Care*, **1**(4), 217–8.

15. Schwartz WB and Joskow PL (1978). Medical efficacy versus economic efficiency: a conflict of values. *New England J Med*, **299**, 1462–4.

16. Palmer RH, Donabedian A, and Povar GJ (1991). *Striving for quality in health care: an inquiry into policy and practice*. Health Administration Press, Ann Arbor, Michigan.

Every hospital should have a plaque in its entrance: there are some patients we cannot help; there are none we cannot harm.

Bloomfield

5.2 Evaluating health care using routine data

John Newton

Objectives

After reading this chapter you should be able to:

* understand the strengths and weaknesses of routine data when used for evaluation*

* develop your ability to design, conduct, and interpret such evaluations.

(For more information regarding *sources* of data, refer to chapters 1.1 and 1.4.)

Introduction

Before deciding what sort of data to use in any evaluation of a service, be clear that:

* evaluation is the assessment of whether a service achieves its objectives

* the objectives of the service being evaluated must always be made explicit and agreed.

Only when you and your team are clear about these points should you then decide if any routine data might serve your purposes.

When should routine data be used for evaluation?

Routine data can and should be used when available datasets are:

* relevant to the objectives of the service being evaluated

* of adequate quality for the purpose.

Routine data are collected for a range of general purposes (see chapters 1.1 and 1.4) which do not normally include evaluation. They are sometimes called secondary data because they are being used for purposes 'secondary' to the one for which they were collected.[1] (Not to be confused with *secondary research*). While such datasets are unlikely to be sufficient on their own for an evaluation they can make a powerful contribution.[2]

* the best evidence of the effectiveness of Alexander MacGregor's public health interventions was a fall in annual child mortality rates in Glasgow from 39 to 10 deaths per 1000 children aged 1–5 years, in the period from 1900 to 1938[3]

* in the 1970s, case-fatality rates after cardiac catheterization were shown to be eight times higher in hospitals that performed fewer

than 100 procedures per year, compared with those that performed more than 400[4]

* introduction of a dermatology liaison nursing service in Oxford, England was followed by a dramatic fall in the number of hospital inpatient admissions for childhood eczema.

'Public health without information is like pathology without a laboratory'.[5]

Scope of routine datasets

The increasing use of computerized databases in all aspects of modern life should increase the availability and scope of routine data sources that could be used for evaluation.

> ### Box 5.2.1 **Important sources of routine data for evaluation**
>
> * vital statistics
> * cancer registration (**see chapter 1.3**)
> * communicable disease notifications (**see chapter 1.2**)
> * hospital activity records
> * primary care records
> * prescribing records
> * insurance claims
> * employment records
> * emergency services records
> * litigation procedures.

Strengths and weaknesses

Routine data do not have to be collected, are retrospective, and cover large populations. However, content is limited and fixed, the

> ### Box 5.2.2 **Strengths of routine data for evaluation**
>
> * large size
> * available quickly
> * multiple uses of data can be efficient
> * 100% ascertainment including subjects that have died
> * prospectively recorded information on past events reduces bias
> * system-wide coverage reduces bias.

researcher cannot specify the data collection methods, and validity may be unknown—although it can and should be tested.[1,6]

> ## Box 5.2.3 **Weaknesses of routine data for evaluation**
>
> * may not include items of interest
> * mostly process information not outcome
> * inflexible
> * access may be difficult to negotiate or expensive
> * analysis can be difficult because of size
> * quality may be variable or unknown.

Limited content frequently prevents firm conclusions being drawn from routine data. For example, lack of adequate data on casemix*, disease severity, and co-morbidity[7] * makes it difficult to interpret observed variations in hospital mortality rates. However, routine sources can also be used as a sampling frame from which to identify a representative sample of cases for further data collection.[6]

Quality and design issues

In deciding whether a data set is suitable for a particular evaluation it is important to consider the following:[1]

As always, start with C.A.R.T. (see chapter 1.1):

* Completeness
* Accuracy
* Representativeness, and Relevance including data content
* Time period covered

Also, take into account:

* size of population covered
* accessibility of data (especially availability, cost, confidentiality, and ethics)
* data format (paper, electronic, file type)
* linkage potential
* adequacy of documentation
* coding systems used and any coding anomalies.

Completeness and accuracy

A suitable comparator should be sought to assess completeness and accuracy, unless this has already been done recently.

- recording of hip replacement procedures in hospital databases can be checked against operating theatre records

- notification of meningococcal infections can be checked against laboratory records

- general practice prescribing records can be checked against records of prescriptions issued by pharmacists.

If more than one incomplete dataset is available, capture–recapture methods can be used to estimate completeness.

It is important to be clear which source is assumed to be most accurate. The prospective nature of routine records means that they are not subject to errors due to recall bias or to knowledge of the hypothesis. Administrative records are assumed to be more accurate than subject interviews for past medical history, diagnostic procedures and prescription drug use.[6]

It is also important to be clear what construct is being measured when comparing sources in a validity test.

Box 5.2.4 **Criteria used in validity check of routine data**

Hospital discharge data record the doctor's working diagnosis at the time of discharge. Patients thought to have had a myocardial infarction would not necessarily satisfy standard objective criteria for a definite infarction such as those developed for the MONICA[†] studies. A validity check of discharge data using such criteria would be bound to show low sensitivity and specificity.

Size matters

In both observational and experimental situations, clinically important effects may only be detectable when the populations studied are very large or are followed for long periods of time. Routine datasets may be the only sources of data that can provide enough person-years of observation for such purposes. For example, the General Practice Research Database covers 3.4 million individuals in the UK and is widely used to quantify the risks of rare adverse events. Very long-term outcomes can only realistically be studied using routine data, for example the relationship between birthweight and heart disease in adults.

....

† **Moni**toring trends and determinants **I**n **C**ardiovascular Disease. (The World Health Organization (WHO) MONICA Project is a ten-year study monitoring trends and determinants of cardiovascular disease in geographically defined populations. Data have been collected from over 100,000 randomly selected participants in 38 populations.) MONICA data only apply to people aged up to 65 years.

Accessibility to data

In the UK, as elsewhere, controls on the use of personal data are increasing. European Directive 95/46 requires informed consent for use of personal data beyond the purpose for which it was collected. Unfortunately, asking patients to consent to the use of their data for research has been shown to introduce bias.[8] Currently, the use of identifiable data for medical research is generally considered acceptable by legislators provided:

- the end clearly justifies the means
- a Research Ethics Committee has approved the specific project.

Anonymous data in aggregated form can also be sensitive if they relate to clinical performance. Negotiating access to such data may take considerable skill and perseverance.

Database custodians may charge users in order to cover their costs. The cost to each researcher is usually much less than the cost of collecting similar data themselves. A good deal of skilled programming time may need to be expended in creating a suitable subset of data from the main database. With luck, a generic program will already have been written for this purpose. These programs may save a great deal of time and effort, but the researcher needs to be very familiar with the constraints on further analysis that they may introduce.

> ### Box 5.2.5 **Commissioning extracts of data**
>
> When commissioning an extract of a large dataset for a particular study, never over-specify your requirements. It is a good idea to request *all* items of data on the sub-population being studied to avoid having to go back for more.

Making routine data more useful

Most routine data sources provide information on processes of care, not outcome. It is therefore important to know how routine process data can be used to evaluate care (see chapter 5.4).

Firstly, process measures, if managed carefully, can be very useful for evaluation[9] and may be the only measures with the statistical power to assess variations in quality.

Secondly, the use of composite indicators, such as complication rates or readmission rates, can be used to convert a group of process measures into more meaningful indicators of quality, if not directly of outcome. Many of these composite indicators require linkage of event-based records (record linkage) to create more meaningful person-based information.

Record linkage can bring an otherwise dull routine dataset to life for the public health practitioner. In the absence of a unique identifier, names, addresses, and dates of birth are used to identify individuals. However, problems frequently arise, for example when married women change their names and when twins live at the same address.

Although there is a small literature on the technical aspects of linkage; it is better to get specific advice from an experienced group. Some of these groups have made their software available for others to use. (Scotland and Oxford both have well-developed systems of record linkage.)

Specific examples of what can be learnt through record linkage:

- linkage of hospital and death data showed that the suicide rate for men in the week after discharge from psychiatric inpatient care was 213 times higher than the general population[10]

- linkage of general practice prescribing data and hospital admission data showed that patients on warfarin had double the admission rate for haemorrhagic conditions compared with age-matched controls

- supermarkets use electronic loyalty cards to link information on individual transactions to customers whose demographic characteristics are known.

Box 5.2.6 **Important outcomes that can be derived from routine data:**

Simple indicators

- mortality rates
- hospitalization rates
- cancer registration rates.

Composite indicators

- complication rates after surgical procedures
- readmission rates to hospital
- inappropriate patterns of care for specific patient groups
- inappropriate combinations of drugs or procedures
- admissions to hospital following an outpatient procedure
- time between events (waiting times, cancer survival)
- route of presentation (interval cancers)

Coding systems and their anomalies

Using routine data for evaluation is made more difficult by, among other things, the vagaries of coding systems. Although the data have already been collected it is essential that the researcher becomes familiar with the precise methods used in order to interpret the results.

Two examples of the importance of coding data correctly:

> ## Box 5.2.7
> When using ICD-9 CM* codes for clinical conditions, trailing zeros are important: the code 716 is used for 'other and unspecified arthropathies' while 716.0 implies 'Kaschin-Beck disease'.

> ## Box 5.2.8
> The process of deriving an underlying cause of death from information on death certificates is governed by 11 rules specified by WHO. One or more of these rules may be invoked when the so-called 'general rule' cannot be applied. A policy of more frequent use of 'Rule 3' by the UK's Office of National Statistics (ONS) led to an apparent 50% reduction in deaths from pneumonia and influenza in England in 1984 compared with 1983.

It is important to know whether the coding system used is hierarchical (i.e. a classification like the ICD systems). Coding dictionaries are usually available as text files, allowing free-text searching for relevant codes. No assumptions should be made about *how* codes have been used until the dataset has been examined. For example, some coders will use a lot of non-specific 'bucket' codes while assiduous coders will be more precise.

Take advice from others who have used the same dataset. Most large datasets have idiosyncratic problems that only become apparent in use.

For datasets that are related to remuneration processes for individuals or institutions, be aware of potential gaming strategies. Ask the professionals involved about these, if there is any doubt.

Summary and conclusions

Using routine data is potentially rewarding and can be very cost-effective. The utility of such data can be increased when composite indicators are used or when the data can be linked. However, care must be taken with the potential shortcomings outlined in this chapter; there are plenty of pitfalls for the unwary. The skills needed are those that often develop with the experiences of dealing with large datasets (especially when trying to assess their utility). The same principles of health data apply. When used with care, and linked, routine data can be highly illuminating in assessing outcomes.

The literature on this form of analysis is small and not particularly up to date. However, a lot can be learned from the experience of others.

Further resources

email listserver www.jiscmail.ac.uk/lists/birthstat/ (accessed 18 August 2000).

Lewsey JD, Leyland AH, Murray GD, and Boddy FA (2000). Using routine data to complement and enhance the results of randomised controlled trials. *Health Technol Assess*, **4**(22), 1–55.

Øvretveit J (1998). *Evaluating health interventions*. Open University Press, Buckingham.

St Leger AS, Schnieden H, and Walsworth Bell JP (ed.) (1991). *Evaluating health services' effectiveness*. Open University Press, Buckingham.

UK Department of Health. www.doh.gov.uk/public/stats3.htm (accessed 18 August 2000).

UK Office of National Statistics. www.statistics.gov.uk/statbase/mainmenu.asp (accessed 18 August 2000).

World Health Organization. www.who.int/whosis (accessed 18 August 2000).

References

1. Sorensen HT, Sabroe S, and Olsen J (1996). A framework for evaluation of secondary data sources for epidemiological research. *Int J Epidemiol*, **25**(2), 435–42.

2. Hanft RS, Sisk JE, and White CC (1990). Special section: measuring health care effectiveness: use of large databases for technology and quality assessments. *Int J Technology Assessment in Health Care*, **6**(2), 181–352.

3. Holland WW and Stewart S (1998). *Public health: the vision and the challenge*. Nuffield Trust, London.

4. Black N and Johnston A (1990). Volume and outcome in hospital care. *Health Services Management Research*, **3**(2), 108–14.

5. Michael Goldacre—personal communication.

6. Armstrong BK, White E, and Saracci RS (1994). *Principles of exposure measurement in epidemiology*. Oxford University Press, Oxford.

7. Roos LL, Sharp SM, and Cohen MM (1991). Comparing clinical information with claims data: some similarities and differences. *J Clin Epidemiol*, **44**(9), 881–8.

8. Yawn BP, Yawn RA, Geier GR, Xia Z, and Jacobsen SJ (1998). The impact of requiring patient authorization for use of data in medical records research. *J Fam Pract*, **47**(5), 361–5.

9. Davies HTO and Crombie IK (1995). Assessing the quality of care: measuring well supported processes may be more enlightening than monitoring outcomes. *BMJ*, **311**, 766.

10. Goldacre M, Seagroatt V, and Hawton K (1993). Suicide after discharge from psychiatric inpatient care. *Lancet*, **342**(8866), 283–6.

5.3 Evaluating health care technologies

Andrew Stevens and Ruairidh Milne

Objectives

Reading this chapter will enable you to:

• explain what Health Technology Assessment (HTA) is

• understand what HTA has to do with public health

• know how it builds on and differs from health care evaluation

• know more about the methods it uses.

Definition: the what, why, and how of HTA

The US Office of Technology Assessment defined Health Technology Assessment (HTA)[1] as 'A structured analysis of a health care technology, a set of related technologies, or a technology related issue that is performed for the purpose of providing input to a policy decision'. In the UK NHS, HTA takes a lead from the NHS Research and Development (R&D) HTA Programme which defines as health technologies the 'activities of all health care professionals [including] the use of pharmaceuticals, health care procedures and care settings'.[2] The HTA programme states that 'HTA considers the effectiveness, appropriateness and cost of technologies. It does this by asking four fundamental questions:

1. Does the technology (treatment, diagnosis, etc.) work?

2. For whom does it work?

3. At what cost?

4. How does it compare with alternatives?'[3]

HTA therefore seeks to meet the information needs of those who make health and policy decisions. It is health care evaluation with an explicit purpose: that is, to improve the ability of health services to meet the objectives of decision makers. These objectives may be efficiency, humanity, choice, or equity—or whatever objectives those who make decisions (who in turn may be managers or health care professionals, but may also be politicians, the public, or patients) seek to pursue.

In considering the 'how' of HTA, it is useful to distinguish two dimensions: methods, which may be primary or secondary; and the focus of evaluation research, where the interest here is particularly on efficacy, effectiveness, economic evaluation, and the broader impact of health technologies (see Table 5.3.1 below). Table 5.3.1 shows that the phrase 'HTA' is most useful when describing those studies relying on secondary data collection and synthesis with a view to measuring:

* effectiveness
* cost-effectiveness
* the broader impact of technologies.

Table 5.3.1 Examples of health care evaluation study types.

	Primary research	**Secondary research**
Efficacy	'Classic' efficacy RCTs	Cochrane review
Effectiveness	Pragmatic RCTs (e.g. funded by HTA programme)	HTA report
Economic evaluation	Pragmatic RCTs including cost data (e.g. funded by HTA programme)	HTA report
Broader impact	A wide range of quantitative and qualitative methods may be appropriate, according to the question being asked	HTA report

The NHS Programme is unusual internationally in including within its ambit both secondary research in which primary data collections are synthesized, often with a cost-effectiveness analysis (a structured comparative evaluation of effectiveness and costs of two or more health care interventions), as well as primary research methods (particularly randomized controlled trials).

Perspectives on HTA

Users and doers of HTA—and the skills they need

A key distinction is between the doers and users of HTA. All public health specialists working in health care are users of HTA. Most are also doers and in many countries public health specialists have played an important part in setting up and running HTA systems and in producing HTA reports.

Users of HTA need skills in finding and appraising HTA reports that are broadly the same as those outlined in chapters 2.3 and 2.4. However, a good HTA search will need to include these two specialist HTA resources, before any visit to MEDLINE*:

* the Health Technology Assessment database, maintained by the NHS Centre for Reviews and Dissemination[4]

- Technology Assessment Reviews commissioned by the NHS R&D programme, information about which is available directly from the internet.[5]

Doers of HTA go to a person or organization needing information and ask three questions:

1. What is the question?

2. How long can you wait for an answer?

3. How much money do you have to spend on getting it?

They will always proceed by deciding what methods are needed to answer the question with the resources available and by finding out what research has already been done in the area.

The HTA patchwork

HTA is not a single process but a multicoloured patchwork. The pieces of this patchwork—the uses of HTA, as well as the funding, levels, and users of HTA—are outlined in Table 5.3.2. The essential outcome of HTA is that it should meet the information needs of decision makers in health care.

Table 5.3.2 The patchwork of HTA.

Level	Components
Uses to which HTA may be put	Licensing Coverage/funding Clinical decision making Informed patient choice
Funding of HTA reports and systems	Explicitly funded or not Privately funded or publicly
Geographical areas at which HTA conducted	Local—Primary Care Organisation, trust, health authority Supra-district/regional National (e.g. HTA programme) International (e.g. INAHTA)
Users of HTA reports	Patients Clinicians Managers Public

The ten steps in HTA

The detail on HTA methods can also be considered to include all the guidance on systematic reviews.[6] However, this had to be extended to include elements of economic analysis and policy relevance.[7,8] These elements include the following ten tasks:

1. Define the question to be addressed clearly to include

- the type of question i.e. is the interest
  - only in effectiveness?
  - in cost-effectiveness?
  - cost-effectiveness and wider e.g. social and ethical and legal implications

  (see Table 5.3.1 above; the presumption is it is the last of these)
- the precise technology under evaluation
- the comparator (pre-existing) technology
- the disease and client group for which it is being assessed
- the outcome measures which are relevant in the assessment. Normally outcomes in health technology assessment are patient-relevant rather than surrogate or proxy outcomes (e.g. AIDS symptoms are preferable to CD4 count).

2. Search for background information

This covers two elements:

- conduct a 'scoping search' to identify issues and perspectives
- ensure the assessment (or a similar one) has not already been undertaken recently elsewhere.

3. Generate a rough 'decision tree'

This is a diagram used to portray the alternative intervention plus outcome options for the chosen population.[9]

4. Find the evidence

(See chapter 2.3.) In short, the review question will dictate the strategy used to search for the evidence. A genuinely systematic approach is vital. Comprehensiveness may not be. Electronic bibliographic databases alone are normally insufficient. Economic evidence is particularly important here if available.

5. Sort and appraise the evidence

(See chapter 2.4.) This includes the elimination of irrelevant material (often by scanning titles and abstracts), the application of study inclusion and exclusion criteria (this will partly depend on the quantity of material uncovered), and a full appraisal of the quality of included studies. If it uses the hierarchy of evidence,[10] and if there is a large amount of material, well-designed randomized controlled trials alone can be used. If there is very little material, even case series, and respected opinions, may be important. Studies should be appraised first for their relevance and quality of execution—and only then for their results.

6. Search for cost information

This is difficult: it should use routine databases, cost studies, a national formulary (e.g. the British National Formulary (BNF)), Netten and Dennett,[11] and pay scales information. Manufacturers, hospitals, and health authorities (contract prices and Healthcare Resource Group* (HRG) unit costs) may be useful.

7. Extract the data

This includes identifying and recording key features and results of included studies. Such data need to be summarized clearly, comparably, and consistently. Statistical summary estimates can be used in the synthesis of data (meta-analysis) where you can be confident there is no publication bias and where studies are relatively homogeneous. Where they are not, the range of effects can be identified; or the best and most relevant study or studies can be selectively used.

8. Perform an economic evaluation

The synthesis of effectiveness information is only half of a cost-effectiveness analysis. Costs need to be calculated too. And if HTA is to generate results which allow comparisons across different technologies in different areas of health care, a cost–utility analysis—in which effectiveness information is translated into generic units of health—will be needed. It may not always be possible to collect new cost data, and the meaning of effectiveness information gleaned from the literature in terms of health utilities may not be clear. Both these calculations can be modelled. The result should be a full decision tree illustrating outcomes, costs, and probabilities of those outcomes. Sensitivity analyses need to be conducted to reflect uncertainty around estimates, probabilities of different outcomes, costs, and utility values (see chapter 2.6).

9. Consider the wider ethical, social, and legal implications

These can be gleaned sometimes from the literature, sometimes from expert contacts, and sometimes from common sense. The knock-on effects of the introduction of some new technologies may be among their most important aspects.

10. Write the report

Use the following headings:

- aims and methods of the HTA
- description of the underlying health problem (epidemiology)
- current service provision (including costs)
- description of the technology to be assessed
- results (both quantity and quality of research available, and the assessment of cost-effectiveness or cost utility)

* wider implications
* options for health care policy makers
* conclusions.

Nobody is perfect but a team can be! (see chapter 8.1). It should be evident from the above that undertaking a health technology assessment requires skills in systematic review techniques (including information science), health economics, statistics and modelling, and clinical and public health expertise. It needs therefore to be the work of a multi-disciplinary team.

Lessons

HTA is still a young discipline, having emerged first in the USA less than 20 years ago. It is closely linked with evidence-based health care and health economics, the other components of the effectiveness revolution, and has great potential for improving the public health.[12] What lessons have we learnt in that time?

(a) Timeliness is important in HTA

HTA reports are a critically timely part of a research system for new technologies (particularly expensive pharmaceuticals). Decision makers need good, understandable information in weeks, and at worst months, rather than years.

(b) HTA is one part of a larger process

HTA is part of a system of research. Typically, therefore, HTA is part of a sequence of data gathering and synthesis (research of all kinds) as follows:

* horizon-scanning for new technologies that are likely to emerge and diffuse within a year or so
* assembly of primary randomized trial data sufficient for licensing by a manufacturer/pharmaceutical company (typically phase II and phase III randomized trials)
* brief reports on the pros and cons of the new technology (bulletins, editorials, and vignettes)—these might be considered as HTA—albeit very brief
* an HTA report—typically rapid systematic review and cost-effectiveness modelling (Development and Evaluation Committee reports are typical here). These are mainstream HTA
* a longer-term Health Technology Assessment or Cochrane systematic review (again mainstream HTA)
* pragmatic randomized controlled trials.

In the case of donepezil, a drug for Alzheimer's disease, only one RCT had been published in full at the time of its launch early in 1997. The HTA programme had at that time considered but not taken forward research in this area, but an editorial was published in the BMJ the week after its launch.[13] A 'quick and clean' review was considered by the UK South and West's Development and Evaluation (DEC) system within three months of the drug's launch[14] helping commissioners decide on the place of this treatment in the management of this important condition. A conventional systematic review was published in the Cochrane library in the summer of 1998[15]; the NHS Executive starting funding a large pragmatic trial (in 2000) on new drugs for dementia.

(c) HTA has to be integrated with dissemination

No matter how sophisticated the HTA process is, it is unlikely ever to be sufficient for managing the introduction of new technologies without some mechanism for ensuring knowledge of, and adherence to, its findings. There is much evidence of slow reaction to research findings in clinical practice (see chapter 6.9). A case study illustrating successful dissemination was in the production of two prostate cancer HTA monographs which were implemented because of a concerted campaign (appropriate to some big ticket issues) and because of links to the UK's National Screening Committee (EL 97 12).

In short, HTA is not a panacea. Generating information that is useful and relevant to health service decision makers does not of itself ensure that that information is acted upon. But it is a necessary first step in the development of a health service that more closely meets the objectives of those who use, fund, direct, or provide that service.

References

1. US Congress Office of Technology Assessment (1994). *Identifying health technologies that work: searching for the evidence.* US Government Printing Office, Washington DC.
2. NHS Executive (1998). *The annual report of the NHS Health Technology Assessment programme.* NHS Executive, Leeds.
3. Milne R and Stein K (1998). The NHS R&D Health Technology Assessment programme. In *Research and development for the NHS: evidence, evaluation and effectiveness,* (ed. MR Baker and S Kirk). Radcliffe Medical Press, Oxford.
4. nhscrd.york.ac.uk/welcome.html (accessed 14 September 2000).
5. www.ncchta.org./htapubs.htm (accessed 14 May 2001).
6. NHS Centre for Reviews and Dissemination (1996). *Undertaking systematic reviews of research on effectiveness.* CRD Report No. 4. University of York, York.
7. Liberati A, Sheldon T, and Banta HD (1997). Eurassess project subgroup report on methodology—methodological guidance for the conduct of health technology assessment. *Int J Technol Assess Hlth Care,* **13**(2), 186–219.
8. Goodman C (1996). A basic methodology toolkit. In *Assessment of health care technologies,* (ed. A Szczepura and J Kankaapaa). Wiley, Chichester.

9. Drummond MF, O'Brien BJ, Stoddart GL, and Torrance GW (1997). *Methods for the economic evaluation of health care programmes*, (2nd edn). Oxford University Press, Oxford.

10. Woolf SH, Battista RN, Anderson GM, Logan AG, Wang E, and the Canadian Task Force on the Periodic Health Examination (1990). Assessing the clinical effectiveness of preventive manoeuvres: analytic principles and systematic methods in reviewing evidence and developing clinical practice recommendations. *J Clin Epidemiol*, **43**, 891–905.

11. Netten A and Dennett J (1998). *Unit costs of community care*. University of Kent, Canterbury.

12. Stevens A and Milne R (1997). The effectiveness revolution and public health. In *Progress in public health*, (ed. G Scally), pp. 197–225. The Royal Society of Medicine Press, London.

13. Kelly C, Harvey R, and Cayton H (1997). Drug treatments for Alzheimer's disease. *BMJ*. **314**, 693.

14. Stein K (1997). *Donepezil in the treatment of mild to moderate dementia of the Alzheimer type (SDAT)*. Development and Evaluation Committee Report No.69. Wessex Institute for Health Research and Development, Southampton.

15. Birks JS and Melzer D (2000). Donepezil for mild and moderate Alzheimer's disease (Cochrane Review). *The Cochrane Library*, **Issue 3**. Update Software, Oxford.

It is always too early to evaluate a new technology, until suddenly it is too late.

Martin Buxton

5.4 Evaluating health care process

Edmund Jessop

Introduction—relating process to health outcome

Many patients are seen but not cured. If 'being seen' equates to process, and 'being cured' relates to outcome and therefore health status, an important rule of evaluating health care *process* is, therefore, that it tells you little about health or health status. A huge number of consultations for anxiety or depression may produce little benefit to individual population health status. A surge in paediatric emergency admissions may reflect no increase in disease incidence or severity but great change in the willingness of parents and doctors to look after sick children at home.

With this limitation firmly in mind, however, some use can still be made of the vast amount of process data generated by most health services. Process data comes cheap, because it can be recorded there and then. (Discovering *outcome* forces you to track down the patient later on.)

More importantly, effective *process* should have an effect on the desired *outcome*. For instance, immunization for diphtheria is highly effective; and so the number of immunizations given is a good (though not perfect) measure of population immunity.

Although it may sound obvious, process only predicts outcome if the process works. Assessing an ineffective process will be entirely unrelated to outcome.

> Box 5.4.1
> Effective process predicts outcome.
> Ineffective process predicts nothing.

so:

- immunization coverage (process) for diphtheria vaccine predicts freedom from diphtheria (outcome)
- number of grommets inserted (ineffective process) gives no information about reduction in disability from hearing loss (outcome).

Process data are worth more when used together with other data. For example, statistics on hospital admission for respiratory disease may tell more if viewed alongside data on air pollution or temperature. Data on geographic variation need to be allied to census information.

Evaluating different stages of health care process

We can think about evaluating different stages of health care process: starting with health promotion, preventive medicine, and screening, through primary care to specialist services.

Health promotion process (see chapter 4.2)

Promoting health requires both work with individuals, for example to stop them smoking, and work within society, for example to ban tobacco advertising. Some process data can be based on the number of people attending events or courses, but evaluating the process of influencing society is not so simple.

Work with *individuals* can be evaluated by simple measures of attendance, augmented by feedback forms on the content of any training or teaching sessions.

Work with *society* is less easy to evaluate. First one needs a framework for a healthy society. If you can get this right the process measures are obvious. One suggestion is, using examples from smoking:

- law or policy: advertising bans, workplace smoking policies
- health protection: age barriers to purchase, consumer protection devices
- common opinion or social consensus: attitudes to passive smoking.

Preventive medicine

Immunization *coverage* is a basic process measure: because the effectiveness of vaccines is known, coverage predicts outcome. Measles vaccine coverage of 95% or more, for example, will result in the elimination of measles, while coverage of 70% or less will result in epidemics.

Similarly, information on clinic *attendance* can suggest population groups in need of special attention. Many teenagers are sexually active by the age of 16, so no attendance by 16-year-old children at family planning clinics should give cause for concern. No attendance by people from ethnic minority groups may indicate that the service is inaccessible or unfriendly. However, the opposite cannot be inferred: clinic attendance does not ensure that people are using contraception correctly and avoiding unwanted pregnancy.

Screening process (see chapter 4.7)

The aim of screening for, say, breast cancer is to avert death from breast cancer. The outcome—reduction in death from breast cancer—is almost undetectable in routine statistics.

However, the elements of an effective screening programme are known and these process measures can be used to evaluate the programme. Population coverage is the obvious first essential. Another measure is the number of unnecessary operations, i.e. biopsies which

Table 5.4.1 Process measures of the UK breast screening programme.

Objective	Criterion	Minimum standard
To maximize uptake	Percentage of eligible women who attend	More than 70%
To achieve optimum image quality in mammogram	Minimum detectable contrast 5–6 mm detail	Less than 1%
To minimize anxiety in women awaiting results of screening	Percentage of women who are sent their result within two weeks	More than 90%

(Source: UK NHS breast screening programme October 1998.[1])

turned out to be benign. The ratio of benign to malignant is therefore a useful process measure. Number of cancers detected can be a useful measure if the number expected in the screened population is known accurately: too few implies cancers are being missed, too many implies over-diagnosis (see Table 5.4.1).

Process measures only work for programmes of proven effectiveness. For much child health screening, effectiveness is in doubt. So beware of screening programmes which simply report the number of abnormalities detected. Knowing that some defect of vision or hearing has been detected by a screening programme gives no information on at least two points:

• was the problem already well known to the parents?
• is it treatable?

In many situations, the answer is yes to the first and no to the second.

Primary care process

Most health care is primary health care: hospital data can be very limited, and mortality data even more so. The burden of low back pain, arthritis, and depression, for example, is barely revealed by mortality or hospital statistics but shows up clearly in primary care consultations.

The common measures (i.e. quantity) of primary care process are:

• consultations
• prescriptions.

The *quality* of consultations is not easy to monitor, though looking at the number and variety of complaints may give some clue. Most people prefer prompt treatment, so waiting times for appointments, or for response to emergencies should be important process data for primary care. These data are not, however, widely used.

Effective prescribing includes the use of preventive medication for asthma, and aspirin for people who have had an acute myocardial infarction. Ineffective prescribing includes using appetite suppressants for obesity instead of advice on diet and exercise. This can form a basis for using prescribing data to judge quality. The total number of prescriptions for appetite suppressants, and the ratio of preventer to reliever for asthma drugs is readily available. Use of drugs for a particular indication (e.g. aspirin for post-myocardial infarct) almost always needs a special audit.

Process data on referrals from primary care to secondary or specialist care is widely used but largely unhelpful because no one knows what constitutes good practice. Are high or low referral rates good, bad, or just random variation?

Good primary care should avert severe asthma or diabetic coma, so admission rates for asthma or diabetic coma have been used to indicate poor primary care.

Acute hospital process

For specialist care, *time spent waiting* is an important process measure.

Surgical operations can be classified into three categories:

- category 1: life saving (e.g. cardiac surgery)
- category 2: highly effective (e.g. cataract removal, cochlear implant)
- category 3: outdated or ineffective in a high proportion of patients (e.g. inserting grommets, diagnostic curettage in young women, radical mastectomy).

This simple scheme allows one—with some caveats—to use process data on operations to form judgements on health care for a population. For example, a very low rate of cochlear implant (less than one per million population) implies failure to provide a highly effective procedure. You need to be sure of data coverage for this work: many country-wide health care data systems (e.g. in the UK) do not capture operations in the private sector, and often miss operations done in the clinic.

Medical specialties are much more difficult than surgical specialties to evaluate through process data; mental health services are most difficult of all. Two key problems:

- *lifelong illness*: surgery is often associated with a cure; medical treatment, however, is often one episode in lifelong illness
- *variation in severity*: major surgery indicates a patient with more disability than minor surgery, but a diagnosis such as bronchitis or depression may conceal disability ranging from minor to total.

Both of these problems apply even more to mental illness. An exception to this is treatment for end stage renal failure. This is an effective process for disease of uniform severity. Geographic variation in treatment rates, put together with information on population and ethnic groups, tells us a lot about access to services.

Summary

+ health care *process* often tells you little about health or health status

+ effective process may predict outcome, ineffective process predicts nothing

+ a huge amount of process data are generated by most health services: process data come cheap

+ undesirable critical incidents can be used to monitor process

+ how closely people adhere to guidance can give an indication of quality of process (see chapter 6.10)

+ being able to show that your process meets defined standards in certain criteria is the basis, not only of audit, but also of clinical governance (see chapter 6.8).

Further resources

A good introduction to UK data on hospital inpatients:
Goldacre MJ (1981). Hospital inpatient statistics: some aspects of interpretation. *Community Medicine*, 3, 60–8.

Two cautionary examples:
Black N (1985). Glue ear: the new dyslexia? *BMJ*, **290**, 1963–5.
Hill A (1989). Trends in paediatric medical admissions. *BMJ*, **298**, 1479–83.

Use of GP attendance data (short but very good):
Fry J, Dillane JB, and Fry L (1962). Smog: 1962 v 1952. *Lancet*, **ii**, 1326.

Process data for needs assessment:
Roderick PJ, Jones I, Raleigh VS, McGeown M, and Mallick N (1994). Population need for renal replacement therapy in Thames regions: ethnic dimension. *BMJ*, **309**, 1111–4.
Smith P, Sheldon TA, and Martin S (1996). An index of need for psychiatric services based on in-patient utilisation. *Brit J Psychiatry*, **169**, 308–16.

Comprehensive use of process and other data to evaluate performance:
NHS Executive (July 2000). *Quality and performance in the NHS: NHS performance indicators: July 2000*. www.doh.gov.uk/nhsperformanceindicators (accessed 21 August 2000).

References

1. National health service breast screening programme (1998). *Guidelines on quality assurance visits*. NHS BSP (Breast Screening Programme) publication No. 40, Appendix 2. NHSBSP publications, Sheffield.

5.5 **Evaluating health care outcomes**

Ray Fitzpatrick

Objectives

This chapter is intended to make it clear that evaluating health care outcomes requires two fundamental kinds of evidence:

* evidence of changes in health status
* evidence that changes in health status can reasonably be attributed to a health care intervention rather than some other cause (either real e.g. coincidental social changes, or methodological e.g. bias in assessment).

Developing a framework for evaluating health care outcomes

A deliberately simplified model (Figure 5.5.1) is intended to underline the essential point that causal connections between one box and the next in the sequence from inputs to health outcomes need to be *demonstrated* rather than assumed. It is outside the scope of this chapter to address relationships between inputs, processes, and outputs. (For example, whether particular forms of financial incentive or level of specialization of the medical profession influence overall rates or quality of investigations and treatments.) The concern of this chapter is with the right-hand side of Figure 5.5.1 and the centrality of the point:

> ### Box 5.5.1 **Processes, outputs, and outcomes**
> Neither processes nor outputs equate with health outcomes.

This point is fundamental: health care systems, whether locally or nationally, can usually only get hold of evidence about processes and outputs, and evidence about the impact of processes and outputs upon health outcomes is both more difficult and more expensive to obtain.

Example

A simple example illustrates the differences between outputs and outcomes. A group of primary care physicians in London and in Boston examined their management of comparable samples of their patients

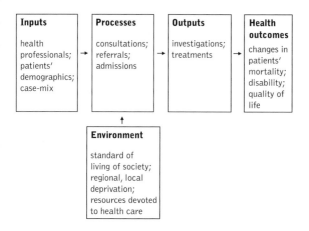

Figure 5.5.1 Simplified model for evaluating health care outcomes.

for hypertension.[1] American physicians found that they carried out more than 40 times more ECGs on their patients than did the London doctors. Other investigations such as X-rays and blood cell counts were between five and seven times more likely to be carried out on Bostonian compared with London patients. There were no detectable differences in health outcome between patients, and the dramatic differences in outputs were considered to be due to medico-legal and cultural differences between health care systems.

Evaluating health outcomes requires careful methodology

Even major innovations in health care produce only modest improvements in health. The dramatic breakthrough produced by antibiotics in the 1940s was rare. Because the size of health improvements that arise from different ways of providing health care tend to be modest (albeit in population terms), it is all too easy to make mistaken inferences about the advantages and disadvantages of innovations. The most likely source of error is that differences (or indeed non-differences) that are observed between alternative treatments are actually due, not to effects of treatments, but to differences in the 'inputs' (in the language of our model in Figure 5.5.1) of patients being treated. Simply put, patients receiving one form of treatment may be different from those receiving a second treatment, either because their presenting health problem is more complex or more severe, or because they have worse health generally ('co-morbidity'*) or have greater social economic or other disadvantages.

It is argued that by using measures of 'casemix'* to assess aspects of patients as 'inputs' that may cause error, and by appropriate methods of statistical analysis, it is possible to make adjustments that reveal the true differences between patient groups that are due to different treatments. However, it is not always possible to know in advance what aspects of patients' health require adjustment. For this and many other reasons, the randomized controlled trial (RCT) has come to be considered the 'gold standard' method for estimating the benefits of one form of health care *intervention* compared with others. It is more likely to take account of both known *and unknown* differences between patient groups that might produce misleading evidence. Kunz and Oxman[2] compared the results of a number of randomized and non-randomized studies examining treatments such as coronary artery surgery, chemotherapy for colon cancer, and control of post-operative pain. They concluded that non-randomized studies seriously overestimated the scale of benefits of treatments compared with RCTs.

The evaluation of health outcomes for most health services is more complex than that of the (relatively) simple intervention such as a particular drug. There are two main reasons for this:

• a drug is a more standardized commodity than most health interventions

• concealing from health professionals ('blinding') which drug a patient receives is easier than with the majority of interventions we study, so that we can more easily reduce possible biases that might creep into drug trials.

The complexity of health care interventions is a particular challenge, when trying to evaluate outcomes.

Box 5.5.2 **Intervention and outcome**

Take care with inferring from the outcome: the cause may not be your intervention.

Imagine that we want to evaluate the advantages of specialist stroke units compared with conventional care for individuals who have had a stroke. Imagine that we perform a RCT and obtain a significant difference indicating benefits to patients who were randomly allocated to specialist units. How can the health service use our results? Our hypothetical trial will have used a large number of specialist units of considerable diversity. What was the 'active ingredient' that helped patients? Access to specialist expertise? The way specialist investigations were so readily available? Particular forms of team work between health professionals? Other methods, such as qualitative research, may be necessary to 'unpack' the results of

RCTs of complex packages of care if we are to learn what worked in terms of effects on health outcomes (see chapter 4.2).

What kinds of health outcomes should be assessed?

There are six basic issues to address in evaluating health outcomes, summarized in Box 5.5.3. We consider each in turn.

> ### Box 5.5.3 **Six issues in assessing health outcomes**
>
> (a) short-term versus long-term outcomes
> (b) surrogate end-points versus target outcomes
> (c) expected versus unexpected outcomes
> (d) whose health outcome? whose viewpoint?
> (e) whose values?
> (f) data sources; how much effort to collect?

(a) Short-term versus long-term outcomes

For some kinds of health interventions, the patient's state is so acute or severe that we are content to examine whether benefits such as survival occur over just a short period of time; for example, new treatments for heart attack or stroke. At another extreme, some interventions may be of little value if their effects last for just a few months; for example, health promotion campaigns may need to demonstrate behaviour change over a longer time period to be worthwhile.

(b) Surrogate end-points versus target outcomes

For pragmatic reasons, it is often difficult to carry out evaluative trials with sufficient size and length of follow-up to examine effects of an intervention on key health outcomes such as death, heart attack, or major disability. In such circumstances, investigators replace target health outcomes with 'surrogate end-points' that are considered meaningful substitutes. Thus a trial might evaluate effects on blood pressure as surrogate for stroke, or CD4 cell counts as a substitute for development of AIDS. Whilst surrogate end-points may make a trial more feasible, they may fail to inform us of likely benefits that matter to patients, and should only be used when there is good evidence that surrogate end-points are consistently related to the health outcomes that are of real concern.

(c) Expected versus unexpected outcomes

Because health is complex and multi-dimensional, it is not feasible to measure all aspects when assessing outcomes of a health care intervention; choices have to be made. In RCTs the choice is very strict indeed because investigators have to choose in advance one primary outcome that is then used to estimate whether a study has sufficient statistical power to detect an impact of the intervention on health. For other kinds of evaluations it is still wise to examine with particular care whether interventions impact on those aspects of health considered most likely to respond. However, a complicating factor is that health care interventions of all kinds may have unexpected (and often adverse) effects. Drug treatments have effects on organs not identified from developmental work. Even behavioural interventions may adversely change peoples' beliefs, expectations, and subsequent behaviour in ways not easy to anticipate. By definition, choice of health outcome measures to assess unexpected events is difficult. Somewhere between the expected and the unexpected are adverse reactions; for example, complications of surgery such as deep vein thromboses or wound infections that need assessment alongside main beneficial effects.

(d) Whose health outcome? Whose viewpoint?

Whilst for the patient's health, outcomes are of primary concern, often the health of others is of importance. In evaluations of treatments for conditions with major demands on carers, for example schizophrenia, dementia, and major physical disability, strains and possibly health consequences for carers may also need to be assessed. A distinct but related issue is that, for some conditions, the patient may not be able to give reliable information about important aspects of well-being and we may turn to the carer to inform us not only of their well-being but that of the patient. Systematic reviews suggest considerable caution in this latter application because of discrepant viewpoints of patient and carer[3] (see 'Whose quality is it?' in chapter 5.1).

(e) Whose values?

Traditional health outcomes implicitly incorporate the issues of importance to health professional practitioners and scientists. Increasingly, as health outcomes such as pain, disability, and health-related quality of life become primary objectives of health interventions, it is essential to have outcome measures in which such dimensions are assessed directly by the patient. A vast array of questionnaires have been developed that permit assessment in these terms, although use should only be made of instruments validated for the purpose at hand.[4] In addition, some health outcomes involve trade-offs between outcomes, most often between possibility of survival traded against short-term deterioration of quality of life (from, for example, toxic drugs). In such instances it is not so much assessments of specific health states, such as pain and disability, that we require from patients as their overall trade-offs and preferences. Although 'preference' or 'utility' measures of outcome have begun to appear to meet this need, they currently require skilled interviewing to administer, which may not always be feasible (see chapter 2.7).

(f) Data sources; how much effort to collect?

Finally, it has to be recognized that, when relating health outcomes to interventions, it is rarely a cost-free activity. There are routinely-collected health status data collected in most societies. However, remembering the caveats with which this chapter began, data on health status cannot be transformed into health outcomes unless the issue of causal attribution is addressed. Thus mortality tends to be the most reliable data available at local and national level. It might be suggested that deaths from potentially avoidable causes, for example, cervical cancer or asthma, could be used as indicators of geographical variations in the quality of services for these conditions. However it is not easy to rule out the role of additional variables such as from the social environment (for example, deprivation) that might be responsible for apparent relationships between health services and outcomes. As one moves along a spectrum of health status from mortality to morbidity, it rapidly becomes less likely that such data are routinely available in ways that allow reliable causal attributions to be made. Hence for accurate estimations of health outcomes it is hard to avoid resorting to the more costly and time-consuming solution of RCTs or similarly robust designs, using specifically-collected and individual, patient-based data on health status, collected before and after intervention where feasible (see 'Trading off dimensions of quality: costs' in chapter 5.1).

Summary

When attempting to measure health care outcome, ensure you address the following questions:

- is there good evidence of health status change?
- can the link be made between the care provided and the outcome? (are you sure that your assumptions about the relationship between outcome and quality will be statistically sound?)
- conversely, is it fair to assume that poor outcomes imply poor-quality care?
- do you know whose outcomes you are measuring?
- does measuring outcomes help *identify* any problems that can be addressed?
- does measuring outcomes itself have a cost?

Although evaluating health care outcomes requires you to be able to measure changes that can be attributed to the health care intervention, this can be one of the most rewarding forms of health care evaluation, as it can provide a direct link between inputs and health outcomes.

With the principles of this overview in mind, the reader can turn to more detailed guides of available health measures.[5,6]

Further resources

Davenport RJ, Dennis MS, and Warlow CP (1996). Effect of correcting outcome data for case mix: an example from stroke medicine. *BMJ*, **312**, 1503–5.

Donabedian A (1992). The role of outcomes in quality assessment and assurance. *QRB*, 356–60.

Orchard C (1994). Comparing healthcare outcomes. *BMJ*, **308**, 1493–6.

References

1. Epstein AM, Hartley RM, Charlton JR, Harris CM, Jarman B, and McNeil BJ (1984). A comparison of ambulatory test ordering for hypertensive patients in the United States and England. *JAMA*, **252**, 1723–6.

2. Kunz R and Oxman A (1998). The unpredictability paradox; review of empirical comparisons of randomised and non-randomised clinical trials. *BMJ*, **317**, 1185–90.

3. Sprangers MA and Aaronson NK (1992). The role of health care providers and significant others in evaluating the quality of life of patients with chronic disease: a review. *J Clin Epid*, **45**, 743–60.

4. Fitzpatrick R, Davey C, Buxton M, and Jones D (1998). Evaluating patient-based outcome measures for use in clinical trials. *Health Technology Assessment*, **2(14)**, 1–74.

5. Bowling A (1991). *Measuring health: a review of quality of life measurement scales*. Open University Press, Milton Keynes.

6. Bowling A (1995). *Measuring disease: a review of disease-specific quality of life measurement scales*. Open University Press, Buckingham.

Impact of health services: reducing distress, disability, disease, and death.

Part 6
Health care assurance

Introduction

This part of the handbook covers the assurance of health care systems, one of the three main tasks of public health practitioners as defined by the Institute of Medicine (assessment, policy, and *assurance*).[1]

Objectives

This part will help you to:

- understand the background to the prioritizing, funding, planning, and commissioning of health services
- appreciate some of the more important dimensions of a quality health care service, such as equity
- appreciate the range of tools available for improving the quality of health services
- identify particular approaches for improving equity, accountability, and the use of evidence, guidance, and frameworks in practice.

Anyone remotely connected with assuring the quality of health care services will appreciate that difficult decisions will always need to be made between competing priorities. Objective data (concerning need, effectiveness, and outcome) are necessary but insufficient in the decision making process. Clarity of thought, and explicitness of assumptions, combined with an inclusive process, are all needed to make the many value-laden decisions in planning and organizing health care at a population level (chapter 6.1).

Like any complex technical, cultural, and political process, variation in the way care is organized and delivered is widespread; however it is also a rich source of learning. The wide international variations in how health care is funded, organized, and delivered are a rich natural experiment. We ignore this evidence at our peril (chapter 6.2).

Health care planning has not traditionally been innovative. Chapter 6.3 highlights the very real advantages of making the planning process flexible, participative, and a learning process in itself. An important function of many health care organizations where public health practitioners work is that of actually commissioning the services necessary. Public health practitioners should have a sound understanding of the general principles of such commissioning (chapter 6.4). This is particularly important not only for services relating to common conditions, but also for specialist services. Commissioning specialist services offers particular challenges and opportunities. A complete perspective of the population need is essential in this area, balancing the needs of the many with the equally important needs of the few (chapter 6.5).

The quality of these commissioned health care services is dependent on the organizational culture of the organizations and teams responsible. Being able to understand this culture, and especially the ways in which it can be developed, is vital if you hope to influence the quality of care being delivered (chapter 6.6). One particularly important aspect of this quality of care, is that of equity, addressed in chapter 6.7.

Central to this process of maintaining and improving the quality of care are the mechanisms that exist within organizations to enhance accountability and promote governance (chapter 6.8). This necessarily involves ensuring that all professional have in place mechanisms for professionally developing themselves, their teams, and their organizations in order to understand, maintain, and improve quality. Only then does it become part of the organizational culture to ensure that the best possible evidence and guidance is used in routine clinical practice. It is only when public health practitioners recognize the importance of quality assurance in health care through the use of evidence-based guidance and frameworks (chapters 6.9 and 6.10) that they can hope to influence this process positively.

References

1. Institute of Medicine (1988) *The future of public health*, and Institute of Medicine (1996) *Health communities: new partnerships for the future of public health*, both available from www.nap.edu (accessed 21 August 2000).

DP

6.1 Setting priorities in health care

Sîan Griffiths, Tony Hope, and John Reynolds

Introduction

Making best use of limited resources—whether it is called rationing or priority setting—is a fact of life. Limited resources need to be made to go as far as possible. This means saying 'no' to some people whilst others benefit. Not a comfortable thing to do, but one in which many people in public health are necessarily involved. Competition may be the result of a new treatment becoming available, demand growing for treatment because of increased patient awareness, or because more people in an ageing population are needing the treatment. The pressures of innovation, public participation/expectation, and demography make priority setting a vital part of public health practice.

Objectives

This chapter will provide practical advice, based on the model of the Priorities Forum developed in Oxfordshire, England, on an explicit process for making difficult choices.

> ### Box 6.1.1 **A Forum for prioritizing**
>
> The Priorities Forum is a whole systems approach, which involves all partners in difficult decision making. As a Subcommittee of the Board, it provides the opportunity to debate the merits of competing priorities for limited resources.

Some examples of competing pressures in the UK National Health Service in 2000:

- beta interferon, a new drug for multiple sclerosis
- cochlear implants, a new treatment for deafness
- increasing waiting list for cataract treatment, because of new technology plus patient demand
- lack of intensive care beds
- government policy to increase cardiac bypass graft operation rates as part of the National Service Framework*
- necessary action to redress the impact of cuts in social services budget for children.

Not everyone can have the funds they request. If there are requests for more funds from a limited budget for all of these, how do you choose between them?

Case study

Example 1

At the year end there was an additional £100,000 available for a hospital. The hospital identified three competing areas for the resource available:

1. The waiting list for cataract operations

   - 1 cataract inpatient operation costs £758
   - 1 cataract day case operation costs £567
   - investment here would mean that 131 in-patients or 176 day cases could be operated on, which would improve the vision for in excess of 130 older people, enabling them to live independently in the community.

2. Children waiting for cochlear implant operations

   - investment here would mean that four children could be helped to hear with a cost of £25k per implant, with maintenance, and that they could then be admitted into mainstream rather than special school.

3. Relapsing remitting multiple sclerosis

   - 20 patients with relapsing remitting multiple sclerosis could be given the drug beta interferon. 30% of those taking the drug would benefit by the disease being slowed down, thus improving their quality of life.

Which would you choose?

   - In the event, the Priorities Forum split the £100,000 50/50 between cochlear implants and ophthalmology.

Key questions

   - how can we be fair when making rationing decisions?
   - how do we account for our decisions?

Key elements

   - ethical framework (see below)
   - open processes
   - involving clinicians.

Using a framework of ethics in making difficult choices

What is an ethical framework and how did it help?

An *ethics framework* is structured around three main components:

- evidence of effectiveness
- equity
- patient choice.

An ethical framework helps to:

* structure discussion and ensure that the important points are properly considered

* ensure consistent decision making, over time and with respect to decisions concerning different clinical settings

* enable articulation of the reasons for decisions that are made. This is particularly important to support any appeals procedure and in the event of a decision coming under legal scrutiny. In such circumstances the courts are likely to consider whether the process and the grounds for making the decision were reasonable. An ethics framework is particularly important in judging the reasonableness of the grounds on which the decision was made.

Evidence of effectiveness

In deciding the priority of a health care intervention, the framework considers that the *evidence of effectiveness is of major importance.* Public health has a key role in providing and critically appraising the evidence, and drawing up practical advice.

This evidence can fall broadly within three categories:

1. There is good evidence that the treatment is not effective.

2. There is good evidence that the treatment is effective.

3. The evidence either way is not good.

Clearly, treatment which falls into the first category should not be funded. Treatments that fall into the second category may or may not be funded—dependent on their relative health impact on the population. Many treatments (or other health care interventions) fall into the third category. In such cases many clinicians may believe that the treatment is valuable, but large well-designed trials have not been carried out. It could be said for treatments in this third category that there is no good evidence for effectiveness. However, they should not be confused with the first category. It is desirable to obtain good quality evidence about effectiveness, and research aimed at obtaining such evidence should be encouraged. However, when evidence is poor then a judgement about the likely effectiveness has to be made in the knowledge that good quality evidence is not available (see chapters 2.3 and 2.4).

Example 2

* beta interferon is a relatively new drug which received its license for use in the relapsing–remitting form of multiple sclerosis, which is the commonest cause of disability for young people. Its impact is to reduce the relapse rate, thereby slowing the disease for 30% of those who are treated appropriately. The cost for a year is around £10,000. The estimated QALYs* gained range from

£750,000 to £5.5 million—with a cost per exacerbation prevented of £61,000

- thus the drug is efficacious but its impact small. Is it worth funding?
- the Priorities Forum believed not and gave available resources to increase quality of care for all patients with MS (multiple sclerosis): more doctor/nurse time and counselling. Over time, political pressure forced the Health Authority to commit some resources to beta interferon. We did not withhold the drug because neighbouring counties were funding it.

Equity

The basic principle of equity is that people in similar situations should be treated similarly. For this simple reason it is important that there is consistency in the way in which decisions are reached at different times and in different settings (see chapter 6.7).

This principle of equity also requires that there is no discrimination on grounds irrelevant to priority for health care.

In developing the principles on which equity is base two broad approaches can be taken:

- maximizing the welfare of patients within the budget available
- giving priority to those in most need.

Neither approach by itself is adequate. The maximization of welfare takes no direct account of how that welfare is distributed between different people. Equity would seem to require giving some priority to those in most need even if this does not produce the greatest level of welfare overall.

These approaches can be balanced using a two-step process:

1. Consider the cost-effectiveness of the intervention under consideration e.g. on the basis of QALYs (see chapter 2.6).
2. If the intervention is less cost-effective than those normally funded, are there nevertheless reasons for funding it?

Having considered approaches, which category does a treatment fall into?

It may be:

- urgent need (e.g. immediately life-saving treatment)
- need for treatment for those whose quality of life is severely affected by chronic illness (e.g. due to a severely incapacitating neurological condition)
- need due to characteristics of the patient, which adds to the cost— these characteristics should not affect the priority. An example is that the same level of dental care should be available to people with learning disabilities as with the normal population, even if it is more costly (less cost-effective) because more specialized services are needed.

Example 3

Beta interferon prevents relapse rates in some patients with MS. In our county there are 25 patients who would potentially benefit but only enough money for 15 to receive the drug. How should the patients be selected? First come first served? Lottery? Using criteria such as age or other features? In our experience we would say there is no perfect way to do this. We would reject the use of personal characteristics as unethical. We would not accept a lottery because it would be unacceptable within our population, but we would accept a first come first served approach on the basis of all patients being referred meeting the criteria laid out in the guidelines, but some being in more urgent need than others. In doing so, the inequity is acknowledged.

Patient choice

Respecting patients' wishes and enabling patients to have control over their health care are important values. (See chapters 2.7 and 8.2). The value of patient choice has three implications:

1. In assessing research on the effectiveness of a treatment it is important that the outcome measures used in the research include those which matter to patients.

2. Within those health care interventions that are purchased, patients should be enabled to make their own choices about which they want.

3. Each patient is unique. Good quality evidence about the effectiveness of an intervention normally addresses outcomes in a large group of people. There may be a good reason to believe that a particular patient stands to gain significantly more from the intervention than most of those who formed the study group in the relevant research. This may justify a particular patient receiving treatment not normally provided.

However, an exception to a decision not to purchase a particular intervention will not be made simply because a patient wishes to have that intervention. This is on the grounds of equity: one patient's choice is another patient's lack of choice.

Example 4

As part of the MS strategy group, patients with multiple sclerosis were given the choice of whether the £200,000 allocated by the Health Authority should be spent on beta interferon for the few or on improving services for all patients by providing more counselling and increased medical and nurse support. This was the preferred option, so patients in the county did not receive the drug whereas others in the next-door county did.

Ensuring the setting of priorities is an open and fair process

To be fair in setting priorities, robust processes need to be made explicit. Using the Priorities Forum as a model, we would suggest the following:

(a) Who needs to be involved?

- those responsible for funding and commissioning (this includes public health, commissioning, non-executive directors, finance . . .)
- representative groups from primary care and family medicine
- hospitals—clinicians, clinician managers, and managers
- public—and lay representatives as appropriate.

> ### Box 6.1.2
>
> In Oxfordshire, the Forum is a *sub-committee of the Health Authority* and reports its decisions to their public meetings. With a membership across sectors and disciplines it is a representative body for the various interests across the county including the public.

(b) What is discussed?

- implications of national policy
- introduction of new drugs
- innovative treatments
- individual exceptional needs.

(c) What is the outcome?

- statements summarizing the debate and decisions go to all general practices
- public reports go to the health authority board meetings
- appeals are heard by the chairman and chief executive of the health authority, who do not attend the meetings
- discussions are fed into the contract negotiations.

Being fair: involving clinicians

Involvement of clinicians in presenting the evidence for their case is important to enable informed discussion. Discussion needs to take place with reference to a defined *envelope of resource*, a notional amount spent on each particular service—often based on historic spend not empirical need. Any change or development needs to consider making the envelope bigger (or smaller!) or alternatively changing the components within the existing envelope. (See 'Priority setting through programme budgeting and marginal analysis, in chapter 2.6.)

Clinicians are asked to consider *three questions*:

1. If you want something outside your current fixed envelope of resource, can it be done by substituting a treatment of less value?

2. If demand for your service is increasing, what criteria are you using to agree the threshold of treatment?

3. If you do not believe that it is possible to either draw thresholds of care or substitute treatment, then which service might you give a smaller resource to in order for you to enlarge yours?

These are not easy questions and the debate is often less structured than this approach may imply, but it is used consistently so Forum members can attempt to be fair.

Example 5 (substitution)
Dermatologists wished to prescribe iso-retitonin for acne. There was no capacity to increase the size of the envelope of resource. They agreed to stop treating hirsutism—deemed to be of lower priority, and resources were thereby made available for acne sufferers.

Example 6 (changing practice to cope with resource limitations)
The cardiology waiting list was increasing, but there were no resources available to pay for more operations. After difficult discussions it was agreed to raise the threshold for intervention, and stricter criteria were laid down as guidelines for admission onto the list, i.e. patients had to be sicker before they received treatment.

Improving the process

The process described is not meant to be a blueprint but reflects development over a period of time. Neither is it a prescriptive process for others to follow. Issues that need to be addressed include:

- more economic evaluation input (see chapter 2.6)
- greater public involvement (see chapter 8.2)
- adapting to a changing world (see chapter 6.3).

The model developed in Oxfordshire, in the UK, was driven by the market culture of the mid 1990s, and in particular the contract culture and extra-contractual referrals. The election of a new government in 1997 has brought with it changes in political philosophy as well as policy. The most important changes that affect this process are:

- *the quality agenda*, particularly the introduction of the 'National Institute for Clinical Excellence'.[1] The two dimensions of quality (see 'Dimensions of quality', chapter 5.1) being given particular attention are equity and access

- *development of the primary care role* in leading the development of health services

- *the changing structure of the health care system*; e.g. the development of the strategic role of health care authorities.[2]

Central guidelines for good practice are welcome—but questions remain about how much this can or will assist local decision making—and also about what values will underlie the guidance. For example, it is easier to calculate the cost of a QALY for a new drug than for a night-sitting service in palliative care—which is of greater value to the patient dying of cancer? What about the choice between lifestyle drugs and counselling in general practice?

Whatever national systems develop, the need remains for local systems of priority set within the context of overall guidance.

Role of public health practitioners and teams

Within the health economies and organizations, public health provides the support to take the overview across the community, and to balance external needs of local communities. This may involve balancing issues concerning community safety, or domestic violence, with needs specific to the health service, such as balancing competing hospital priorities.

The skills of needs assessment, critical appraisal, application of evidence-based care, and management of risk, which are key to public health, are all needed to develop this role.

Whatever changes occur to the structure of the health services, local clinicians will continue to make decisions on a patient-by-patient basis, guided by accepted good practice guidelines. The difficulty of balancing resources can be assisted by clear processes and common ethical values, with the development of appropriate decision making frameworks within which trade-offs can be made. To do this requires open and mature debate.

Further resources

Coulter A and Ham C (ed.) (2000). *The global challenge of health care rationing*. Open University Press, Buckingham.

Hunter D (1998). *Desperately seeking solutions*. Longman, Harlow.

International society on priorities in health care. spp3.bham.ac.uk/isociety (accessed 14 September, 2000).

Klein R (1995). Priorities and rationing: pragmatism or principles? *BMJ*, **311**, 761–2.

Klein R, Day P, and Redmayne S (1996). *Managing scarcity: priority setting and rationing in the NHS*. Open University Press, Buckingham.

Mechanic D (1995). Dilemmas in rationing health care services: the case for implicit rationing. *BMJ*, **310**, 1655–9.

New B (1999). *A good enough service—values, trade-offs and the NHS*. King's Fund and IPPR, London.

New B and LeGrand J (1996). *Rationing in the NHS: principles and pragmatism*. King's Fund, London.

Smith R (1995). Rationing: the debate we have to have. *BMJ*, **310(6981)**, 686.

Wennberg JE (1990). Outcomes research, cost containment, and the fear of health care rationing. *N Engl J Med*, **323(17)**, 1202–4.

References

1. Department of Health (1997). *The new NHS: modern, dependable*. Chapter 7: The National Institute for Clinical Excellence. Cm.3807. The Stationery Office, London. More details: www.nice.org.uk (accessed 14 September 2000).

2. Hope T, Hicks N, Reynolds DJ, Crisp R, and Griffiths S (1998). Rationing and the health authority. *BMJ*, **317**, 1067–9.

Rationing: delay, discrimination, deterrence, diversion or deflection.

Smith R (2000). *BMJ* 321, 1364.

6.2 Learning from international models of funding and delivering health care

Jennifer Dixon

Objectives

This chapter aims to help you learn about international models of health care by appreciating the three key aspects of a health system:

- the different models of *funding* health care
- the different models of *organizing and delivering* health care
- the different approaches and objectives of health care *reform*.

The best literature in these areas focuses on a few key aspects of funding and delivery, makes international comparisons, and does so in a systematic way (e.g. though organizations such as the Organization for Economic Cooperation and Development (OECD)).

Models of funding health care systems

The most useful evidence concerning international comparisons of health care funding focuses on five aspects, and compares these across nations in a systematic way:

- what is the overall *level* of funding?
- what is the *source* of the funding? (government, workplace, individual . . .)
- who actually *purchases* the health care?
- how are funds *distributed* to these purchasers?
- what are the *methods* used by these purchasers to fund the *providers*?

Overall level of funding

The overall *level* of funding is important because it gives some indication of the extent (range, quality, and volume) of health care benefits available to the population.

Health care benefits can be viewed in terms of:

- range (diversity)
- quality (see chapter 5.1)
- volume.

The level is usually expressed as the total amount of expenditure on health care as a proportion of gross domestic product (GDP), by country. If possible, distinguish between public expenditure (e.g. from taxation) and private (e.g. from private health insurance).

Even better, show the figures for *per capita* expenditure expressed in terms of 'purchasing power parity'—reflecting what the expenditure could actually purchase in each country to allow more meaningful cross-country comparisons.

Figure 6.2.1 gives an example.

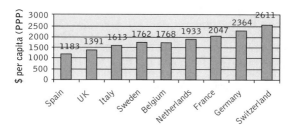

Figure 6.2.1 Total expenditure per capita PPP[†] ($) 1997. (OECD data, published 1999)[1].

Comparisons in overall health care expenditure between countries are not straightforward, because all countries have different definitions of what constitutes health care, as opposed to, for example, social care. Literature in this area should at least acknowledge this, or ideally contain broad definitions.

Source of funding

The *source* of financing is important, because it gives some indication of the extent to which the state (national or local government) can control the distribution of heath care resources, as opposed to private concerns (for example the medical insurance industry).

In Western Europe, where the state plays a major role in financing health care, the state has acted to ensure that those least well-off in society have adequate access to health care. (In the USA, the OECD country with the largest proportion of private financing of health care, over 17% of the population do not have health insurance, and access to health care is often limited.)

There are three main sources of funding health care:

• *General or local taxation.* For example, the UK National Health Service (general taxation), and Scandinavian countries (local taxation). These countries have adopted the so-called 'Beveridge' model of health care, in which the state not only finances but also

....

† PPP: 'purchasing power parity' the notion that a dollar should buy the same amount in all countries.

provides health care. The state, as in Britain, can control the distribution of resources directly. By doing so, the state can put a limit on health care expenditures in what is known as a 'global budget' and effectively limit health care expenditures. For example the level of National Health Service expenditure in the UK is set by Government, and has risen at approximately 3% in real terms per annum between 1980 and 2000.

- *Employers and employees (via compulsory taxation).* This is usually in the form of a compulsory payroll tax, for example as used in many western European countries, such as France and Germany. This is the so-called 'Bismark' or 'social insurance' model, in which the state ensures that there are tax revenues to pay for health care, and that the population has access to adequate state-sponsored health insurance, but does not necessarily provide health care through state-owned providers (hospitals may be privately owned). The state funds social insurance for those who are not employed. Since Governments set the level of compulsory tax, the total level of health care expenditure can be controlled. Since the tax is compulsory, the whole population is covered.

- *Private sources.* In most countries with a sizeable proportion of total health care expenditure coming from private sources, the bulk comes from employers who pay for private insurance on a voluntary basis for their employees. Employees usually contribute a percentage of salary towards the cost.

Most countries require users of health care to pay a user charge typically towards the cost of prescriptions, and also for consultations with physicians—this is also classified as private funding. The scope and level of expenditure on user charges is low in the UK NHS; in 1998/9 2.3% of revenue was from user charges—a figure which has changed little since 1948. Most countries use a combination of these three systems of financing.

Who purchases care, and what are the incentives?

Who purchases, and what their incentives are is important because it suggests the extent to which purchasers of care (e.g. Governments, Sickness Funds, private insurers) keep within budget and can purchase cost-effective care.

In most health care systems, the main funders of health care do not usually purchase health care directly for individuals. This is done by an intermediary using a budget devolved from the main funder, for example Sickness Funds in Germany,[2] health authorities in the UK,[3] and health maintenance organizations in the USA.[4]

The *size of budget* controlled by this purchaser is important—bigger budgets lend more purchasing clout when negotiating prices with providers. The *incentives for staying within budget* are also important—in capitated budgets for example (in which purchasers have a lump sum per year with which to purchase care for each person covered) a proportion of end of year savings are often allowed to be kept by the purchaser.[4] The *incentives on clinicians to be cost-conscious* are also crucial—clinicians who run or own purchasing organizations, such as medical groups in the USA[5] and primary care groups in the UK,[6] or who have direct financial incentives to stay within budget, have more incentives to be cost-conscious in their decision making.

How are state funds distributed to purchasers?

In publicly-funded systems, the way that resources are allocated to purchasers is important to consider because it has implications for equity, and the possibility of 'selection bias'.

Most countries allocate funds to purchasers on the basis of a capitation formula, which usually takes into account the health care needs of the population covered—the UK NHS has a very well-developed system in this respect.[7] An inaccurate formula can result in a distribution of resources away from need, and can lead purchasers (for example private insurers) to select healthy patients to cover–selection bias.[8]

> 'The NHS is funded out of public expenditure, primarily by taxation. This is a fair and efficient means for raising funds for healthcare services'.[9]

What methods are used to fund providers?

The *method of funding providers* is important because it indicates the extent to which expenditure on health care can be controlled in some way.

There are many different ways of paying providers. These include:

- *fee-for-service*. For every item of service provided to an individual patient. This method of payment is associated with relatively high growth in health care expenditures because providers have the incentive to provide more services to attract more fees. Countries using a fee-for-service method of paying providers attempt to keep costs down by fixing the level of fees paid

- *casemix*. A fixed payment is made for a package of care provided to an individual according to diagnosis, based on average costs of all patients treated with that diagnosis or related diagnosis. Payment to providers is made according a measure of 'casemix' or severity of illness—using 'diagnosis-related groups' (DRGs)* (a term used in the USA) or 'healthcare resource groups' (HRGs)* (the term used in the UK) of the patient.[10] Providers have the incentive to provide care within the fixed payment of the HRG

- *block contract*. A fixed payment is made to providers to provide care for a population of patients in a specified time period (e.g. a year), whatever the use of care. This way all risk is transferred to the providers. Some block contracts specify 'ceilings and floors' to activity outside of which the contract can be renegotiated.

These methods of paying providers are frequently combined with other features designed to prevent cost growth, and encourage the provision of cost-effective care. For example:

• utilization review, in which a third party reviews the appropriateness of services provided

• national setting of payment rates for fees paid to providers

• publication of costs charged by providers, and freedom of providers to compete for funds from purchasers. Both, in theory, stimulate providers to keep costs down.

Don't confuse the different methods of funding providers (as organizations), with the different, but related, methods of remuneration of doctors (as individuals) i.e. fee-or-service, capitation, salary.

Which method of funding is best?

This is hotly disputed. The only way to answer this question properly is to examine carefully the objectives of the health care system. If the objective is to have a high level of overall funding, the US model (in which a relatively high proportion of funding comes from the private sector) clearly is the best model. If, as is more usual, the objective is to provide comprehensive benefits to the whole population at a reasonable cost, then the 'social insurance' model (as seen in France and Germany) or the Beveridge model (as seen in the UK and Scandinavia) is the most appropriate. If the objective is to provide comprehensive benefits to the whole population *fairly* (that is on the basis of equal access for equal need regardless of ability to pay), then the Beveridge model is likely to be most appropriate. Each method has benefits and drawbacks.

Methods of delivering health care

The models and methods of *delivering* health care can be categorized using different perspectives:

• by setting

• by profession, discipline, and skill mix

• by the different mix of professions, disciplines, and skills in each setting

• by the methods and incentives by which people, and patients, move between the professionals who deliver the care, and the settings in which it happens.

Internationally, there is a wide range in the type, and relative amount, of health care facilities and staff available, and the way in which health care is delivered. Self-care, primary and community health services, secondary care, and tertiary specialist care are available in all countries, although exact definitions of these differ. Similarly the number of staff, their different roles, and the proportions working in different settings varies considerably.

Learning from the different models of care is best done by comparing four key areas:

- what is the broad distribution of resources across sectors?
- how (if at all) are people registered with a primary care service?
- what factors influence all aspects of access to secondary and specialist care?
- at what level (national, local . . .), and by what mechanisms (central planning, local markets . . .) is health care organized?

There are a huge number of areas for comparison, and the literature contains endless detail. *It is useful to focus on four key elements*:

(a) What is the broad distribution of resources across sectors?

This is important because there is an international desire to transfer resources from secondary and tertiary care to pre-hospital care (particularly primary care) where it is cost-effective and appropriate. In reality it has been difficult to achieve this aspiration because of the political power of hospitals.

(b) Are the public registered with a general practitioner/ family doctor?

In many countries, such as the UK, patients are registered with a general practitioner (GP), and generally cannot easily shop around to other GPs for care as they can for example in New Zealand or France. This is likely to increase continuity of care, ensure more cost-effective care, and allows an easier mechanism whereby GPs and their staff can be allocated a capitated budget with which to purchase care for their registered population. The incentives for GPs to keep patients well, using effective preventive measures are also enhanced. The general practitioner has a dual (and sometimes conflicting) role of being an individual patient advocate as well as a guardian of resources for his/her registered population.

(c) How does the public access secondary and specialist care?

Can the public access secondary care directly, or do they have to be referred by a general practitioner or family doctor—a 'gatekeeper'?

This is an important feature. Allowing the public direct access to specialists is unlikely to be the most cost-effective way of using health care resources for the population as a whole. However, direct access to specialists might allow individual patients more choice over their provider.

(d) To what extent is the availability of health care resources planned?

How far health care facilities are planned and co-ordinated geographically is important to maintain access to care for the population, and to avoid unnecessary duplication of expensive facilities. Even the least centrally-planned health system in the developed world—in the USA—has some influence on the volume and distribution of big capital projects.[11] In the UK, capital and staff numbers are planned centrally.

Health care reform

Demands are outstripping health care resources across the world. In response, many countries are reforming the key elements of funding and delivery mentioned above, to curb the rise in expenditures while maintaining coverage, comprehensive benefits, and quality of care. Key elements of health care reforms include:

- *increasing efficiency*. For example encouraging more cost-effective health care, by making more information available about the relative costs and effects of treatments, and giving incentives to purchasers and providers to use the information (for example through 'capitated' budgets). This can be combined with utilization review as described above

- *managing demands on health care resources better*. For example by increasing user charges, curtailing health care benefits available to the public, introducing priority scoring systems in which the most severely ill have greater access to care,[10] reducing the level of fees paid to providers, encouraging payments to providers on a 'capitated' basis, and introducing utilization reviews

- *managing public expectations*. For example by encouraging a fuller debate about the limits to health care, and health care resources.[13,14]

Summary

It is important to note that the four major powerful stakeholders in health care in each country—the government, the professions, the public, private industry—often have differing objectives for health care, and its reform. For example the medical profession is likely to be concerned with income levels of its members (e.g. the levels of fees paid, and opportunities for private practice), curbs upon its freedom to practice, and the quality of care. Governments are likely to be interested in providing adequate benefits for the population, which are fairly distributed, keeping the costs of health care down (for example by managing demand and increasing efficiency), and reducing variation of quality of care between providers. The public is interested in greater access to affordable health care, greater consumer choice, and responsiveness of providers. Employers and private insurers are interested in keeping costs down and profits up.

The reader could use any of these criteria to assess different international models of care.

The ability of any country to reform health care depends upon the relative strengths and bargaining power of each stakeholder. Given the competing objectives, and the complexity of health care, there is no model that is ideal for all. Every 'solution' is likely to create further, often unintended, problems and opportunities. Most countries therefore have shied away from, and been unable to implement, 'big bang' reform; hence, 'incremental' reform is the norm.

Further resources

Newhouse JP (1993). *Free for all? Lessons from the RAND health insurance experiment*. Harvard University Press, Cambridge MA.

World Health Organization (2000). Chapter 5, Who pays for health systems? *World Health Report 2000*. WHO, Geneva. filestore.who.int/~who/whr/2000/en/pdf/Chapter5.pdf (accessed 3 August 2000).

References

1. Organization for Economic Cooperation and Development (1999). www.oecd.org/els/health/ (accessed 21 August 2000).
2. Freeman R (2000). Social insurance systems, France and Germany. In *The politics of health in Europe*. Manchester University Press, Manchester.
3. Mays N and Dixon J (1996). *Purchaser plurality in UK health care*. King's Fund, London.
4. Robinson R and Steiner A (1998). Chapter 1: Models and techniques in managed care. In *Managed health care, US evidence and lessons for the NHS*, (ed. R Robinson and A Steiner). Open University Press, Milton Keynes.
5. Robinson JS and Casalino LR (1996). Vertical integration and organised networks in health care. *Health Affairs*, **15**, 7–22.
6. Department of Health, (1997). *The new NHS: modern, dependable*. Cm. 3807. The Stationery Office, London.
7. *Resource allocation: weighted capitation formulas 1999/2000*. The Stationery Office, London, 1997.
8. Glennerster H, Matsaganis M, and Owens P (1994). Countering the risk of biased selection. In *Implementing GP fundholding: wild card or winning hand?* (ed. H Glennerster). Oxford University Press, Oxford.
9. *The NHS Plan: a plan for investment, a plan for reform*, Principle 7. Cm. 4818-I, July 2000. HMSO, London.
10. UK Department of Health. www.doh.gov.uk/nhsexipu/strategy/archive/1992/infrastr/hrg.pdf (accessed 21 August 2000).
11. Starr P (1982). *The social transformation of American medicine*. Basic Books, New York.
12. Tudor Edwards R (1999). Points for pain: waiting list priority scoring systems. *BMJ*, **318**, 412–4.
13. Cummings J (1997). Defining core services: New Zealand experiences. *J Health Serv Res Policy*, **314**, 131–4.
14. (AJ Dunning, chairman) (1992). *Choices in health care: a report by the Government Committee on Choices in Health Care*. Ministry of Health, Welfare and Cultural Affairs, Rijswijk, The Netherlands.

6.3 **Strategic approaches to planning health care**

Philip Hadridge

Objectives

This chapter considers the latest thinking on what makes for an effective strategic planning process—in a way that seeks to demystify this whole area. The principles introduced are relevant to strategic work in all sectors and for all topics. This chapter unashamedly introduces some theory and concepts—for these are guides to planning that are designed to make a real difference.

Why is this an important public health issue?

Public health practitioners are often very well versed in the evidence on a particular topic. This knowledge needs to be coupled with skills in implementing the evidence through techniques such as strategic planning; a knowledge of effectiveness with skills in strategic planning make a powerful combination in creating effective change.

Definitions

There are many different definitions used in the planning world.[1] For the purposes of this chapter, planning is concerned with:

- developing and achieving a vision
- ensuring the values and purposes of an organization are explicit
- understanding some of the wider drivers of change
- a process that is flexible in light of these changes
- a process that is achievable in light of the resources available
- a vision that is, importantly, implementable
- a process that can be continuously reviewed as part of a learning process.

A strategy can, therefore, be defined as a methodological framework for achieving a vision in the face of changing circumstances with a finite set of resources (see chapter 7.6).

Strategic planning seeks to help a service or organization develop in a way that is in harmony with a fast-changing world/environment, at a macro level (e.g. deciding whether to close an existing hospital, or commission a new one), or at a micro level (e.g. improving the processes of patient care along a care pathway). This chapter focuses on the former—i.e. deliberate, large-scale planning interventions— though the principles introduced are relevant to all efforts seeking to bring about change.

Traditional rational planning vs. strategic planning

Traditional, rational planning is based on three deceptively simple and seductive questions:

* where are we?
* where do we want to be?
* how do we get there?

However, the problem with this approach concerns the assumptions about the predictability of the issues outside the control of the planner. The consequences are that there are at least six severely limiting features of traditional rational planning:[1,2]

* a tendency to treat the issue in question as an isolated phenomenon (cf. whole system approach)
* a dangerously narrow focus on quantitative analyses at the expense of other complementary methods (e.g. qualitative methods) that can help understand the issues
* an assumption that the future can be predicted by extrapolation
* the production of blueprints (i.e. detailed linear plans)
* a failure to acknowledge that many important issues are outside the control of the traditional planners
* an inability to cope with increasing organizational change and environmental uncertainty.

Strategic planning involves recognizing problems as they emerge, and designing processes to address them as being emergent. The importance of emergent planning is a direct response to the problems with rational planning outlined above.[3]

The characteristics of emergent planning include:

* recognizing that change is inevitable and necessary
* having a clear vision based on explicit and shared values
* acknowledging and embracing uncertainty, and designing systems and processes accordingly
* acknowledging the value of creativity and lateral thinking as well as quantitative analysis
* valuing participation with all those involved in the funding, delivery, and receipt of service (funders, technical, users).

Principles for a successful planning process

The following principles should be checked:

* the problem identified
* the people involved
* the process used
* the resources available.

Get the problem, the people, and the process right

Three elements are essential in any strategic planning process:

* ensure the right question or dilemma is the focus of a planning initiative
* ensure the right people are in the team (see below)
* ensure it is a learning process that helps key players debate things that matter.

When we are given the opportunity to see our world (and our biases) afresh, we can develop new ideas and commitment for action.[4,5] It needs to be a learning process both for individuals and for organizations. It is rarely possible to be sure of all the issues or questions at the start of a specific project. It is often necessary to tailor the planning methods in light of initial investigations. The modern planner needs to be able to redesign the process continually in a way that moves the whole process forward, without feeling that it is undesirable to change one's mind. Focus on strategic direction and modify tactics along the way.

Who should lead and who should be involved in the planning?

In large complex systems (such as health care) in which many people have a strong interest, a centralized steering group should be established. It is important that this group leads, commissions, oversees, and manages an *inclusive* process—it should lead the process, not seek to second-guess the ideas of colleagues (see chapter 7.1). Many different internal and external stakeholders are involved in most planning problems. These people need to be genuinely involved. A poorly-designed process that excludes a few key stakeholders will almost undoubtedly slow the overall process, if not stop it completely.

There are two important risks here that must be addressed. They both refer to poor early involvement of others:

1. It may appear that early involvement of many people will slow the process down. This is common. Do not be tempted to rush this part of the process. The basic tenet of 'participative' planning is that the time spent in participation speeds implementation.

2. This involvement needs to be planned carefully if others are to feel the planning exercise is meaningful and worthy of their best efforts and energy.

What are the resources available?

The effort put into the planning processes will be determined by the size of the problem and the resources available. It is essential to match the size of the problem with the resources that are going to be used to address it. This is crucial both in the planning *and* in any implementation phase (see chapter 8.4).

Strategic planning is a learning process

Strategic planning puts a great emphasis on the process of learning as an integral part of the planning process. Table 6.3.1 highlights the comparisons. If your organization is not in or moving toward the right column there is a very real chance that your efforts will come to nothing.

Table 6.3.1 The changing nature of strategic planning.

Planning as a *traditional* process	Planning as a *learning* process
Main value is the plan of analysis and action	Main value is in the process of generating the plan of analysis and action
The value is in the product	The value is in both the process and the product
Quantitative analysis is given more prominence than ideas	Ideas are as prominent as numbers
Assumptions about the future are not raised or questioned	Assumptions about future are explicit and questioned
The role of executives is to delegate the planning to planners	The role of planners is to facilitate the strategic thinking of executives
A single person generates the plan	People who need to own (and ultimately implement) the plan are all genuinely involved
The plan is an instrument for budgeting and contracting	The plan is an instrument for turning a vision into reality

Summary

A more chaotic and unpredictable world needs planning approaches to match.

Modern strategic planning processes need to be . . .

* *emergent*
* *participative*
* *learning*

. . . avoiding assumptions, hierarchies, and an over-reliance on any one particular analytical technique. The methods used need to be open and shared and flexible in accordance with the learning which is an integral and beneficial part of the process.

The planning approach adopted by an organization is an intervention that is influenced, and influences, the culture of the whole organization, health care system, or community. It is best considered as an organizational development technique, a learning opportunity, rather than a rational fix.

Health care organizations that adopt and adapt modern planning processes identify real issues and problems, generate the right vision, involve the right people and processes, and ultimately survive, develop, and deliver.

References

1. Whittington R (1993). *What is strategy and does it matter?* Routledge, London.
2. van der Heijden K (1996). *Scenarios: the art of strategic conversation.* Wiley, Chichester.
3. Mintzberg H (1994). *The rise and fall of strategic planning.* Prentice Hall, Hemel Hempstead.
4. de Geus AP (1986). Planning as learning. *Harvard Business Review*, **66(2)**, 70–4.
5. Senge P (1991). *The fifth discipline.* Doubleday, New York.

6.4 Commissioning health care: general principles

Nick Payne

Objectives

After reading this chapter you should understand the general principles of commissioning health care.

Definitions

In this chapter the word 'commissioning' is used to mean a process by which those responsible for the planning and organization of health care come to a clearly-defined agreement with the providers to ensure that services for a defined population and a defined clinical area are available. (The terms 'contracting' and 'commissioning' are often used synonymously. However, it is generally understood that commissioning represents a less adversarial, more collaborative process, with less implied competition between health care providers.)

Background

To some extent health care has always been 'commissioned'. In the UK, this process became established on an institutional rather than an individual-to-individual basis with, for example, the establishment of the Poor Law in 1601, by which local parishes arranged for the provision of residential 'hospital' care. The National Health Insurance Act of 1911 established the commissioning of primary care services by the state from general practitioners for groups of patients (usually working males). Those commissioning these services set out some statement of *what sort of care* should be provided *for whom*.

Health care systems around the world have always contained elements that are directly managed and elements that are commissioned. For instance, when the National Health Service was established in the UK in 1948, hospitals and community health services were largely provided on a directly managed basis. Conversely, primary care services (family doctors, dentists, opticians, pharmacists) were provided by independent contractors who entered into contractual arrangements with a local body who commissioned these areas of health care.

During the last 20 years of the twentieth century, however, many Western countries instituted changes in their health care systems that moved commissioning centre stage, making the process much more explicit. Drawing on the example and analysis from the private industrial sector, it was postulated that a division between health care 'purchaser' and health care 'provider' would:

• increase quality

• drive down costs.

The belief was that this would lead to greater efficiency or cost-effectiveness. Competition between providers and the power of the market were assumed to be the agents by which these changes would occur. In Britain, the suggestions made by the American economist, Alan Enthoven,[1,2] were taken up by the government of the time and incorporated in the series of changes set up following the publication in 1989 of the UK government's White Paper *Working for patients*.[3]

Local health authorities no longer directly managed hospitals and community health services, but were expected to purchase/commission these services from providers. These providers (e.g. hospitals and community units) were allowed to develop an independent status as *Trusts*. The public health objectives were that the local health authorities would be responsible for assessing need (see chapter 1.5), and then commissioning care from those best able to provide the quantity and quality of health care service necessary. This was the 'internal market', which was supposed to lead to greater efficiency, with money following the patients to pay for their care.

Although a new government came to power in 1997 with the commitment to end the internal market, many elements remained. Provider trusts were still fundamentally independent of the health authorities, services were 'commissioned' not 'purchased' and, although primary care fundholding was abolished, there are now specific primary care organizations ('Primary Care Groups' and 'Primary Care Trusts') whose responsibilities are to:

• provide care

• commission care

• collaborate with other agencies to promote health.

These are taking over the health care commissioning functions of the health authorities for all except a minority of specialized services (see chapter 6.5).

Provision of health care by commissioning services, as opposed to direct management, while to some an appealing idea, was never formally evaluated on a prospective basis. There is no clear binary distinction between a commissioned health care system and a directly managed one. To some extent each in practice is comprised of features of the other. There is a complex relationship between the use of markets in health care and the consequences in terms of process and outcome. The advantages can be that many implicit assumptions are made explicit and that the objectives of the system can be made absolutely clear. However, markets in health care often fail to deliver the expected benefits for the following reasons:

- the consumers, whether the patients or their advocate (the doctor), rarely have all the relevant information to hand (lack of true 'consumer sovereignty')

- there is rarely an easy choice to be made between two local comparable providers

- it is only in highly commercial health care systems that it is politically acceptable to let health care providers collapse due to market forces.

However, the commissioning or purchasing process does tend to ensure that some of the important stages in planning health care services are clearly defined. In theory it does allow for a better relationship between what is needed and what is provided, helping to ensure that it is the needs of the population, rather than simply the aspirations of the providers, that determine health care provision.

Assessing the needs of the population

Commissioning health care begins with the assessment of need (chapter 1.5). The most difficult part of such as assessment is deciding exactly which individuals or sub-populations require a given type and level of health care within the available resources (chapters 2.6 and 6.1). What should be commissioned can be determined by an epidemiologically-based needs assessment. This assesses the:

- size of the underlying population

- incidence or prevalence of the disease status concerned

- effectiveness of the interventions available

- relative cost-effectiveness of those interventions

- prioritization process that maximizes health gain across the population as a whole.

In practice, many of these key sources of information are unavailable. Therefore, the needs assessment process often has to move away from this ideal approach. Two other methods can be used:[4]

- comparing what is already in place with what is provided elsewhere in the country and attempting to redress any obvious mismatches (comparative needs assessment)

- taking advice on the population's health needs from expert and lay groups (corporate needs assessment).

Given that almost no health care area begins with a clean slate of zero provision, that all the information is rarely available for the epidemiological approach, that experts and lay groups will always tend to make their views heard, and that comparisons are always likely to be drawn, in practice, a combination of needs assessment methods is almost always used.

Involving the right staff and skills in commissioning

The commissioning process requires a broad range of skills and experience. Genuine team work is essential (see chapter 8.1). Sometimes these can all be embodied in one person, but this is rare, and usually a team-based multi-disciplinary process works best. The key skills are listed in Table 6.4.1.

Table 6.4.1 Skills, people and tasks needed in commissioning health care services.

Skill	Person or discipline	Tasks
Epidemiological	Epidemiologist, public health practitioner	To use data (e.g. mortality, demographic, surveys, case registers); To analyse these data to determine the actual and potential health problems in the population
Health technology assessment	Health economist, public health practitioner	To evaluate critically the (cost)-effectiveness of health care interventions; To highlight gaps in information where further research is needed
Negotiation and conflict management	NHS manager, all members	To negotiate skilfully, matching what the commissioner believes is required and the provider wishes to offer
Financial	Accountant, NHS manager	To handle complex finances (services are rarely costed comprehensively and in a way that readily allows comparison)
Clinical	Public health clinician, GP, specialist clinician, nurse	To understand the specialist clinical aspects of the services being offered and provided. (Beware: like any input, specialist clinical advice can be biased—more general clinical advice, for example from primary care practitioners is often equally or more important)
Experience of the wider health system	NHS manager, public health practitioner	To appreciate how the individual services fit in with the wider health care provision of the locality or region—experience and understanding of the wider health service is essential
Information	Information specialist, operational research, epidemiologist	To understand health information systems (information systems are complex and not always designed specifically to serve the commissioning process); To understand issues such as casemix measurement, relationships between casemix, costs and prices; To understand how the provision of health care should be matched to predictions of need

Establishing the formal agreement or contract

Commissioning health care can be done informally with unwritten agreements between commissioner and provider, or using only minutes of meetings as a record of decisions taken and agreements reached. More usually, however, there is some form of written contract, which sets out the nature and scope of care to be provided. These will need to be contracts in the legal sense if commissioner and provider are from separate organizations.

There are at least six issues that should be covered in a contract:

(a) Who? (who is entering into the contract?)

Parties entering into the contract—for example, 'The contract is between the North West Health Care, 'Any Locality Commissioning Group' and 'Bethesda Hospital' for the provision of unplanned (emergency) and elective orthopaedic surgery services'.

(b) What? (a general descriptive statement of overall process)

General statement describing the services to be provided and the duration of the contract. This could be quite specific, e.g. unilateral cataract surgery for 100 named patients. Alternatively, and perhaps more usually, it will cover a whole area of care such as emergency and elective general medical services, nursing services, etc.

(c) How much care? (the *quantity* of health care commissioned)

Measures of activity and provision of information about the *quantity* of health care to be provided. It is, however, an important component particularly because it provides an opportunity to agree and document key components of the health care service and is often used, in addition, to describe the limits of what is and is not included in the services to be commissioned.

(d) How good? (the *quality* of health care commissioned)

(see chapter 5.1)

Measures of quality and specifications should be to agreed quality standards. This should include specifications for the process of audit and clinical governance. It is difficult to be prescriptive about what should be included in this service specification section, but six examples illustrate the sort of topics that can (and often should) be addressed:

• is the service for elective, emergency, or both types of care?

- how is the population service described—is it those registered with the authority, those who are subscribed to a particular health insurer, those living in a defined area, those who simply present as emergencies at an emergency room?

- how is the access secured—by referral from another doctor only or by patient self-referral?

- what are the major elements of the service?—for example coronary artery surgery, valve replacement, and cardiac transplantation in cardiac surgery?

- are there specific agreements about certain elements—for example about which implants to use in hip and knee replacement surgery; first line drugs to be used in the management of schizophrenia; x% of cataract operations to be performed as day cases; use of cholinergic-agonist treatment in Alzheimer's Disease should only be in the context of an agreed national clinical trial?

- where should services be provided?—e.g. should there be outreach clinics from the main hospital to community hospitals or primary care centres?

(e) How much money? (funding details)

Payment arrangements need to be agreed carefully. In addition, there needs to be an agreed process regarding the action that would be taken if the quantity or quality of the service differs from agreed limits. Contracts can be 'block'—with an amount payable for the provision of a service irrespective of, for example, numbers of patients treated. Conversely contracts can be 'cost per case' with payment linked strictly to the activity provided at full cost. In between are 'cost and volume' contracts, where an overall payment is made but under- or over-activity results in adjustment to payment at a lower (marginal) cost rather than at full (unit) cost.

(f) What if? (arbitration arrangements)

Arbitration arrangements in event of the parties concerned failing to reach agreement about the delivery of the contract.

New health care service developments

Contractual arrangements often allude to the objectives for the service over an agreed period of time (e.g. next two or three years). This is particularly important with any agreed procedure for dealing with new service developments. This may be part of the commissioning documentation or may be separate. Commissioners of health care usually find themselves being asked to commission new developments such as new diagnostic and/or therapeutic procedures (e.g. new screening tests, diagnostic services, pharmaceuticals, operations, etc.).

Specialist clinicians are usually well aware of new developments in their particular clinical area and often press for the introduction before adequate objective evidence is available of their effectiveness and cost-effectiveness.

Commissioners need an established mechanism for assessing new service developments. The mininum information that should be sought is:

- a clear description of the intervention (including intended population and outcome)
- an assessment of the size of the population that would benefit
- a critical assessment of the effectiveness.

(See chapter 5.3.)

Problems and hazards of commissioning

The issues below should be used as a check-list of issues to be addressed in discussions between commissioners and providers:

- there is often a gap between what is commissioned and what is actually delivered. Targets for quantity, quality, and efficacy can be set but not achieved—there can even be a gap between what the providers agree to do and what their clinicians actually do in practice
- while it is relatively easy to determine the quantity of what is provided overall, its quality is harder to assess. The efficiency and effectiveness of the care provided is relatively easy to investigate for a small number of interventions, but hard to address for the totality of care within an average contract. Moreover, the casemix of interventions actually provided may not match with what was intended. Casemix is a measure of the variety and scope of interventions provided—thus, for example, surgical care might in practice include more complex and time-consuming procedures than the mix the commissioner of the service was expecting. Conversely, there might be a financial incentive, in a block contract, to carry out less expensive procedures. Even in a casemix-adjusted, cost per case contract there is an incentive to re-code procedures into ones that have a higher price. Thus, although careful contract monitoring is likely to be required, it is perhaps even more important to develop a good level of trust between commissioner and provider
- even if the casemix was what was intended, commissioners may need to ask if it is being delivered to the population for whom it

was intended? Health care services have a habit of being used most by those living close to where they are available and to affluent middle-class groups at the expense of the underprivileged

- finally, even if all these problems are addressed, and perhaps especially if they are, there are transaction costs associated with commissioning services, which can be substantial. There is little evidence to suggest that a commissioner/provider arrangement is either more efficient than other systems, or that it alone is capable of making substantial changes to health care delivery.

Conclusion

Commissioning of health care services is not a new process in any health care system: it has been in operation for as long as health systems have existed. There is, moreover, no absolutely clear distinction between commissioning and direct management and, in most health systems, each contains elements of the other. Commissioning health care is not an exact science and needs a variety of different skills and disciplines. The important skills are to combine an epidemiological approach with a practical understanding of the comparative and corporate approaches to assessing need. With this as a firm foundation, make every decision and agreement as specific as possible, using all the negotiating skills of the team.

Further resources

Øvretveit J (1994). *Purchasing for health: a multidisciplinary introduction to the theory and practice of health purchasing.* Open University Press, Buckingham.

Muir Gray JA (1997). *Evidence-based health care.* Churchill Livingstone, London.

Rosnick M (1998). Building public health goals into the purchasing process: managed care perspective. *Am J Preventive Med*, **14**, 78–83.

Stevens A and Raftery J (1994). *Health care needs assessment.* Radcliffe Medical Press, Oxford.

Stevens A and Raftery J (1997). *Health care needs assessment: second series.* Radcliffe Medical Press, Oxford.

References

1. Enthoven A (1985). *Reflections of the management of the National Health Service.* Nuffield Provincial Hospitals Trust, London.
2. Enthoven A (1989). NHS review, words from the source: an interview with Alan Enthoven. *BMJ*, **298**, 1166–8.

3. UK Department of Health (1989). *Working for patients*. Department of Health, London.

4. National Health Service Management Executive (1991). *Assessing health care need*. Department of Health, London.

6.5 **Commissioning health care: specialized services**

Caron Grainger

Objectives

This chapter will help you organize and influence commissioning arrangements for small numbers of patients with more complex needs.

Background

Many health services around the world are responsible for commissioning services on behalf of their resident population. Although many routine health care services can be commissioned with only moderate public health input, specialized services need the application of many public health skills to make the process work well. Specialized services are usually provided by a small number of providers and usually serve multiple commissioners. The public health consequences of this may be that unnecessary inequalities in commissioning arrangements develop between commissioners—patients will receive different levels of treatment or access to treatment depending on where they live: classic geographical inequity.

To overcome some of these difficulties, commissioning arrangements for specialized services need to be *collaborative*, with multiple commissioning organizations working together to assess need and contract for services.

Defining specialized services

There is no one agreed definition of specialized services, but they all tend to exhibit some or all of the following characteristics:

(a) Commissioning for a very large population

The population on behalf of which you are commissioning is much larger than that of a single commissioning organization. This is because patient numbers are *small* and *often unpredictable*, and a *critical mass* is required at each centre to ensure:

- optimum outcomes for patients (e.g. sustained training and clinical competence for specialized staff)
- optimum use of resources (e.g. to ensure cost-effectiveness of provision, making the best use of scarce resources including clinical expertise, high technology equipment, donor organs, etc. e.g. cardiac surgery services.)

(b) Commissioning for rapidly-developing high technology services

Services develop very quickly, and often involve high technology, where research and development need to be supported, and where the introduction of new technologies need to be managed (e.g. bone marrow transplantation services). In these situations, note that the evidence for effectiveness is often emerging rather than established, making commissioning decisions on the basis of complete evidence difficult.

(c) Commissioning services with prominent ethical dimensions

High profile ethical issues, for example around equity of access, require commissioners of health care to balance the high cost needs of the minority against the needs of the majority e.g. the use of recombinant blood products for patients with haemophilia, secure psychiatric facilities (see chapter 2.8).

(d) Commissioning collectively

Occasionally, it makes logistical sense to commission high volume, low cost services on a collective basis, simply because, for example, there is only one local provider, strategic re-configuration is required, or there are issues around the standardization of clinical care. Such services are unlikely to exhibit the above characteristics.

Levels of commissioning for specialized services

The key to effective commissioning of specialized services is the population base necessary to plan services appropriately. This depends on three factors:

- the incidence and/or prevalence of a condition
- the number of providers
- issues concerning geographical access.

Commissioning organizations therefore need to work together to purchase specialized services in the most effective manner, with some services commissioned by a single body, others by three or four, and yet others by a dozen or so organizations. The following levels of commissioning can work effectively:

- *population base 15 million plus.* These are a very small number of extremely specialized services affecting perhaps 5–10 people per million population. They include such services as treatment of choriocarcinoma, and major cranio-facial surgery. In the UK, these services are commissioned through the National Specialist Commissioning Advisory Group (NSCAG)
- *population base 5–10 million.* Again a relatively small number of services, affecting perhaps 30–100 people per million population.

Examples include bone marrow transplant services, haemophilia services, spinal injury services, and medium and high secure psychiatric services

• *population base 1–2 million.* For some of these conditions, incidence will be low, but because of the chronicity of the condition, prevalence will be quite high, leading to a relatively large pool of patients requiring ongoing treatment. Such services include renal replacement therapy (incidence approximately 80 per million population, prevalence approximately 400 per million population). Other services in this category have a relatively high incidence but patients come into contact with the service on a single/occasional basis only. Examples include cardiac surgery (incidence 600–800 per million population), plastic surgery, and burns services

• *population base ¼–½ million.* Services here fall into two main categories:

  • rare but subject to rationing e.g. gender reassignment services, tertiary infertility services

  • more common but requiring specialized treatment e.g. eating disorder services.

Understanding the essential stages

The strategic element

This work involves up to six steps:

1. Agreeing the most appropriate arrangements for commissioning specialized services on the basis of population need and service configuration (the 'level of commissioning' identified above).

2. Prioritizing developments, both within specialized services, and between specialized services and the general portfolio of services. This needs to consider:

   • multiple high-cost advances in specialized services that must be balanced against the need for development in other, less specialized areas

   • the consequential effects of changes both within specialized services and within more general services e.g. access to cardiac angiography and catheterization will result in increased referrals for cardiac surgery; access to transplantation requires long-term follow-up of patients.

3. Ensuring that service development takes place within a framework that allows provider stability and maintenance of the research and education/training base within the provider unit.

4. Managing risk across organizations (see Box 6.5.1).

5. Ensuring commissioning arrangements are open and transparent and lines of accountability are clear.

6. Ensuring appropriate performance management and review of the commissioning of specialized services.

Box 6.5.1 **Managing and sharing risk with specialized services**

A very important reason for the collective commissioning of specialized services is sharing risk. This is because of the small numbers and relative unpredictability (both across time and geography) of patients requiring these services.

There are three major types of risk involved:

1. *Financial risk*, shared in three main ways:

   - within a single service, across multiple commissioners. Each commissioner shares a proportion of the costs involved in treating a patient, irrespective of where the patient lives. This is effectively an insurance policy arrangement, resulting in a fairly predictable premium for all commissioners rather than an infrequent high cost for an individual commissioner. Most specialized services commissioners share risk in this way

   - across multiple services, within a single organization, where either a commissioner or a provider offsets potential high costs in one area against other more predictable areas within the same organization. This is often a short-term response to problems and is generally neither desirable nor appropriate long term. It may also be contrary to financial guidance on cross-subsidization

   - across time. This involves regular payments, sometimes called subscriptions, to a fund that over a given period of time will finance an infrequent event, which is predicted to occur within the time-frame. Unfortunately it is not possible to predict when in the time-frame the event will occur, which may result in surpluses when activity is low and insufficient funds to meet the costs when activity exceeds plan.

2. *Clinical quality risk*—ensuring a critical mass of patients are treated in one area, maintaining clinical expertise, allowing for appropriate audit and comparison of outcomes, etc.

3. *Organizational risk*—preventing the destabilization of a small number of providers with consequences for the research and development base and training base, resulting in fewer scientific advances in an area, or lack of appropriately-trained staff to deliver operational service.

The operational element

Those involved in the operational level need the following skill/professional bases—public health, finance, commissioning, information, clinical, plus access to experts in research and development, training, and education. In addition staff will need to be skilled in involving users in the planning of services (see Figure. 6.5.1).

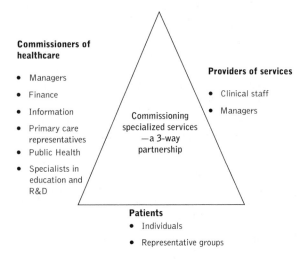

Commissioners of healthcare

- Managers
- Finance
- Information
- Primary care representatives
- Public Health
- Specialists in education and R&D

Commissioning specialized services —a 3-way partnership

Providers of services

- Clinical staff
- Managers

Patients
- Individuals
- Representative groups

Figure 6.5.1 Who is involved in specialized commissioning?

The following functions are required:

(i)   assessment of need (including a service review) (see chapter 1.5)

(ii) commissioning and the performance management of the services

(iii) appropriate user involvement (see chapter 8.2)

(iv) appropriate clinical involvement

(v)   business planning (see chapter 8.4).

More details of each of these operational steps are set out below. Note that many of the elements of commissioning specialized services overlap with each other and with work in more generic fields.

(i) The assessment of need (including a service review)
This involves:

• assessing needs, based on both quantitative approaches (epidemiological, comparative, and corporate) and, if appropriate, more qualitative approaches, considering both met and unmet need. It may also involve complex modelling to predict alterations in the pool due to changing incidence or survival among the affected population (e.g. patients with end stage renal disease)

- reviewing current provider performance and clinical outcome, and, where appropriate, comparing it with national or international outcomes (audit, performance management, and quality assurance/ clinical governance processes)

- reviewing, where possible, the evidence base for interventions, including evidence of clinical and organizational effectiveness, and, where appropriate and possible, cost-effectiveness

- reviewing training, educational, and R&D needs to ensure future provision of the service can be planned for, and to ensure that other staff have some knowledge of specialized services

- ensuring appropriate quality standards/assurance arrangements are in place.

(See chapter 1.5.)

(ii) Commissioning and the performance management of the services

This involves commissioners and providers agreeing:

- levels of activity
- quality standards for care
- plans for service development, including training, development, and R&D work
- mechanisms for monitoring of the services through routinely collected and specially collected (e.g. audit) data, and agreeing the process and frequency of monitoring arrangements
- a contract reflecting all these details.

(See chapter 6.4.)

(iii) Appropriate user involvement

Patients come into contact with specialized services through two main routes:

1. They live with a long-term disorder requiring ongoing medical care. Patients in this group may:

   - have an in-depth knowledge and expertise of their condition
   - be involved in active patient groups, sometimes with considerable lobbying power
   - be abreast of new developments in the treatment of their illness
   - have multiple members of the family affected.

   (Examples include haemophilia, renal replacement therapy, spinal injuries, and specialized mental health services such as secure psychiatric services.)

2. They require short-term access to specialized services, often as part of a more general service. Care must however be seamless. (Examples of these types of specialized services would include bone marrow transplant, the management of high risk pregnancy, specialized pathology services, specialized services for infectious diseases such as drug resistant TB or viral haemorhagic fevers, specialized cardiology/cardiac surgery.)

(See chapter 8.2.)

(iv) Appropriate clinical involvement

1. *Specialized providers.* Given the nature of specialized services, most expertise rests with providers of services, not commissioners of services. Any decisions related to the planning of services, prioritizing developments within services, etc. will therefore need especially close involvement of clinical staff. In addition, clinical staff are sure to provide an early alert mechanism for major clinical advances that will impact on the service. Commissioners will need to find the most appropriate mechanisms to access this expertise.

2. *Primary care.* It is important to involve primary care professionals in commissioning decisions about specialized services when possible, because the long term care of the patient ultimately rests here.

(v) Business planning

It is important to work within an appropriate business planning process known to both commissioners and providers of services. This is important for identifying:

- the timetable for reporting and reviewing services
- changes to the specialized services portfolio
- clinical/service developments
- clinical advice to commissioning decisions

(See chapter 8.4.)

Summary: principles and pitfalls for commissioning specialized services

Principles

- commissioning should be based on need and be, as far as possible, evidence-based
- patients with equal need should have equal access to treatment
- providers should have a secure financial base, enabling them to develop both the appropriate research and development infrastructure, and a training and education base

- provision should be as cost-effective as possible
- commissioning should take place as close to the patient as possible, but within a strategic framework
- clinical staff and patients need to be genuinely engaged in the commissioning process.

Pitfalls

- large-scale risks—especially financial, staffing, and infrastructure
- destabilization of providers with knock-on consequences for training, research, and development
- high profile media interest
- 'postcode' purchasing
- managing the introduction of new and expensive technologies
- rationing debate can destabilize rational decision making
- political interest in commissioning decisions
- lack of evidence base for making rational commissioning decisions
- difficulty in defining and monitoring these services.

Further resources

Black N (1997). Commissioning specialist services in the NHS. *BMJ*, **315**, 1323–4.

Ham C and Donaldson LJ (1996). Population-centered and patient-focused purchasing: the UK experience. Maintaining excellence: the preservation and development of specialized services. *Milbank Quarterly*, **74**, 191–214.

6.6 Improving the health care system: overview

Nicholas Hicks

Objectives

This chapter will help you to:

• assess the potential for improving the quality of health services
• plan and implement such improvements
• identify and use a contextually appropriate set of tools and methods.

Why is this important to public health practice?

The practice of public health

Improving the health of populations requires:

• an understanding of the determinants of health
• an understanding of which determinants you/your team/your organization can influence
• an understanding of the effective methods for doing this.

As a public health practitioner, you will not make much of an impact on the health of populations if you spend your professional career trying to influence determinants of health for which there are no effective interventions. Nor will you have much impact on the public's health if you spend your time trying to tackle determinants of health over which you (or the organization for which you work) have no influence.

By contrast, you do have a responsibility to use effective interventions to improve those determinants of health for which you (or your organization) have direct responsibility and influence. For the many public health practitioners who work in or with services, that means we have a responsibility to make the health care system as effective a determinant of health as possible.

Health care is a determinant of health

As is made clear throughout this handbook, there are many determinants of health which have nothing to do with health care and health services. Health care itself is an important and often underestimated determinant of health.[1] Many developed countries, including the USA, Australia, and the UK, have experienced dramatic (30–50%) reductions in age-specific mortality from coronary heart disease in the past two decades. About half of this mortality reduction is attributable to health care and half to changes in exposure to risk factors (e.g. smoking, physical inactivity, elevated serum cholesterol). In addition, there are other very good reasons why health care is an important area for public health practice:

- the persistent documentation of widespread variations in clinical practice and the imperfect reflection of research results in practice imply that there is considerable potential to improve health gains for individuals and populations

- medical errors are common and lead to much avoidable ill-health and expense[2] (see chapter 5.1)

- the quantity and accessibility of valid, relevant evidence about effective health care interventions is increasing rapidly (huge advances in information technology and management allow the rapid delivery of relevant and usable evidence in ways that were unimaginable 20 years ago) (see chapters 2.3–2.5)

- the last 20 years have seen the development and application of methods for improving organization and interpretation of evidence (e.g. the development of the science of systematic review, and the recognition of the role of evidence-based medicine/health care)

- research has led to a more sophisticated understanding of how to influence professional behaviour (individually and institutionally) (see chapters 6.9 and 6.10)

- there is an increasing public expectation that nations' substantial investments in health care should deliver good value (where value is defined as improvements in health per pound spent)

- there is a professional acceptance that clinicians and institutions should be held accountable for the quality and effectiveness of the services they provide (see chapter 6.8).

The improving understanding of the scientific basis of medicine, the potential for improving practice, a knowledge of how to intervene, and a political mandate to act, mean that public health practitioners who have responsibility for, or work within, a health care service have a huge opportunity to make a real difference to the health of individuals and communities.

Three key principles

Whenever you are faced with improving the quality of health care it is helpful to remember three key principles:

(a) improving the quality of health care implies change

(b) health care quality is multi-dimensional

(c) health care quality is the product of individuals working with the right attitudes in the right systems and organizations.

(a) Improving quality implies change

Improving quality of care implies *change* in a way that is not implied by the phrases 'assessing quality' and 'assuring quality'. You need to be *practical and driven by results.* Beautifully written plans, theoretical perfection, elegant presentations, publication in high quality journals are not enough if there are no improvements in the quality of service that individuals and population receive.

(b) Quality of care is multi-dimensional

There are many facets/dimensions of quality of care. These dimensions can be conceived and classified in many different ways. A practical classification that has proved enduring was first proposed by Robert Maxwell in 1984[3] and revisited in 1992.[4] He originally identified the following dimensions of quality (see chapter 5.1):

* effectiveness
* efficiency
* acceptability
* access
* equity
* relevance.

It is important to be clear which attributes of quality matter most especially to those who *use* the services and to those who *pay* for the services (the two groups to whom, ultimately, public health practitioners in this sector are accountable). Although you may often be right in your assumptions about the relative importance of different dimensions of quality, it is important to test these assumptions with others.

(c) Health care is the product of systems

The quality of health care depends not only on the *quality of interaction between clinician and patient* but also on the *quality of organization and management of the environment/institution* in which care is delivered. Most health care problems are due to bad systems of care rather than to bad individuals. Too often, the public only receive high quality care because excellent clinicians practise well *despite* the system. Your aim should be to create systems in which a range of clinicians can deliver excellent care *because* of the system.

An important implication is that the greatest improvements come from changing systems rather than by changing within systems. Always examine the system of care and not just the performance of individuals within it.

Starting the process—competencies and tools

Arm yourself with a systematic approach. There are many to choose from, but few are as practical and well-tested as that proposed by Langley *et al.*[5] and recommended by Don Berwick.[6]

First ask, and get agreement, to the following three questions:

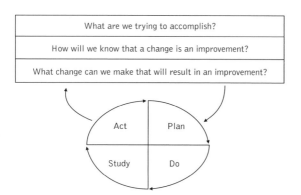

| What are we trying to accomplish? |
| How will we know that a change is an improvement? |
| What change can we make that will result in an improvement? |

Figure 6.6.1 Framework for improving the system. (Taken, with permission from the BMJ, from Berwick[6])

1. *What are we trying to accomplish*? (remember Maxwell.)

2. *How will we know that a change is an improvement*? (defining specific measures of success will help clarify what's really important as well as provide you with a tool for monitoring change.)

3. *What change can we make that will result in improvement*? (be receptive to ideas derived from experts, from science, from experience, and from theory.)

Now embark on and test the ideas in practice. Do so by actively learning and reflecting on the consequences of your actions, and those of your team.

Competencies

If you are to be successful you will need to be able to harness a range of competencies. Very few people possess all the necessary competencies themselves. To be successful you should recognize the importance of each of them, be able to identify the competencies that others possess, and be able to harness those competencies through team work (see chapter 8.1).

You will (through your own efforts and those of others) need to:

• *create a culture* where quality matters; in which everyone has a shared and passionate commitment to the pursuit of quality

• *motivate* those who deliver and manage clinical services to want to improve (and to recognize that things can always be better than they are)

- *be bold and ambitious*—ask 'What should this service be like from a patient's perspective?' and encourage people to think how this could be possible, not just what the difficulties might be

- *challenge the status quo*

- *focus on the needs and want of those who use the services*—patients, families, communities. Make a grid from either Maxwell's dimensions of quality[3,4] and/or Donabedian's classic structure–process–outcome approach[7] to health care evaluation, and map the potential actions on these grids

- *set specific aims* and make sure that the *whole team understands and supports* these aims. If you are not explicit, it's very likely that different groups—nurses, doctors, managers, porters, and others—will be pulling in different directions

- demonstrate *technical competence*. This includes the ability to measure relevant aspects of quality and to apply an understanding of how to influence the behaviour of individuals and organizations

- *harness relevant resources*—including energy, skill, time, tools, and money. (Improving quality often requires some early investment but can often reduce costs in the long run)

- apply good *organization and people skills*. Identify shared goals and claim the moral high ground—the reason for change is to improve the health of individuals and the public. Remind people of the specific agreed aims if they begin to create new barriers

- *don't let the best be the enemy of the good*. If you wait until you have a plan for perfection you will never begin

- get *senior and powerful commitment* to change

- *be analytical*. Make a diagnosis of specific barriers to change. Identify all the relevant stakeholders. Consider who might be winners and losers (and hence supporters or antagonists). Can you make more people winners? How will you answer the 'What's in it for me?' or 'Is it really worth the effort?' questions?

- *plan* how to get round the barriers and use all the *practical tools for changing the performance of a clinical system* (see below).

Tools

Here is a check-list of practical tools that you can use to change the performance of clinical systems:

(i) Develop your personal qualities

- leadership skills (see chapter 7.1)

- knowledge

- attitudes

- role model (enthusiasm, past success, etc.).

(ii) Understand and use the organization

Understand its:

* structure and management—especially the methods of performance management
* culture
* incentives and sanctions
* distribution of power (both formal and informal), including the agenda of those with power.

(iii) Harness and co-ordinate mechanisms specifically aimed at improving the quality of team and individual performance

Such as:

* audit and feedback
* education and continuing professional development
* clinical decision support systems e.g. prompts and reminders
* guidelines (see chapter 6.10)

(iv) Genuinely involve the public and patients

* increase public knowledge and expectations
* increase patient knowledge
* listen to patient groups (and arrange for other members of the team to hear what they have to say)
* involve users in defining the aims for the service
* show the public how things are improving (or not)
* make special efforts to hear the views of those least likely to offer them—the elderly, the frail, those with limited access, those with learning disabilities, the illiterate. You will often be surprised at the new and relevant insights that they bring. Use every mechanism available to involve the user perspective (e.g. a patient advocacy liaison service (PALS)[8]).

(See chapter 8.2.)

Being an external change agent

Often, as a public health practitioner, you will not be part of the team responsible for delivering care. You may have been invited in or (more threateningly, sent in) to improve a service. Once you have helped to create the improvements you will leave to tackle another problem.

You will have failed if the improvements evaporate after you leave. You should aim to have created a system of *continuous improvement*. If you are successful then not only will the improvements you helped to create be sustainable, but they will also be the foundation for further improvement.

In practice that means you must have (or develop) some other skills, competencies, and qualities that are not necessarily required of those left providing the service. These include:

- the *self-confidence* to give others the credit (even when you think the credit should be yours) and to take the blame (even when it is not your fault): acting as an external scapegoat can be a valuable social role that can help teams to function better

- the ability to identify a *product champion* who can lead and sustain change once you have gone.

Finally, don't be afraid to *celebrate success*. Most people enjoy favourable publicity. Recognition and success breed further success. Publicizing good practice is not just self-glorification, it's good public health practice: if you have improved the health of your local population by improving the quality of care in an innovative way, you can multiply the public health benefits by helping others learn from and emulate your success.

References

1. Bunker JP (1995). Medicine matters after all. *J Roy Coll Phys London*, **29**, 105–12.
2. Kohn LT, Corrigan JM, and Donaldson MS (ed.) (2000). *To err is human: building a safer health system*. National Academy Press, Washington DC.
3. Maxwell RJ (1984). Quality assessment in health. *BMJ*, **288**, 1470–2.
4. Maxwell RJ (1992). Dimensions of quality revisited: from thought to action. *Quality in Health Care*, **1**, 171–7.
5. Langley GJ, Nolan KM, and Nolan TW (1992). *The foundation of improvement*. ABI Publishing, Silver Spring MD.
6. Berwick DM (1996). A primer on leading the improvement of systems. *BMJ*, **312**, 619–22.
7. Donabedian A (1980). *The definition of quality and approaches to its assessment*. Health Administration Press, Ann Arbor MI.
8. *The NHS Plan: A plan for investment, a plan for reform*. Cm. 4818-I, July 2000. HMSO, London.

6.7 Promoting equity in health care

Anna Donald

Definitions

Promoting equity involves minimizing inequity. Inequity means a difference (inequality) which is unfair. Promoting equity is centrally involved with promoting social justice: a foundation of all public health activities around the world. This chapter is concerned with *minimizing unfair inequalities in health care*. These are defined as differences in the distribution of health care goods and services for people with the same health need. Note:

• it is important to distinguish inequalities in health care from the larger issue of inequalities in health, to which inequalities in care contribute

• typically, socially marginal and economically deprived groups have the greatest overall need for health care but are least able to obtain it—e.g. because they are poor or cannot speak the dominant language, described by Tudor Hart as the 'inverse care law' (Box 6.7.1). Other groups may be independently affected, however, such as by age, sex, and geography

• strictly equal provision of goods and services *per capita* results in inequitable distribution according to health needs, because some sub-populations have systematically greater needs for health care

• the words 'inequality' and 'inequity' are often used interchangeably. However: *inequality* is a broader term, meaning 'unequal' or a 'difference in size, degree or circumstances'[1] *inequity* is a more specific and moral term, meaning 'lack of fairness or justice'.[1]

> Box 6.7.1 **The inverse care law**
>
> 'The availability of good medical care tends to vary inversely with the need for it in the population served.'[2]

Why are inequalities in health care an important public health issue?

Reducing inequalities and promoting equity in health care is one of the most important political imperatives in many countries today. Unequal health care is important because it reinforces poverty, causes social injustice, and increases overall rates of morbidity and mortality. For example, in the USA, access to physicians by low-income children can vary by almost 200% depending on which state they live in.[3] Reducing inequality in health care, however, is in everyone's interest, rich and poor alike, as those creating Britain's National Health Service recognized. Inequality in health care is usually associated with considerable administrative and political costs, as well as social ones. For example, the USA spends about 33% of its health budget on administrative costs, due to the large billing apparatus needed in a multi-payer system, compared with Britain's 10%. The spectre of drug-resistant infectious disease, such as tuberculosis, also makes accessible health care desirable for the whole population, not just the poor.

What are the main causes of inequalities in health care?

Inequalities in health care can result from several factors, including:

(a) Unequal distribution of health care resources

Unequal distribution of health care resources either results from unequal resource allocation at the level of central planning (more typical in single-payer systems[†] such as those of the UK or France) or from unequal coverage of people (more typical of multi-payer systems, such as that of the USA). At a global level, the main cause of inequalities in health care is the way in which health care systems are financed and regulated. Not surprisingly, health systems that mandate universal coverage regardless of income tend to have more equal health care in all respects than those that do not mandate universal coverage. Even in single-payer systems, however, services and staff tend to become unequally distributed in the absence of policy to ensure location in less desirable areas. For example, Australia and the UK have long had policies to ensure that health professionals practise in rural and poorer areas, as well as in urban and wealthy areas. Family doctor services, as well as specialist cancer and surgical centres, are not evenly distributed in the UK, due to weak enforcement of policy designed after World War II to ensure more equitable distribution.[4]

(b) Unequal access to care

Access should be considered as an integral part of the health care 'package' rather than extraneous to it. For example, services that can be reached only by car; through the dominant language; or by filling in forms, usually reduce access for more deprived groups.

....

† Single-payer health systems are those where one actor—usually the government—purchases health care on behalf of the whole population.

(c) Different treatment of different groups with the same health need

This may result from:

- ignorance and poor training (for example under-treating women with heart disease) or active discrimination against a particular group, either embedded in policy (for example, women in Afghanistan under the Taliban) or due to individual prejudice

- different perceptions and preferences of care by different social groups[5] (for example, some migrant groups' preferences for traditional medicines over Western ones).

Identifying and assessing inequalities in health care

Identifying and assessing inequalities in health care can be achieved by comparing expected use of health care based on health needs assessment with actual use of health care. The four steps of assessing health inequality are:

(a) measuring health need

(b) measuring service use

(c) measuring health care supply

(d) appreciating health care demand.

(a) Measuring health need

Health needs can be assessed using routine or specialized survey instruments (see chapter 1.1). Where information is plentiful, health needs assessment can specify levels of disease and population subgroup. If information is sparse and difficult to obtain (for example, in countries that do not collect routine health statistics), needs assessment can be simpler, using estimates of death rates standardized roughly by age and broad disease category.

(b) Measuring service use

Actual use of health care can be measured in several ways, including routine statistics, specialized surveys, and stratified sampling of a common 'basket' of procedures. Linking service use to social groups of interest (for example, people with low income) may need additional data or routinely collected proxy measures, such as zip-code/postcode.[6] If resources are scarce, it may be possible to confine assessment to a few, key goods and services. Many countries have their own indicators of poor quality and use of health care use. Common indicators include: higher rates of hysterectomy and tonsillectomy; lower rates of treatment for high blood pressure; elective hip replacement, coronary artery bypass operations, child immunization, and breast and cervical cancer screening. Utilization statistics often need to be reformulated (or even re-collected) to reflect service use per capita of defined populations, rather than service use per clinic.

(c) Measuring health care supply

In assessing equality of health care, it can help to get a summary, graphic overview of roughly who gets how much. The curve in Figure 6.7.1 (Lorenz curve[‡]) helps to measure equity of *supply* of health

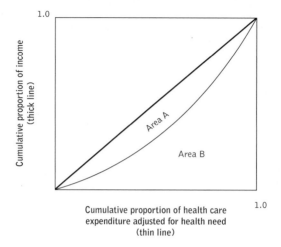

Figure 6.7.1 Lorenz curve for displaying the distribution of health care expenditure by income group.

care. The straight line represents an equal health care expenditure across the five quintiles of the population (e.g. quintiles by income) (see sample data in Table 6.7.1). The degree of unequal distribution of health care expenditure can be represented by the size of area A. A health-related 'Gini' coefficient[§] can be calculated as the proportion of the total area A+B made up by area A. The larger A/(A+B) (a value between 0 and 1) , the more unequal the resource distribution.

....

‡ A Lorenz curve is a graph on which the cumulative percentage of some variable (e.g. income or health care expenditure) is plotted against the cumulative percentage of the corresponding population (ranked in increasing size of share). The extent to which the curve sags below a straight diagonal line indicates the degree of inequality of distribution. (M Lorenz— American statistician, b. 1876.)[1]

§ A Gini coefficient is a measure of how dispersed (or unequal) is a set of values (e.g. income distribution, health care expenditure, etc.) in a specified population. The value is derived from a Lorenz curve, as shown in Figure. 6.7.1. (C Gini—Italian demographer and economist, b. 1884.)—see Last.

(The techniques can be extended to control for the greater need that is associated with poorer income groups—see Goddard and Smith 1998.[7]) More details concerning Lorenz curves can be found in Stilgitz.[8]

(d) Appreciating health care demand

Measuring inequalities in use of care should also take into account *demand*-side factors—people's preferences and perceptions of health care. Further measures that may help to define these include measures of patient preferences and perceptions of treatment.[9]

Table 6.7.1 Example of data needed to draw a Lorenz curve and calculate a Gini coefficient.

Quintile	Income (as percentage of total population income)	Cumulative population	Cumulative income
1st	5	20	5
2nd	10	40	15
3rd	18	60	33
4th	26	80	59
5th	41	100	100
	100		

Addressing inequalities in health care

(a) General measures

Generic steps in planning include:

- identify the size and nature of the problem and what might be causing it (see above)
- prioritize potential solutions according to:
  - severity of the inequality and disease burden it places on the under-served population
  - resources available
  - feasibility of solutions
- set realistic time scales. Some may involve staggered programmes or policies that take years or even generations to see to fruition, particularly if the programme's immediate impact is on children or young health professionals (for example, see Rabinowitz *et al.*[10])
- identify potential political (and other) barriers. If reform is politically contentious, then it can help to present it differently to make it more palatable. For example, fluoridating water (a good way to improve poorer people's dental care) can be presented as

'clean teeth for all' (which is, of course, true—just more true for the poor!).

(b) Specific measures

Specific strategies are likely to vary depending on the level at which you are working. Often, solutions for unequal distribution of regional or national resources lie at a macro-policy level, but more piecemeal solutions can be effective in addressing inequalities arising from biases in particular services.

- whatever level you are working at, *make equality of care according to need an explicit policy criterion*. For example, against such a criterion, hospital closure policies would need to be assessed for how they affect overall equality of access to services

- develop measurable outcomes of equitable health care distribution and access, monitor them (either continuously or sporadically) on a population (rather than service**) basis, and use them to performance manage health services

- identify and address individual or systematic prejudice against particular groups. This may involve changes to legislation, guidelines, political mobilization, helplines, simple anonymous feedback forms, ombudsmen, media, or educational programmes

- provide policies, incentives, and regulations to ensure that health workers and services are distributed according to health need. For example, ensure that health commissioners for different areas (who tend to serve different social groups) are required to purchase care according to health need rather than according to other criteria that will tend to bias care away from those who need it most

- save time and money by replacing political 'horse-trading' arrangements (whereby political representatives vie for health resources for their area according to political favour) with explicit allocation formulae that weight resource allocation according to health need (for example, by age, sex, geography; particularly for expensive conditions, such as HIV infection)

- provide better access to services for those who need them most. For example, it might be possible to improve public transport or translation services; to relocate services or provide 'satellite' clinics (including in supermarkets, schools, public malls and the

....

** The problem with basing outcomes on service use, rather than per head of a defined population, is that you end up without a denominator for estimating service use *rates*. That is, the figures do not mean anything. For example, if one hospital has 10 operations and another has 25, it is impossible to say much about distribution of operations across the population unless you know how many people in total (the population denominator) were being served by both hospitals.

like), and to provide opportunistic health care at times conveni-
ent to clients (for example, using a community nurse's routine
home visit for a new baby to give influenza vaccine to an elderly
relative)

• similarly, ensure that the treatment-at-point-of-use is the same
for people with similar health needs. For example, alert health
workers to under-served groups or adapt treatments for easier use
(for example, providing tablets in easy-to-open bottles or in once-
daily doses instead of in multiple doses for the frail elderly, or providing instructions in the patient's own language)

• empower under-served groups to demand the care they need.
Empowerment could involve media campaigns to ensure that
under-served populations are aware of services and their rights of
access (for example, antenatal and immunisation services);
collaboration with advocacy groups and distribution of health
information with routine information (for example, local council
leaflets, electricity bills, supermarket receipts, or newspapers).

Measuring success in addressing inequalities in health care

There are many ways of measuring the gap and how it might be
changing. Ideally, use several measures at the same time ('triangu-
late'), ensuring they make sense in the context you are working in.
They do not all need to be quantitative; qualitative data can say a lot
about the distribution of health care. Examples of measurement
include:

• mapping the distribution of health care activity (for example
clinics, doctors, or procedures for conditions that are more common in poorer groups, such as coronary bypass surgery) against a
map of income distribution (for example electoral wards). Does
density of activity correspond to density of decreasing income?
Or, at the very least, is health care activity evenly spread, with a
bias towards being more dense in poorer areas?

• comparing quality of care indicators for different groups. What
is the distribution of failed hip replacements? Peri-operative
deaths? Readmission rates for operations? Waiting times for heart
surgery?

• describing and comparing premises in different areas. What are
waiting rooms and building maintenance like in different sectors
of the community?

• critical incident/exception reporting. How often do rare, serious
events, such as maternal mortality, deaths for minor operations,
or anaphylaxis in people known to be allergic to a drug, happen in
different sections of the community?

If some of these measures are designated important criteria, measured, and followed over time, then you are performing an 'equity audit', like any other audit. This can help you communicate what you are doing to others as well as keep track of how the situation is changing around you. Clearly the change and your interventions may be unrelated, but the importance of serial measurements should not be underestimated. If nothing else, the high profile you give this can keep it high on the political agenda, an important outcome in itself.

Health and health care

It should be noted that addressing inequalities in health care is unlikely to redress completely inequalities in *health*. It is difficult to calculate how much health care inequalities contribute overall to inequalities in health, particularly as causal factors interrelate. Nonetheless, more general measures, such as improving education, employment, and housing, usually predict health outcomes more strongly than most health interventions. They are likely to have larger effects on health outcomes because they can dramatically affect the incidence of disease onset and death rather than affecting the course of disease once it has begun.[11]

Further resources

Acheson D (1998). *Independent inquiry into inequalities in health report*. The Stationery Office, London.

Benzeval M, Judge K, and Whitehead M (1995). *Tackling inequalities in health—an agenda for action*. King's Fund, London.

Bulletin of World Health Organization 2000, **78**(1), 1–152. Special theme issue: Inequalities in health.

Jacobson B, Smith A, and Whitehead M (1988). *The nation's health. a strategy for the 1990s*. King's Fund, London.

Macintyre S (2000). Modernising the NHS: prevention and the reduction of health inequalities. *BMJ*, **320**(7246), 1399–400.

Povertynet. World Bank resources on inequality, poverty, and socio-economic performance. www.worldbank.org/poverty/inequal/index.htm (accessed 28 August 2000).

Saving lives: our healthier nation. (White Paper). The Stationery Office, London, 1999. Available at www.ohn.gov.uk (accessed 14 September 2000).

Shaw M, Dorling D, Gordon D, and Davey Smith G (1999). The widening gap: health inequalities and policy in Britain. The Policy Press, Bristol.

The NHS Plan: a plan for investment; a plan for reform, Chapter 13: Improving health and reducing inequality, Cm. 4818-I. July 2000. HMSO, London.

References

1. *The new Oxford dictionary of English*. Oxford University Press, Oxford, 1998.
2. Tudor Hart J (1971). The inverse care law. *Lancet*, **696**, 405–12.
3. Long SH and Marquis MS (1999). Geographic variation in physician visits for uninsured children. *JAMA*, **281**, 2035–40.

4. Benzeval M and Judge K (1996). Access to health care in England: continuing inequalities in the distribution of GPs. *J Publ Hlth Med*, **18**, 33–44.

5. Le Grand J (1984). Equity as an economic objective. *J Appl Phil*, **1**, 39–51.

6. Danesh J, Gault S, Semmence J, Appleby P, and Peto R (1999). Postcodes as useful markers of social class: population based study in 26000 British households. *BMJ*, **318**, 843–5.

7. Goddard M and Smith P (1998). *Equity of access to health care*. University of York, Centre for Health Economics, York.

8. Stiglitz JE (1993). *Economics*. W.W. Norton and Co., New York.

9. Pencheon D (1998). Matching demand and supply fairly and efficiently. *BMJ*, **316**, 1665–7.

10. Rabinowitz HK, Diamond JJ, Markham FW, and Hazelwood CE (1999). A program to increase the number of family physicians in rural and underserved areas. *JAMA*, **281**, 255–60.

11. Wilkinson R (1996). In *Health and social organization: towards a health policy for the 21st century*, (ed. D Blane, E Brunner, and R Wilkinson), pp. 109–22. Routledge, London.

6.8 Governance and accountability

Cameron Bowie

Objectives

By reading this chapter you will be better able to appreciate:

- the ways professional health staff are accountable for their actions
- the limitations of the concept of individual responsibility in modern health care
- how health institutions use systems of governance to safeguard the quality of services they provide
- how a public health practitioner can influence the quality of health care provided to a population.

Definitions and issues involved

A useful definition of clinical governance is 'the means by which organizations ensure the provision of quality clinical care by making individuals accountable for setting, maintaining, and monitoring performance standards'.

The essence of accountability is 'the identification and acceptance of the role and responsibility of each clinician and manager'.

A *clinician* is responsible for providing individual patient care of high quality and being able to demonstrate this by setting and monitoring acceptable standards. This will require joint standard setting and monitoring where care is provided by more than one clinician.

A *health institution* is responsible for:

- providing services of high quality
- demonstrating this by setting and monitoring standards of the systems set up to provide the services
- ensuring that clinicians deployed by the institution are fulfilling their individual responsibilities.

Why is this an important public health issue?

Public health practitioners, especially those with a clinical background, are well placed to develop a clear understanding of the interactions between clinicians and institutions in the pursuit of quality care. The identification of systems and incentives to monitor and constantly improve the quality of care is an essential role for public health practitioners working in health care settings. Assurance is one of the three key public health tasks identified by the Institute of Medicine.[1]

The challenges of promoting accountability, responsibility, and governance

Delivering clinical care is complex. There are five specific challenges that need to be addressed in creating a system with the necessary mechanisms and incentives to maintain quality:

(a) applying population-based evidence to individual patients

(b) managing the multi-disciplinary nature of modern clinical care

(c) empowering clinicians in a receptive environment

(d) coping with the changing nature of professional practice

(e) maintaining openness.

(a) The professional application of population-based evidence to individuals within a limited budget

Clinical care has features distinct from financial and other service industries that demand a particular approach to governance. Its relative complexity is because:

- the needs of each patient are different and often multiple, requiring individual professional assessment and intervention. Although good evidence must come from populations, it has, ultimately, to be applied to individuals with individual needs

- the social, economic, and biological context of each patient results in variable outcomes requiring sophisticated approaches to evaluation

- technology and medical science are changing increasingly rapidly, requiring up-to-date clinicians and their teams to be highly responsive to new evidence and new approaches to service provision

- resources are limited, requiring judgements about their most effective and efficient use.

The consequence of these features, with respect to quality and accountability, is that specialist professionals at the point of service delivery, and not the managers, are the ones who know what standards are possible, how they can be measured, and what changes in practice are possible to make improvements. Indeed, top-down standard setting does not seem to work in health care without strenuous efforts made to persuade clinicians of their appropriateness.[2] Bottom-up standard setting is more likely to encourage ownership. However, clinicians need to earn the right to set their standards by making them realistic, open, and likely to achieve continual improvement. Top-down standard setting very rarely has an impact as an isolated intervention.

(b) The multi-disciplinary nature of modern clinical care

It is rare for one individual clinician to satisfy the health needs of a patient. Usually an array of people and services are needed. Each individual clinician is responsible for contributing to high quality teamwork.[3] The institution providing the service has a *corporate* responsibility of ensuring that the system of service provision is well organized and of high quality despite the usual resource constraints.

The consequence is that in health care organizations both the individual and the institution have separate and complementary responsibilities for ensuring the quality of clinical care. The clinical governance responsibilities of institutions in many systems have not, until recently, been delineated. This changed in the UK with the 1999 Health Act, which included clause 13(1): *'It is the duty of each Primary Care Trust, and each NHS trust, to put and keep in place arrangements for the purpose of monitoring and improving the quality of health care which it provides to individuals'*.

There is now for the first time in the UK a *statutory duty* not only to maintain quality but to have in place adequate processes for continually improving it:

- individual clinical virtuosity is important but not sufficient; good teamwork is paramount
- there is a *corporate* duty to maintain and improve quality
- this duty can be statutory.

Both staff and institution will need to be able to demonstrate the reasonableness of the standards set, the monitoring arrangements used, and actions taken to remedy poor quality provision. Medical specialization is so developed that for some aspects of care clinicians can only assess themselves by comparing their performance to that of colleagues from other institutions. Professionals will be expected to participate in internal and external peer review.[4] Comparison with the mean is not going to be sufficient; comparison with the best possible will be increasingly the norm. Internal audit by itself is insufficient—some external audit is also required.

(c) Empowering clinicians in a receptive environment

The challenge for management is to empower clinicians with full-time clinical responsibilities, helping them to feel more, not less responsible for providing quality care. This means promoting a supportive culture, and not one where name, blame, and shame are the methods of dealing with under-performance. In so doing, the role of management changes from a passive to an active partner in the delivery of the quality component of care. Managers must be as interested in *quality* of care as they are in *quantity and cost* (see chapter 6.6).

(d) The changing nature of professional practice

The social environment in which health professionals work is changing with profound effect on the nature of clinical practice.[5,6] Patients demand more say in decisions about their own care and have their own perceptions of reality in a postmodern environment.[7] Staff must be encouraged to address these issues through continuing professional development programmes. Professional autonomy and clinical freedom are in retreat: patients are demanding empowerment not paternalism.

(e) Maintaining openness

The public is demanding more openness. Professional organizations are responding hesitantly. Complaints about health care increase by the decibel. Staff tend to adopt defensive postures to criticism. Governments are determined that standards in their national health services rise. This conflict between professional protectionism and public scepticism requires an appropriate response from health care organizations. What is required is an environment in which self-criticism is possible because professional confidence is high.

To create such an environment health organizations will need to:
- empower clinicians
- encourage team work and collaborative standard setting
- develop shared information to monitor standards
- use an appropriate mix of incentives and sanctions
- respond to consumer criticism in a positive way
- help clinicians respond to the changing social environment
- be open about the real risks of health care.

How to respond to these challenges

A public health practitioner will encourage clinical colleagues and managers to develop clinical governance methods that are sensitive to these complexities as well as setting the highest standards individually.

The building blocks of clinical governance

There are five essential building blocks of clinical governance:[8]
- *clinical effectiveness* (knowing what works)
- *clinical audit* (making sure what is agreed is actually done, with quality criteria and standards)
- *risk management* (appreciating the risks and benefits of every decision)
- *quality assurance* (being explicit about errors, criteria, and standards, and having processes in place to deal with them)
- *organizational and staff development* (acknowledging the most important resource of the organization).

The role of the public health practitioner

There are four important areas within health care systems that require public health practitioners to contribute to the accountability process for clinical quality.

* health programmes
* inter-sectoral services
* whole health system
* statutory and formal responsibilities of a clinical nature.

Remember that this role involves both standard setting *and* the monitoring of performance against these standards:

Health programmes

There are three particular sorts of health programmes where public health practitioners have a special responsible to promote accountability for quality:

(i) Disease programmes

Where patient care is provided by different health care organizations, although each one is responsible for ensuring individual standards are set and monitored, the public health authority is responsible for ensuring that the standards set by the various organizations involved are compatible, coherent, and where necessary jointly agreed. There may be standards of organizational quality such as a 'seamless' service to users and carers that will be the prime responsibility of the authority to set and monitor. Examples include diabetes, hypertension, maternity, cancer care, and severe mental illness.

(ii) Screening programmes

Screening programmes, such as breast cancer, neo-natal, cervical cancer, and child health screening, will require the setting of local standards in health districts, in collaboration with the involved clinicians (see chapter 4.7).

(iii) Preventive programmes

There are a number of preventive programmes that are the primary responsibility of the health authority. Examples are accident prevention, vaccination and immunization, alcohol and drug education, anti-smoking campaigns, and nutrition and good parenting programmes.

Inter-sectoral services

Many patient services are dependent on organizations outside the health service. Public health practitioners are often responsible for establishing and monitoring common standards with these other organizations. Examples include:

* welfare/social services for child protection and mental health

- the criminal justice system for prisoners' health problems such as AIDS and drug addiction
- local government services concerning housing and environmental health.

Health systems

There are many ways in which standards are set and maintained in a health care system if it is to provide and be assured of quality care, notably information systems, where the data provide evidence of the quality of care. There is always debate about the value of routinely-collected data for quality control purposes (see chapter 5.2). Systematized, ongoing long-term data collection to allow casemix, intervention, and outcome analysis is the ideal. However, focused *ad hoc* studies addressing specific issues can often be more cost-effective.

Statutory and formal public health responsibilities

There will always be critical public health functions that need epidemiological and public health skills:

- infectious disease control
- environmental hazard investigation
- emergency planning.

Not only will you need to set appropriate standards and measure your performance against them, but you will need to demonstrate the rigour of the process and outcome, often under stressful conditions (e.g. in front of the media).

How will you know if you have been successful?

You will know when you are being successful in promoting accountability, responsibility, and governance when:

- your health care providers address the most important clinical quality issues using technically sound clinical governance methods in an open and self-critical way
- your public health authority has joint audits with a wide range of welfare agencies and health care providers, looking at jointly identified and agreed problems
- you participate in a regular public health department clinical governance programme with documentary evidence of results and actions agreed in response to findings
- you have improved on Shakespeare. 'Yet I can make my audit up' *Coriolanus*, Act 1, Scene 1.

Further resources

Allen P (2000). Clinical governance in primary care: accountability for clinical governance: developing collective responsibility for quality in primary care. *BMJ*, **321**, 608–11.

Black N (1998). Clinical governance: fine words or action? *BMJ*, **316**, 297–8.

Dawson S, Garside P, and Moss F (ed.) (1998). Organisational change: the key to quality improvement. *Quality in Health Care*, (7) **Supplement**.

Donaldson LJ (1998). Clinical governance: a statutory duty for quality improvement. *J Epidemiol Community Health*, **52**, 73–4.

Huntington J, Gillam S, and Rosen R (2000). Clinical governance in primary care: organisational development for clinical governance. *BMJ*, **321**, 679–82.

Lugon M and Scally G (ed.) (2000). *Clinical Governance Bulletin.* Royal Society of Medicine Press. www.roysocmed.ac.uk/pub/cgb.htm (accessed 10 September 2000).

McColl A and Roland M (2000). Clinical governance in primary care: knowledge and information for clinical governance. *BMJ*, **321**, 871–4.

Millenson ML (1997). *Demanding medical excellence: doctors and accountability in the information age.* Chicago University Press, Chicago.

Pringle M (2000). Clinical governance in primary care: participating in clinical governance. *BMJ*, **321**, 737–40.

Scally G and Donaldson LJ (1998). The NHS's 50 anniversary. Clinical governance and the drive for quality improvement in the new NHS in England. *BMJ*, **317**, 61–5.

The European Foundation for Quality Management (EFQM). www.efqm.org/ (accessed 22 August 2000).

Walshe K and Dineen M (1998). *Clinical risk management; making a difference?* The NHS Confederation, Birmingham. www.nhsconfed.net/ (accessed 22 August 2000).

References

1. Institute of Medicine (IOM) (1988) *The future of public health*, and IOM Health Communities (1996) *New partnerships for the future of public health*, both available from www.nap.edu (accessed 22 August 2000).

2. *The new NHS Charter—a different approach (Report on the new NHS Charter by Greg Dyke.)* UK Department of Health, December 1998. www.doh.gov.uk/charter.htm (accessed 14 May 2001).

3. General Medical Council, London (1998). *Maintaining good medical practice.* www.gmc-uk.org/standard/good/good.htm (accessed 22 August 2000).

4. Treasure T (1998). Lessons from the Bristol case. *BMJ*, **316**, 1685–6.

5. Freidson E (1989). *Medical work in America.* (Essays on health care.) Yale University Press, Newhaven CT.

6. Krause E (1996). *Death of the guilds: professions, states, and the advance of capitalism, 1930 to the present.* Yale University Press, Newhaven CT.

7. Muir Gray JA (1999). Postmodern medicine. *Lancet*, **354**, 1550–3.

8. *Clinical Governance in the London Region.* www.doh.gov.uk/ntro/links.htm (accessed 22 August 2000).

6.9 Improving the use of evidence in practice

Jeremy Grimshaw, Jeanette Ward, and
Martin Eccles

Objectives

By reading this chapter, you will be able to:

- identify opportunities for research transfer in clinical and public health settings
- apply a systematic approach to research transfer, including the selection of evidence-based strategies to promote professional behaviour change.

Key concepts

'Evidence based medicine should be complemented by evidence based implementation.'[1]

- public health practitioners are well placed to facilitate the implementation of research findings
- these strategies are intended to encourage clinicians to change their own clinical practice in line with research evidence
- research in this area has generated knowledge about effective strategies to change clinical practice
- evidence from this research should inform research transfer.

Why is research transfer an important public health responsibility?

There is an increasing evidence base to inform both clinical and public health practice. However, the findings of clinical and public health research will not change population outcomes unless health services and health care professionals adopt them in practice. Information overload, pressures of work in health care systems, and other factors can result in mismatches between important research findings and delivered care (Box 6.9.1). As a result, the potential benefits of research based health care are not achieved. Public health practitioners are well placed to promote the use of evidence in practice because they are often involved in setting local health care strategies and they have been trained in the methodological tools to critically appraise research evidence and to assess the quality of care. The population perspective, paramount in public health, suggests that research transfer is a public health responsibility.

Box 6.9.1 **Examples of failure in research transfer**[2,3]

A range of different interventions have been shown to improve survival following myocardial infarction, however the median proportion of eligible patients in 11 European countries receiving appropriate management was:

- thrombolysis 36% (range 13–52%)
- beta-blockers 46% (range 31–77%)
- aspirin 87% (range 72–94%).

A systematic approach to research transfer

A systematic approach is needed if the potential benefits of research are to be maximized. This will be facilitated if the health care system and local health care organizations value evidence-based approaches and continuous quality improvement.

There are three interrelated stages to promote research transfer:

- identifying and prioritizing problems for research transfer
- developing an implementation plan for research transfer
- monitoring the impact of research transfer.

Whilst these stages represent a logical, ordered approach, in practice they can overlap or occur contemporaneously.

Identifying and prioritizing problems for research transfer

Problems with research transfer may often become apparent when:

- population health surveillance reveals poor outcomes
- critical incident analysis reveals more general problems
- stakeholder or professional opinion perceives a gap between evidence and current practice
- the publication of new evidence, systematic reviews, or guidelines identifies opportunities for improving current performance.

Problems with research transfer are likely to be complex and multi-faceted. Typically, there are limited resources for interventions to promote research transfer. Therefore, the problems need to be prioritized by an explicit process which considers the following questions:

- what are the variations in outcome?
- what are the explanations for the variations?
- could research transfer achieve better population outcomes?
- where is the maximal health gain most likely if research transfer is effective?

- how does the clinical topic fit with other local or national priorities?
- is there momentum or vehicle for local initiatives to enhance research transfer?

The prioritization process should identify a limited and achievable number of topics for research transfer at the local level. Once prioritized, public health practitioners proceed with a systematic approach to each topic.

Developing a plan for research transfer

(i) Creating local coalitions for action

Research transfer requires co-ordinated action by a range of local organizations and health care professionals at national and local levels. Creation of a local multi-disciplinary coalition of stakeholders will support this process. Creative thinking with due attention to local politics, power-bases, and champions for innovation is critical.

(ii) Developing local evidence messages

Research evidence is usually not presented in a format that is easily accessible to professionals. It is usually necessary to synthesize and translate research findings into a simple format (for example, an evidence-based guideline). Local health care organizations and individual professionals are unlikely to have the necessary skills or resources required for rigorous guideline development. As a result, it is preferable to identify and adapt existing systematic reviews or valid guidelines. This local adaptation process should involve a multi-disciplinary group (with adequate technical and administrative support) (Box 6.9.2).

Box 6.9.2 **Example of multi-disciplinary group for microscopic haematuria referral guidelines**

- general practitioners
- urologist
- nephrologist
- anaesthetist
- theatre nurse
- specialist nurse
- public health specialist
- manager
- patient representative.

Identifying barriers and facilitators to change

It is important to identify local barriers and facilitators to inform the choice of implementation strategies. Within any individual setting, there are likely to be a number of different barriers and facilitators operating at different levels (Box 6.9.3). Individual professionals in any target group may vary in their preparedness for change and face different barriers and facilitators. Different 'segments' in the target group may be identified and may need different implementation approaches. A variety of methods can be used to elicit information about barriers, ranging from informal discussions with key professionals to representative surveys and focus groups.

> ### Box 6.9.3 **Where are the barriers to evidence based practice?**
>
> * within *the health care system*—e.g. if the method of reimbursement provides perverse incentives to professionals
> * within *the health care organization*—e.g. if there is an inappropriate skill mix or if the organizational culture does not encourage innovation
> * within *local professional peer groups*—e.g. if the desired behaviour change is counter to prevailing norms and attitudes
> * within *individual professionals*—e.g. if individual professionals lack knowledge about research findings or skills to perform a procedure
> * within *professional–patient consultations*—e.g. within busy consultations, professionals may overlook important items of care.

Choosing strategies

There is an emerging evidence base to help you select a suitable strategy for research transfer (Box 6.9.4). There are 'no magic bullets'; most interventions are effective under some circumstances, but none are effective under all circumstances. Passive dissemination strategies (such as educational materials or mailing guidelines) are generally ineffective and should not be solely relied on. Active approaches are more likely to be effective. Multifaceted interventions targeting different barriers to change are likely to be more effective (but more costly) than single interventions.

At present there is little empirical evidence to guide the choice of intervention when faced with specific barriers and facilitators. However, in general, the choice of strategy should reflect: the current evidence of its effectiveness; the perceived barriers (Box 6.9.3); the

Box 6.9.4 **Findings from implementation research**[4,5]

(a) Generally ineffective strategies

- didactic educational activities
- distribution of educational materials (including guidelines).

(b) Strategies of variable effectiveness

- audit and feedback
- local consensus process (e.g. developing local guidelines)
- local opinion leaders
- patient-mediated interventions.

(c) Generally effective strategies

- educational outreach visits or academic detailing
- reminders (manual or computerized)
- interactive educational workshops
- multifaceted interventions.

available resources for its implementation, and practical considerations—for example:

- political interventions resulting in macro health reform may be necessary if the barriers relate to the health care *system*
- specific organizational interventions may be necessary if the barriers relate to the local health care *organization*
- social influence approaches (local consensus processes, educational outreach, opinion leaders, marketing, etc.) may be useful when barriers relate to local *professional peer groups*
- audit and feedback may be useful when health care professionals are unaware of sub-optimal practice and to reinforce change
- educational approaches may be useful where barriers relate to health care professionals' knowledge, skills, and attitudes. In general, interactive educational activities are more likely to lead to research transfer. Passive dissemination approaches (e.g. mailing guidelines to target professionals) are unlikely to lead to changes in behaviour by themselves but may be useful for raising awareness of the desired behaviour change
- reminders and patient-mediated interventions when barriers relate to information processing within consultations

• evidence about the effectiveness of different interventions is being synthesized by the Cochrane Effective Practice and Organization of Care group (Box 6.9.5).

Box 6.9.5 **Cochrane Effective Practice and Organisation of Care group[6]**

This international group aims to undertake systematic reviews of the effects of:

• professional interventions (e.g. continuing medical education, quality assurance strategies)

• organizational interventions (e.g. professional substitution)

• financial interventions (e.g. reimbursement mechanisms)

• regulatory interventions (e.g. statutory requirements).

(Reviews and the specialized register are published in the Cochrane Library.[7])

Research transfer requires adequate resources for the development of local evidence messages and implementation activities. Decision makers may need to adopt less than optimal implementation strategies in the face of limited resources (for example, interventions addressing a limited number of barriers or groups of professionals). In these cases, public health practitioners are encouraged to adopt a population perspective. Even low rates of participation with implementation strategies may result in small changes in behaviour sufficient to shift a population outcome. Even if only a third of GPs adopted a systematic approach to smoking cessation advice, the resulting numbers of successful quitters would have a substantive public health impact.

Furthermore, research transfer may not incur substantial additional costs if existing structures can be harnessed to support it. For example, quality improvement departments within hospitals, primary care, and community-based organizations may include individuals with appropriate technical skills to support local guideline development and implementation. Existing postgraduate educational mechanisms can be exploited to support dissemination and implementation activities.

Evaluating impact

Ultimately, it is changes in the population outcome of interest which will vindicate a planned approach to research transfer. To guide implementation decisions, however, performance indicators can be developed to monitor progress. Thus, process and outcome indicators can be used together.

Key issues

As in any emerging discipline, the evidence base for research transfer is as yet patchy and often of uncertain generalizability. Public health practitioners who apply the same critical processes to the appraisal of published research reporting successes and failures in implementation will benefit from an evidence-based approach. Public health practitioners should demand a comparable knowledge base to inform their efforts in research transfer as clinical professions do in determining individual clinical treatment options for patients.

Further resources

Grol R and Grimshaw JM. Towards evidence-based implementation. *Joint Commission Journal on Quality Improvement* (accepted for publication).

Haines A and Donald A (ed.) (1998). *Getting research findings into practice*. BMJ Publishing, London.

Haynes RB, Sackett DL, and Tugwell P (1983). Problems in the handling of clinical and research evidence by medical practitioners. *Archives of Internal Medicine*, **143**, 1971–5.

References

1. Grol R (1997). Beliefs and evidence in changing clinical practice. *BMJ*, **315**, 418–21.
2. Ketley D and Woods KL (1993). Impact of clinical trials on clinical practice: example of thrombolysis for acute myocardial infarction. *Lancet*, **342**, 891–4.
3. Woods KL, Ketley D, Lowy A, *et al.* (1998). Beta-blockers and antithrombotic treatment for secondary prevention after acute myocardial infarction. Towards an understanding of factors influencing clinical practice. The European Secondary Prevention Study Group. *Euro Heart J*, **19**, 74–9.
4. NHS Centre for Reviews and Dissemination (1999). Getting evidence into practice. *Effective Health Care Bulletin*, **5(1)**, 1–16. Royal Society of Medicine Press, London. Also available from www.york.ac.uk/inst/crd/ehc51.pdf (accessed 22 August 2000).
5. For description of interventions see Bero L, Grilli R, Grimshaw JM, Mowatt G, Oxman AD, and Zwarenstein M (ed.) (1999). Cochrane Effective Professional and Organisation of Care Group. *The Cochrane Library*, **Issue 3**. Update Software, Oxford.
6. EPOC web site www.abdn.ac.uk/public_health/hsru/epoc/index.htm (accessed 22 August 2000).
7. The Cochrane Library www.update-software.com/cochrane/cochrane-frame.html (accessed 22 August 2000).

6.10 Using guidance and frameworks

Gene Feder and Chris Griffiths

Objectives

By reading this chapter you should be better able to:

- understand, appreciate, and identify issues where guidance and frameworks could help
- identify existing relevant clinical guidelines
- assess their validity
- adapt them to local circumstances
- support clinicians in their implementation.

Why is the implementation of clinical guidelines an important public health activity?

Clinicians and public health professionals are inundated by a tide of guidance and frameworks. These are often in the form of clinical guidelines and service frameworks, and come from government, national and international health agencies, professional colleges, health care funders, and the pharmaceutical industry. Guidance on effective clinical practice is necessary because most clinicians do not have the time to go back to search and appraise the primary research, or even systematic reviews, for the majority of practice decisions. Public health professionals have a vital role to play in helping clinical colleagues use guidance, both in day-to-day practice and in development of clinical policy. In this chapter, we focus on the use of clinical guidelines as an example of the application of guidance or frameworks in practice. Guidelines themselves are only tools designed to help clinicians and managers; they need to be integrated into broader clinical or management systems.

Definition

Although the principles of clinical guidelines use can also be applied to health care policy guidelines, we deliberately do not address guidance linked to financial rewards/penalties (e.g. cervical smear targets in the UK) or obligatory frameworks (e.g. managed care requirements in the USA) (see chapter 6.2.)

Box 6.10.1 **Clinical guidelines defined**

'Systematically developed statements to assist practitioner and patient decisions about appropriate health care for specific clinical circumstances.'[1]

Identifying specific skills needed to fulfil this role

In order to bring added value to the process of guideline implementation, there are six important competencies that you need to either have yourself (unlikely) or have in the team (more likely)— see Box 6.10.2.

Box 6.10.2 **Competencies needed in guideline implementation**

- collaborating with clinicians and other stakeholders to define policy issues
- searching for relevant guidelines
- appraisal of guidelines' validity and applicability to local context
- adaptation of guidelines
- analysing and addressing obstacles to implementation
- assessment of guidelines' impact.

What are the stages in a guidelines implementation project?

Like any complex process involving different groups of people with different perspectives, it is important to manage the process of guideline implementation carefully. There are at least eight identifiable stages in the process. Some of these will overlap; and it is important to appreciate the potential barriers that may occur at any of these stages before you and your team begin.

Identifying a clinical issue

To justify devoting resources to guidelines adaptation and implementation, a clinical issue must be important. Ideally, at least three criteria should be fulfilled:

- the condition or issue should have a large impact on public health or health care resources
- there should also be demonstrable and unjustified variation in its clinical management
- there should be evidence for what constitutes good practice (see Box 6.10.3).

Box 6.10.3 **Example of suitable issue for guidelines implementation**

In a local audit of survivors of a myocardial infarction, it was found that although 92% were using aspirin six months later, only 30% were using beta-blockers, with a range of 12–72% in different general practices. Secondary prevention of coronary heart disease is an obvious subject for guidelines implementation, with a large health impact and unjustified variation in clinical management.

Box 6.10.4 **Realistic and unrealistic objectives for local guidelines development**

Realistic objectives

- develop local guidelines on use of beta-blockers after myocardial infarction
- identify national or international guidelines on use of beta-blockers after myocardial infarction
- if none found, identify systematic reviews of use of beta-blockers after myocardial infarction
- appraise guidelines or systematic reviews and choose most valid one
- adapt to local context and circulate to target clinicians for comment
- develop implementation programme with general practitioner leaders and consultant physicians.

Unrealistic objectives

- develop local guidelines on primary and secondary prevention of cardiovascular disease
- search for relevant randomized controlled trial evidence
- appraise individual trials and summarize
- formulate recommendations directly based on trial evidence.

Although these are necessary, on their own they are not sufficient. Discussion with clinicians is crucial; they also need to think the issue is important and so worth their commitment to an implementation project. The genuine involvement of opinion leaders (which increases the likelihood of implementation) is likely to be more successful if initiated at an early stage. Potential barriers to improvement should also be considered early. If these are judged to be insurmountable, then another issue should be prioritized.

Forming a local guidelines group

Choose no more than a dozen people. This should include three sorts of people:

• clinicians, managers, and others who will be implementing the guidelines on the ground

• 'content' experts (people who know the *subject* well)

• someone with the competence to identify, appraise, and summarize guidelines or systematic reviews.

The group will need to have a chair who has all the usual management skills for guiding the process. The group's objectives must be clear and not too ambitious.

Identifying pre-existing national or regional guidelines

National and regional guidelines are increasingly accessible via the internet and may be identified on bibliographic databases, although they are not necessarily indexed in the commonly available databases. Some of the better-developed guideline web sites include full-text versions or abstracts (Box 6.10.5). If in doubt, ask more than one person who has good experience of searching for guidelines.

Appraising the validity of guidelines

When you have identified relevant guidelines, you need to appraise their validity before choosing which to adapt for your own use. Adopting recommendations from guidelines of questionable validity may harm patients or waste resources on ineffective interventions. Within the UK, appraising the validity of existing guidelines will be helped by the recently established NHS Appraisal Centre for Clinical Guidelines and by the establishment of guideline development programmes, which use rigorous methods and include formal appraisal within the programmes. Examples include the Scottish Intercollegiate Guidelines Network (SIGN) and the work proposed under the auspices of the National Institute for Clinical Excellence in England and Wales.[2] If (explicitly) appraised guidelines are not available, you can do your own appraisal using a validated appraisal tool (Box 6.10.6).

Adapting guidelines to fit local circumstances

This is an essential part of the process. For example, if a guideline recommends a drug not licensed in your country or an investigation that is not available, then the guidelines recommendation clearly must be changed. Development of a local version also allows information about local services and referral pathways. If the

Box 6.10.5 **Identifying national or regional guidelines**

Search terms for common bibliographic databases

• MEDLINE and Healthstar 'guideline' (publication type) and 'consensus development conference' (publication type). Healthstar includes journals not referenced in Medline and grey literature such as AHRQ guidelines

• CINAHL 'practice guidelines' (publication type). Includes full text version of some guidelines, including AHRQ guidelines

• EMBASE 'practice guidelines' (subject heading). This is used for articles about guidelines and for those that contain practice guidelines; the term was introduced in 1994.

Useful web sites

• Agency for Healthcare Quality and Research. Full-text versions of guidelines, quick reference guides, and versions for patients can be downloaded from text.nlm.nih.gov/ftrs/dbaccess/ahcpr (accessed 23 August 2000) or ordered from the AHCPR website, www.ahrq.gov/cgi-bin/gilssrch.pl (accessed 23 August 2000)

• Canadian Medical Association Clinical Practice Guidelines Infobase. Index of clinical practice guidelines, includes downloadable full-text versions or abstracts for most guidelines: www.cma.ca/cpgs/ (accessed 23 August 2000)

• Scottish Intercollegiate Guidelines Network (SIGN). Full-text versions of guidelines and quick reference guides: www.show.scot.uk/sign/home.htm (accessed 23 August 2000).

Box 6.10.6 **UK guidelines appraisal tool**

This is a 37-item instrument that can be applied to guidelines. It is not intended to give a pass/fail assessment, but does allow a judgement of validity and comparison of different guidelines on the same clinical topic. The tool can be viewed on the web site of the Health Care Evaluation Unit and St George's Hospital Medical School, London: www.sghms.ac.uk/phs/hceu/clinguid.htm (accessed 23 August 2000).

Other appraisal tools are available.[3]

'source' guideline is more than a couple of years old, you should update it by identifying recent systematic reviews from bibliographic databases and sources like the Cochrane Library. Lastly, there is the important issue of local ownership. Those clinicians whose practice will need to change in line with the guidance will need to be convinced that the guideline is relevant to them.

Piloting and identifying barriers to implementation

Once the development group has agreed on a draft guideline it is advisable to pilot the guidelines in real-life practice settings: recommendations may turn out to be impossible to implement, no matter how much thought the team has invested. This also gives an opportunity to identify barriers to implementation. These may relate to:

- *people*: target clinicians (skills, knowledge, attitudes, rules, or norms about roles)
- *culture*: the organizational context (e.g. style of management, an openness to change within general practices)
- *structures*: structural and resource issues can stall perfectly logical guidance for purely practical reasons (e.g. lack of resources for prescribing or extra staff).

Failure to clarify and specifically address these with implementation strategies will result in failure or weakened impact.

Dissemination and implementation strategies

The previous stages will be wasted if guidelines are not used in practice. Research on the implementation of guidelines and other sources of evidence gives us a basis for designing strategy at this stage (see chapter 6.9). Passive methods of giving guidelines to clinicians (e.g. just through the post) are unlikely to be effective. Multifaceted programmes, especially those that explicitly tackle obstacles to implementation, engage clinicians face-to-face and build in reminders or prompts into the consultation are more likely to work. Tailor your strategy to address the barriers identified.

Monitoring impact of guidelines

Set up some form of routine data collection to assess whether the guidelines are used in clinical practice. Where guidelines make prescribing and referral recommendations this is relatively straightforward when data are stored electronically. In the UK, the introduction of clinical governance means that health care trusts and primary care groups have a statutory obligation to monitor performance through these methods (see chapter 6.8). Linking performance measures back to evidence-based guidelines makes them more likely to seem credible to clinicians, particularly if they have been involved in the guidelines programme.

What is actually involved in getting something done?

The importance of managing the process

Implementing a guideline is like any other development work: it needs to be carefully designed and managed. Regular reviews of progress are vital, perhaps by a steering group consisting of the multi-disciplinary panel that adapted the guidelines. The group needs to monitor progress of implementation (particularly when a labour-intensive approach such as outreach visits is being used), watch for new or unforeseen barriers, and check data on expected change in practice. Like all monitoring and evaluation, it is important to decide early on what are the standards and criteria you are going to use, and at what level you will see them as success.

Embedding into organizational structures

Always take the opportunity to embed any change process within a larger context. Implementation may be more easily achieved by including it within local organizational structures (e.g. clinical governance in UK primary care, or an integrated care pathway in secondary care).

Potential pitfalls

Mismatch between guidance and available resources

Lack of resources will hinder implementation if recommendations require extensive new tasks outside clinicians' usual roles, or prescription of medication where clinicians may be penalized for excessive spending. Barriers such as clinicians taking on new roles and prescribing resources should be addressed at the outset. Think carefully if resources are likely to be a big problem. The art of successful implementation often feels like identifying and minimizing every possible barrier. In purely practical terms this is equivalent to making it as easy as possible for those engaged in the process of clinical care to actually use the guidance to improve care.

Insufficient attention to implementation and review

Effective implementation will always demand time, enthusiasm, and resources; choosing implementation methods that are likely to give the best return on available investment is vital. You are unlikely to bring about change in other people's practice if you appear ambivalent about it. Even when the guidance appears implemented, don't assume that change will follow automatically without review of progress and, if necessary, changes in strategy.

Myths

There are many myths associated with guideline development and implementation. Three of the most important to be aware of:

Clinicians do not use guidelines

Although clinical guidelines often get a bad press—for instance, because of suggestions that they limit clinical freedom—research shows that carefully chosen strategies do result in effective guidelines implementation both in primary and secondary care settings.

Guidelines should always be developed locally from scratch to ensure local ownership

There is a commonly-held assumption that adaptations of national guidelines don't work. It is very inefficient to start the complete search and appraisal process from the beginning for each locality. Nationally- and internationally-generated evidence needs to be checked for validity and then adapted locally. Nationally-developed guidelines do have sufficient credibility, especially if adapted to local circumstances by respected opinion leaders.

Guidelines lead to litigation

Although the legal status of guidelines varies between different countries, overall they have not been used to override expert opinion in courts of law. On the other hand, if clinicians implement faulty guidelines it is they, rather than the authors of such guidelines, who are likely to increase their liability in negligence. The relationship between guidelines and clinician liability will vary between countries and is likely to evolve over the next few years.

The increasing importance of governance means that every team, clinician, and policy maker needs to be able to justify their professional practice (see chapter 6.8). An evidence and a value base should underpin every decision and action (see chapters 2.7 and 6.9). At an individual level, there may always be good reasons not to follow blindly guideline recommendations for a particular patient. What is essential is that significant deviation from guidance be justified.

Pitfalls

Two randomized trials of guidelines implementation in east London general practices illustrate some of the difficulties in working with guidelines:

- despite using a multifaceted strategy to implement diabetes and asthma guidelines (outreach visits, consultation prompts, and audit with feedback), we found that general practices with poor organization (e.g. no practice manager), or with internal conflict between clinicians, failed to implement guidelines. The lesson we learned is that such practices need organizational support before guidelines can take root
- a trial tested the use of postal reminders concerning guidelines sent to patients discharged after a myocardial infarct, *and* to their

general practitioners. The results indicated that some general practitioners did not see it as their responsibility to address secondary prevention in patients discharged from hospital. Furthermore, whilst practice nurses could have played a larger part in providing secondary prevention, this part of their role was poorly encouraged. The lesson here is that roles and responsibilities of target clinicians may need to be addressed before attempting to change clinician behaviour.

Key determinants of success

Six important actions are associated with the success of guideline development and implementation.

* setting priorities clearly
* setting clear and attainable objectives
* collaborating early with stakeholders
* identifying and targeting barriers to change
* choosing as powerful an implementation strategy as resources will allow
* ensuring a rigorous project management approach is used.

Summary

The challenge of this area is that you are dealing with the most powerful human emotions: experience and prejudice. You need every piece of evidence to help to make guidelines an effective way of improving clinical care.

Further resources

Black N (1990). Medical litigation and the quality of care. *Lancet*, **335**, 35–7.

Feder G, Eccles M, Grol R, Griffiths C, and Grimshaw J (1999). Using clinical guidelines. *BMJ*, **318**, 728–30.

Grol R (1997). Personal paper. Beliefs and evidence in changing clinical practice. *BMJ*, **315**, 418–21.

Hurwitz B (1999). Legal and political considerations of clinical practice guidelines. *BMJ*, **318**, 661–4.

Hutchinson A and Baker MR (1999). *Making use of guidelines in clinical practice*. Radcliffe, Oxford.

McDonald CJ and Overhage JM (1994). Guidelines you can follow and can trust—an ideal and an example. *JAMA*, **271**, 872–3.

Newman L (2000). AHRQ's evidence based practice centres prove viable. *Lancet*, **356**, 1990.

NHS Centre for Reviews and Dissemination (1999). Getting research into practice. *Effective Health Care*, **5**, 1–12.

Setting priorities for clinical practice guidelines. Institute of Medicine, Washington DC, 1995. www.nap.edu/books/0309052475/html/index.html (accessed 4 August 2000).

Thomson R, Lavender M, and Madhok R (1995). Fortnightly review: how to ensure that guidelines are effective. *BMJ*, **311**, 237–42.

References

1. Marilyn J, Field MJ, and Lohr KN (ed.). *Clinical practice guidelines: directions for a new program*. Committee to Advise the Public Health Service on Clinical Practice Guidelines, Institute of Medicine, Washington DC. books.nap.edu/books/0309043468/html/38.html (accessed 4 August 2000).

2. National Institute for Clinical Excellence. www.nice.org.uk (accessed 14 September 2000).

3. Hayward RSA, Wilson MC, Tunis SR, Bass EB, and Guyatt G (1995). Users' guides to the medical literature. VII: How to use clinical practice guidelines: are the recommendations valid? *JAMA*, **274**, 570–4.

Breaking through the culture of contentment is essential if real change is to happen.

Galbraith, JK

Part 7
Personal effectiveness

Introduction

The whole of this handbook is aimed at increasing your effectiveness. Sometimes that means careful self-examination of your personal effectiveness. That is the focus of this part.

Leadership and management are critical for effective public health practice. These attributes can and should be distinguished, although both are needed for effective collaboration. Developing relationships is the key to managing change with people and groups as diverse as colleagues, vulnerable communities, or the Minister's office. These settings are explored in chapters that apply particularly to your work as an individual public health practitioner. The appeal of chapters 7.1–7.6 will vary according to the stage of your career, but all of us have a responsibility for continually improving our own professional practice (chapter 7.7).

Professional isolation is a hazard that takes many forms. Consider yourself, for example, as the report writer, or as an expert working on a consultancy contract (chapters 7.3 and 7.6). All authors in this section suggest ways to connect, communicate, and collaborate with colleagues more productively.

Public health sometimes has a reputation for being well-intentioned, but meddlesome. Giving unsolicited advice can fall into this category. If you are providing advice, at least remember to be brief.†

CSG

---

† After Horace, Roman poet (65–8 BC).

7.1 **Developing leadership skills**

Fiona Sim

Objectives

This chapter should equip the reader with many of the complementary skills which are necessary to make your public health practice more *effective*.

Definition

Leadership

Great leaders are traditionally characterized as highly charismatic, high profile individuals—Churchill, Mandela, Thatcher, Hitler—some we may wish to emulate, others not. They shared attributes of immense power to influence, to communicate a clear vision which would be attractive to their followers, and the ability to deliver that vision.

In your workplace or community, you could probably identify someone, not necessarily charismatic or extrovert, or even very senior, who has been the architect of a substantial change and who has made it happen. This is often a more useful characterization of leadership.

Public health leadership

This is the application of such characteristics to the cause of improving the health of a given population or community. In order to achieve what has become known as the Acheson definition of Public Health—to prevent disease, prolong life, and promote health through the organized efforts of society[1]—competent leadership must be exercised in order for those efforts to be deployed effectively.

A former Chief Medical Officer for England described leadership in the following terms in December 1998:

- knowing where you want to go and setting the direction of travel
- taking people with you on the journey in spite of their differences in views and methods, working background, and rates of travel
- giving sufficient time and energy to the process of changing things for the better—learning to do things in a different way.

(Source: Calman[2])

Aims of public health leadership

These include:

- attributable improvement in the health of a population or community

* better inter-agency working
* higher profile for public health
* greater efficiency in health decision making.

Is leadership different from management?

Leadership complements and differs from management in some important respects. Whilst an effective manager requires planning and problem-solving skills to produce largely predictable, desirable results, a leader will go further *to establish the vision* and take it forward, usually by motivating and developing others, to produce significant, sometimes dramatic, change. Table 7.1.1 illustrates these distinctions.

Table 7.1.1 Comparing management and leadership.

Manager	Leader
Coping with complexity	Coping with change
Ensuring order and consistency	Delivering change
Planning and budgeting	Setting direction—developing a vision
Organizing and staffing to accomplish objectives	Aligning people
Problem solving	Motivating and inspiring

(Source: Kotter[3])

Why is leadership an important public health attribute?

For a public health practitioner to be effective, *technical skills and knowledge are essential but not sufficient*. Imagine absorbing all the information in this handbook and yet being unable, in the face of opposing views, to articulate and implement your sound, professional, evidence-based advice?

Every public health practitioner must to be able to exercise leadership skills, even if his/her role is not explicitly a 'leading' one. For instance, it may at some time be appropriate for the public health member of any team to take the lead, with the agreement of the team.

A programme of work around public health leadership

Virtually any piece of work in public health lends itself to scrutiny of the public health leadership element. For example, if you were expected to implement a local screening programme, you would set yourself objectives, based on your professional competence and integrity.

Review of this task will reveal aspects that require competent public health leadership:

• having a clear vision of what you were trying to achieve and why
• working across organizational boundaries by communicating appropriately and effectively
• understanding and gaining the trust of service users
• persevering in the task through to implementation and evaluation
• demonstrating professional integrity—and thereby moral courage.

Competencies for leadership

It is easy to see that technical knowledge and skills lead to technical competence; for public health leadership, however, whilst acquisition of relevant competencies *should* lead to competence, the evidence to date is largely circumstantial. This is due in part to a lack of research in this area and partly because the competencies comprise skills and attitudes, some of which we may acquire at an early age, while others can be learned later.

Box 7.1.1 **Competencies usually associated with effective public health leadership**

(a) Knowledge
• good grasp of the core knowledge base required for public health practice.

(b) Skills
• ability to define and articulate a clear vision
• ability to share the vision so that others are influenced to adopt it
• resilience and perseverance towards the vision despite difficulties
• maintenance of professional integrity.

(c) Attitudes
• self-esteem combined with critical self-appraisal
• a degree of humility to allow one to acknowledge that someone else is right
• an understanding of and respect for others' beliefs and perceptions, which may differ from one's own
• personal values including a passion for public health.

Orientation and execution of leadership tasks

• public health leadership requires the participation and commitment of other people

• many public health practitioners have little formal power in the traditional sense, such as control of substantial budgets or a large, directly employed workforce. It is essential, therefore, that they are able to achieve commitment to their vision by others. A 'command and control' model of leadership becomes redundant

• leadership is important at different levels in public health practice:

  – *personal*: for effective leadership, the public health practitioner should have a clear understanding of his/her own strengths and weaknesses, personality type, and preferred leadership styles

  – *organizational*: to be an effective public health leader within an organization, the practitioner must understand fully the organization's structure, its culture, key players to be influenced, financial position, and decision making processes

  – *community*: for public health leadership to be effective within a community, the practitioner must understand its culture and history, and be able to identify and engage its key members, who may include community leaders, politicians, and journalists, for instance. He/she must work *with and through* leaders of other relevant organizations in order to effect changes which will improve the health of that community.

• the public health vision *and* the role of the public health leader must be clearly articulated. In an established public health system, these may be obvious. But in developing systems, the practitioner will need to deploy the appropriate leadership skills and demonstrate the attitudes most likely to result in success. We can be inspired by pioneer public health leaders, including Snow, Chadwick, and Simon, who created their own vision and persevered to achieve their societal goals.[4]

Potential pitfalls

• recognizing a public health challenge and producing a technically competent project plan to address it is necessary, but not sufficient

• neither vision nor professional expertise alone will lead to change—political skills including diplomacy, communication, and timing are just as important

• leadership may not always be from the front. Exercising different styles of leadership in different circumstances is necessary—in leading an outbreak investigation, getting local industry to take seriously your vision for workplace health, or introducing changes in clinical practice

• avoid appearing pious in your enthusiasm to do good. Understand that others may not share the vision unless it is explained explicitly in terms of the evidence and values upon which it is based.

Unpicking dogma

* 'Leaders are born and not made.' This assertion is not based upon fact or evidence. It appears from the evidence that there are few inherent attributes of leadership, other than intelligence, courage, and aptitude. Much of the research on this subject has been based on military leadership, so aptitude has been found to comprise features such as the ability to respond rapidly in warfare. In public health, a quick mind to respond to debate and challenge under pressure, and a willingness to learn continually and from every situation are more clearly important

* it has been suggested that physical height lends itself to leadership: history refutes that assertion

* that a particular personality type is likely to make a better leader is often discussed. It is the case that when leaders have been studied, the majority have 'extrovert' personalities, according to widely-used personality type inventories. So some people may have a natural potential for leadership. This does not, however, rule out the possibility of other people becoming effective leaders, and many do so

* 'What is your leadership style?' is a commonly asked question at interviews. The effective leader may well have a preferred style, but will have a whole battery of styles to suit different situations[5]

* 'Leadership is just a fancy term for management.' Well, it is neither fancy nor the same, as described earlier.

Determinants of success

Clarity of vision and the perseverance to ensure its implementation by engaging all relevant parties is most likely to lead to success. There will often need to be flexibility in the vision—the world is a dynamic place and what is clearly appropriate today may need some amendment in the near future.

Successful leadership requires imagination and plenty of energy and perseverance, in addition to sound technical skills and a commitment to professional integrity and respect for the views of others.

How will I know if I have been successful?

Success may take several years. If the vision is based on evidence, it should be possible to monitor progress towards objectives. This will serve to support the vision as well as to encourage those involved with implementation that the direction of travel is correct. Objectives set at the outset might include qualitative as well as quantitative measures of success, the latter including the extent of involvement of partner organizations, amount of positive media coverage, or knowledge of the initiative among the local community.

The practicalities of acquiring leadership skills

Consider the following in your personal plans for continuing professional development:

* understand your personality type, the way you operate, your personal and professional strengths and weaknesses. You will gain a clearer understanding of how you operate, how others see you, and how they operate or could be developed. Many well-known tools, such as the Myers Briggs Type Inventory (MBTI) can be helpful.[6] Whilst the theory provides an interesting and informative read, consult a personal development consultant or your Human Resources department for expertise in interpretation of your personal profile

* make better use of the mass media. The media are very effective at conveying to the public either positive or negative health messages. Most people can benefit from media training, which is available from many sources. Your organization's Press Office would usually be a good starting point. Establish a rapport with the local reporters, so that next time a public health issue is about to hit the headlines, existing trust will help counter any tendency to inflate or bias a story (see chapters 3.5 and 7.4)

* know and respect your partners, both within and outside your organization. Remember, it may be just as important to engage a major budget holder within your organization as to form an alliance with a chief executive of another body, or a community leader, so remember partnership working 'inside and out'

* be confident about your public health skills, competencies, and attitudes and your understanding of the local scene; not only its demography and epidemiology, but also its key players, culture, politics, and its priorities outside health. This means acquiring and maintaining a high standard of professional practice. The public health message is more likely to be understood and respected if articulated clearly and accurately, whilst using language suited to the audience. Different modes of communication are effective with different audiences, so it is worthwhile exploring and becoming familiar with techniques not often taught formally to professionals, like story telling. A little humility is also valuable: professional arrogance has no place in the specialist practice of public health.

Further resources

Adair J (1993). *Effective leadership*. Pan, London.

Barger N and Kirby L (1995). *The challenge of change in organizations*. Davies-Black, Palo Alto CA.

Grainger C and Griffiths R (1998). For debate: public health leadership—do we have it? Do we need it? *Pub Hlth Med*, **20**, 375–6.

Griffiths S and McPherson K (1997). We need strong public health leadership. *BMJ*, **314**, 685.

Kotter J (1996). *Leading change*. Harvard Business School Press, Boston.

Leape LL and Berwick DM (2000). Safe health care: are we up to it? *BMJ*, **320**, 725–6.

Mann JM (1997). Leadership is a global issue. *Lancet*, **350(Suppl III)**, 20–7.

Novick LF, Woltring CS, and Fox DM (ed.) (1997). *Public health leaders tell their stories*. Aspen, Gaithersburg MD.

Pencheon D and Koh YM (2000). Leadership and motivation. *BMJ*, **321** (**7256**), S2.

UK Department of Health (1997). *The new NHS*: modern, dependable. Cm. 3807. The Stationery Office, London.

UK Department of Health (1999). *Saving lives—our healthier nation*. Department of Health, London.

US Centre for Health Leadership. www.cfhl.org (accessed 10 September 2000).

Wright K, Rowitz L, Merkle A, Reid WM, Robinson G, Herzog W, Weber D, Carmichael D, Balderson TR, and Baker E (2000). Competency development in public health leadership. *Am J Public Health*, **90(8)**, 1202–7.

References

1. Acheson D (1988). *Public health in England, the report of the Committee of Inquiry London. the Future Development of the Public Health Function*. Cm 289. HMSO, London.

2. Calman K (1998). Lessons from Whitehall. *BMJ*, **317**, 1718–20.

3. Kotter J (1990). *A force for change*. Harvard Business School Press, Boston.

4. Holland WW and Stewart S (1997). *Public health: the vision and the challenge*. (The Rock Carling Fellowship.) Nuffield Trust, London.

5. Goleman D (2000). Leadership that gets results. *Harvard Business Review*, 78–90.

6. Briggs Myers I and Myers P (1980). *Gifts differing, understanding personality type*. Davies-Black, Palo Alto CA.

Go to the people. Live amongst them. Start with what they have. Build with them. And when the deed is done, the mission accomplished, the people will say 'We have done it ourselves'.

Lao Tze, 600 BC

7.2 **Effecting change at meetings**

Edmund Jessop

Introduction

All meetings are negotiations. Whether it is a ten-minute meeting with your boss, a regular meeting with colleagues, or a twenty-minute presentation to a committee, you are trying to alter or modify what someone else thinks. They start the meeting with one set of views: you want to move them nearer to your point of view. So there are two essentials for any meeting:

- *you*: know what you want to achieve from the meeting
- *them*: find out as much as you can about them.

Before the meeting

Think about your aims

Public health is about changing the way other people think. Meeting people face-to-face is an important way of achieving that goal. Most people hate meetings, but part of the reason for this is that they see meetings as a chore, not an opportunity. Of course some—even many—meetings are tedious and unproductive. But if you don't go into a meeting knowing what *you* want out of it, you certainly won't get it.

Like any negotiation, sort out in your own mind beforehand:

- what would be the best result for you (opening position)
- what is the minimum acceptable (your fall-back position).

For example, your opening position is probably complete acceptance of your policy; but as your fall-back, would you rather have partial acceptance or decision deferred till later? What points are you willing to compromise on? How much are you prepared to change your views? Distinguish between changing your views through weakness or lack of clarity on your part and changing your views through mutual respect and genuine learning. Trading perspectives and explicit mutual respect can be a powerful way to elicit respect for your point of view.

Research before the meeting

Find out as much as you can about the other people who will be there. It is especially important to find out:

- what other people might believe
- what other people might want to achieve.

Of course, you need to ask these questions of yourself first.

Even if the meeting is with someone you know well, what is he or she likely to think about the issue you want to raise with them today?

If you are attending an unfamiliar meeting, find out about the people who will be there. Do they like the big picture or the detail? Should you be thorough or quick? Will they be impressed by government policy or dismissive of it? Sometimes quoting the opinion of a medical academy or expert society will impress, sometimes it will antagonize. Use your friends and colleagues to get the inside information on the people who will be at your meeting.

A successful negotiation is one in which you get what you want and they get what they want—at least to some extent. Listen hard and long: find out as much as you can about what they want. You can't do that if you haven't questioned thoroughly and listened carefully.

Most people are reasonable, but people want different things in life. No one deliberately seeks (except in war) to damage other people's health by *commission*, but many of us do it unwittingly by *omission*. So if it seems to you that other people are not working for public health, there must be a reason which is important to them. Maybe it seems trivial, irrelevant, or outrageous to you: but it is stopping you from changing the way they think. So you need to find out what that reason is. Only then can you start to resolve the difference between you.

Sell the benefit not the proposal

Focus on how they will benefit, not what you want to do. And concentrate on benefits that are relevant to them. Of course you can only do this if you've already found out what they want.

Remember that differences often exist in the mind, not in reality

To resolve a conflict of opinion, you need to address the other person's mind, not the 'objective facts'. Scientifically trained workers find it hard to understand why people don't respond to objective data. But if you lived next to a toxic waste dump, and your child developed leukaemia, no amount of scientific evidence on exposure, doses, latent periods, and so on would convince you that the waste dump was safe. The same is true in any meeting, from a discussion of where to put the coffee machine to agreeing on a multi-million pound budget.

The relationship is more important than any one meeting.

Build the relationship

Public health work takes time. So the people you are meeting today will be people you have to work with again in the future.

So sometimes you need to lose gracefully and come back next time. As Dale Carnegie said: 'no one ever wins an argument'. If you have an argument and 'win', the other person is left feeling bruised and battered. This is always damaging to a long-term relationship. You can't afford that kind of ill-will in public health work. Your success depends on other people, so you need other people to be on your side. Exploring assumptions nearly always improves the quality of relationships and the overall outcomes of meetings (see chapter 2.7).

Setting up your own meeting

When you set up a meeting, good administration is important. If people arrive flustered, or unprepared, or can't come at all, you won't achieve your aim.

Timing

Give people plenty of notice that you want to meet them. It is difficult to generalize, but four weeks' notice for a half-day meeting and six weeks or more for an all day meeting is about right for senior people. People of national importance may need six months' notice or more.

Be aware of committee cycles: find out regular dates, for example budget setting meetings. You may need to map a sequence of meetings (e.g. ethics committee before grant committee, or personnel committee before finance committee).

Venue

The venue is important, so get the best you can afford. People who are cold, sitting in uncomfortable chairs, and have had a long, difficult journey will not be paying attention to you. Think about parking, wheelchair access, and refreshments.

Should you invite other people to your office or go to visit them; or meet on neutral territory? For one-to-one meetings it is more polite to put yourself out by going to them; for big meetings you have to be the host. If conflict is severe, neutral territory is best.

If you are expecting conflict, don't sit people who are likely to disagree directly opposite each another. It reinforces the feeling that it's 'us' against 'them'. In public health everyone is facing a common problem: death and disease. Have everyone facing a screen or board on which the problem you have in common—an outbreak, an overspend, whatever—can be described. You can do this even in one-to-one meetings: never sit across a desk from someone.

Agenda

Send out an agenda so that everyone has the chance to prepare for the meeting. Most people *won't* prepare, but if you don't send an agenda they *can't*.

Help them to know which are the important items, perhaps by indicating on the agenda how long you expect to spend on each item. It is wise to allow 10–15 minutes for people to settle in with small or routine items before tackling the major topic.

During the meeting

Meetings are the live theatre of public health: exciting, exhilarating, and unpredictable. Actually of course most meetings are very boring, but if you have thought beforehand what you want out the meeting, your time will not have been wasted completely. But remember:

Build the relationship: you'll be meeting again!

Listen: don't speak

Even if you've been invited just to give a presentation, you need to listen first. So get there early to gauge the mood of the meeting, and find out who is asking what.

If you're the first to speak on a topic, human nature ensures that the next two or three speakers will oppose what you said, if only to show they can think for themselves. So bide your time and present your ideas towards the end of discussion on an item. Sometimes this will mean not revealing your own opinion in any briefing paper you have circulated before the meeting.

Words matter: use them carefully

You will not build the relationship by giving offence. If in doubt, find out beforehand from a colleague what terms are acceptable to your audience. Most people become disproportionately irritated by the use of certain words and phrases. If you know what these preferences are before meetings, it can only help.

If you've achieved your objectives, stop arguing

After you've achieved your objectives, anything else you say can *only* make things worse, so shut up! Of course this means you need to be listening hard to know when you have won. But all too often people throw away victory by continuing to argue their case and alienating people who have already been won over.

Use summary statements

With more than five people in a meeting, normal conversation is impossible and special tactics are needed. If more than eight people are present, you will not get more than one chance to speak on any topic. Often a summary statement ('soundbite')—a single phrase or sentence which puts across a message or creates an image—will be more effective than a speech in helping other people to change their minds or modify their views. Avoid soundbites that sound good and mean nothing.

Instead of 'We are aiming to change the culture from one where doctors are treated deferentially in a hierarchical structure, to one where they are open to request and enquiry from patients and colleagues in a more responsive manner', try 'Doctors should be more on tap than on top'.

Don't read or refer to papers in the meeting

If you are reading you are not listening. In the meeting, it is more important to concentrate hard on what is going on in the meeting than to read some point of detail. If someone asks a detailed query the correct response is to say, 'I'll get back to you after the meeting', and carry on with more important business of listening hard to the discussion. If you read the papers beforehand (even if you only skim them), there will be much less need to read *during* the meeting.

After the meeting

After the meeting always follow through.

After formal meetings, send out notes of what was decided and who agreed to take what action.

Even informal meetings are worth written follow-up to ensure no misunderstanding (and no reneging on agreements): see Box 7.2.1.

Box 7.2.1 **'A follow up letter'**

Dear Jim

This is to confirm that you Fred and I agreed yesterday to write a 1500 word paper together entitled 'Waiting List Solutions that Work' within the next two weeks. I will let you have the statistics by Thursday, and you will do the first draft within five working days. We agreed to meet next on Wednesday 30 March at 3 pm in your room.

Julie

cc Fred

Further resources

Fisher R and Ury W (1982). *Getting to Yes. Negotiating agreement without giving in*. Hutchinson Business, London.

The world is run by the people who turn up.

David Foxcroft

7.3 **Writing to effect change**

Edmund Jessop

Introduction

The most important thing to remember when you write is that no one *has* to read what you write. You can't force people to read—you have to tempt them. Never think that because what you write is important, people will read it: they won't. Consider for a moment how much material you have not read in the past two weeks.

If what you write is difficult to read, people will simply give up. So you must do everything in your power to make it easy for your readers. In essence, you can't force people to read: you have to tempt them.

Objectives

This chapter should help you make your writing more enjoyable to create and to read. Consequently, it should be more effective in initiating and sustaining appropriate change in others.

Writing has three stages: before, during, and after. The most important stage is before.

Before you write

Know who you are writing for

Are you writing for:

- your boss?
- co-workers?
- a committee?
- the general public?

This seems obvious, but it is the key to success. If you are going to tempt people to read, you must know who they are and what they like. Always keep the reader in mind. It is sometimes easier to think of some person you know rather than a whole group: if writing for old people, write for your aunt. If writing a committee paper, think of one typical member of the committee and write for him or her.

Give them what *they* want to *read*—not what *you* want to *write*

Never fall into the trap of thinking people *should* read what you write; they may not. Even if it is telling them about their own pay rise, there will always be some people who won't read it. So give them your message in the form they want it—make it easy for them.

Most people don't want scientific methodology: so don't give it to them. If you do, they'll probably just give up and move on to something easier. And if *they* have stopped reading, *you* have stopped persuading.

If your readers (e.g. a grant-giving committee) have asked you to complete a form, *complete the form*. Don't leave items out. Don't add pages of extra material. If it says do it in 12 point type, don't try to cram more in by using a smaller font. Your aim is to help them to understand your way of thinking; and failing to heed their instruction will not achieve that aim. You must start with where your audience is, not where you think it should be or might be.

Be active in finding out what your readership wants; if writing for a committee, ask to see previous committee papers. Speak to the secretary of the committee.

Give it to them on time

'You want it good or you want it Thursday?' The classic response of the newspaper reporter. A report or paper which arrives after the decision is made is worthless. So find out when decisions will be made. And remember that the formal meeting at which, say, budgets are agreed is often a formality: all details may have been sorted out long before. So you need to check if minds will be made up *before* the formal decision.

Hit the deadline—even if it means your paper isn't perfect. And never 'table' a paper—i.e. give the paper out for the first time at the meeting at which you want it discussed. No one can read it properly, so the only correct course of action for a chairman if you do this is to ignore your paper completely. Worse still, people may assume you are lazy or devious or both.

Allow time for all stages of writing, review, and distribution to hit the deadline.

Be aware of their constraints

The usual constraints are:

- people's attitudes, prejudices, way of life
- local regulations, law, or policy
- precedent
- available funding.

Think what each may mean for your readers. You may be able to alter constraints but if not you must at least show awareness of them.

Think before you write

If your thoughts are woolly your writing will be woolly. Each piece of writing should have a single aim, and the whole structure of your piece should lead to this aim. Spend time thinking this out.

Write down your aim. Make it short and clear. e.g.:

* to persuade this school to adopt a no-smoking policy
* to persuade this committee to give me a research grant.

The next stage is to decide what are the individual messages that are most likely to sell your idea. This may need further thought. For a school smoking policy it could be:

1. Smoking causes cancer in non-smokers; *or*

2. Smoking is a fire hazard.

Message 1 may seem more important to public health workers but message 2 was what got the ban on smoking throughout the London underground transport system. Choose the message which will achieve your aim, not the one you most want to put.

Do all your homework before you put pen to paper (or finger to keyboard)

This usually means:

* key statistics
* research literature
* law and government policy
* local precedents (what have they done before on this or similar issues?).

Make sure you can prove every assertion you make. You may not want to fill the text with scientific references, but truth matters: don't rely on memory! Readers will increasingly want to check references online, so give internet web site references (URLs*) when you can. Ensure you make clear the date of access, as the internet is a very dynamic medium.

Write a framework

When you have all the facts in your head, write a framework for your piece. This needs to give:

* a major heading for each two or three pages (2–3000 words)
* minor headings per half page (500–1000 words)
* a main point for each paragraph (100–200 words).

Start with the major headings, then fill in the minor headings, and finally the points for each paragraph. This rule applies however short or long your piece—be it a three-page letter or a 10,000-word report. If you don't do it, your reader won't find it easy to follow your line of thought and will probably give up trying.

Make a word budget

Make a word budget for each section. For example:

1. Introduction: 300 words.
2. Evidence base: 500 words.
3. Local situation: 500 words.
4. Recommendations: 250 words.

You now have a clear line of thought for your piece, be it a one-page memo or a 10,000-word report.

When you are writing

Don't write anything until you have the shape of your entire piece clear in your mind and/or sketched out on paper

Cut and paste is easy with computers but it is lazy and destroys the clarity of thought both you and your readers need. A pencil and paper can encourage structure in a way that computers often do not.

Use short words

Think what you would say in conversation: 'he had a stroke' not 'he had a cerebrovascular accident'. Sometimes the short word loses precision—'heart attack' may mean acute myocardial infarct or ventricular fibrillation; if so always consider: does this distinction matter to my readers? If not use the short word.

There is one exception to this rule: don't give offence. More on this below.

Use short sentences

Whenever you are about to write a comma: don't. Put a full stop and start a new sentence.

Don't give offence

Words such as leper and cretin have technical meanings but they give offence and have been replaced by 'person with Hansen's disease' and 'person with congenital hypothyroidism'. This is an exception to the 'use short words' rule. It may look odd, but if you give offence people will stop reading and your writing will not achieve its aim (quite apart from common decency).

Don't use abbreviations

People read word groups, not individual letters or words, so in reading (unlike speaking) readers don't get slowed up by a lack of abbreviations. Abbreviations, because they are all capitals, *are* difficult to read. If you must abbreviate, spell it out in full the first time e.g. acquired immune deficiency disease (AIDS).

Use headings and subheadings

Most people don't read: they skim. So help them to skim. Headings can be extremely useful in telling the reader something.

If there is a house style use it; readers are familiar with it and anything different is a distraction. Even if you think your style is better: do not use it. Give the readers what they are used to. If there is no house style, keep to a standard format for the font size, underlining, and so on.

Structure your piece

A good general structure for a briefing paper is as follows:

- table of contents (if more than ten pages long)
- summary
- purpose or aim
- background
- precedent or local/national policy
- current issues (i.e. why now?)
- options including implementation
- cost
- politics
- recommended option and why
- document control—authorship, reason (for info, action . . .) sent to whom, date, version . . .

It can be very helpful to number the paragraphs of a document—this can help readers refer to particular passages in meetings or correspondence.

Use lists

Lists are easy to skim. More than three of anything demands a list. Use bullets for up to four items but, for more than that, consider numbers, especially if the order of the points is important.

Use graphics

Try to put a chart, graph, or picture in to break up the text. Newspapers do it to attract readers—so should you. It is easy enough to insert graphics into text with modern software, though considerable effort may be needed to generate a good graphic.

Electronic mail

With e-mail the message header may be the *only* thing people read, so use the header for your message not the topic. Try this sample:

- 'Read your papers before tomorrow's meeting' vs. 're: Tomorrow's meeting'

- 'Telephone message for you' vs. 'Home called: no dinner tonight'
- 'Latest health statistics' vs. 'Teenage pregnancy rate lowest ever'.

Remember that some people never read their e-mail. If they want it as paper, send it as paper.

Advertising

Advertising copy is a special form of writing not used by most public health workers. However, advertising techniques can be extremely useful. Techniques include: slogans, phrases, and campaign titles. Advertisers and public health practitioners have much in common. They are in the business of using data effectively to change behaviour and action—usually via a response that has an emotional or subjective element. The power of phrases to change thought and action can be profound. 'Add life to years, as well as years to life' is a good example.

Advertisers are often heard to say 'If you to have explain your policy, you're dead'.

After you write

Don't send it off

Once your paper is written, mull it over. Never send a paper out as soon as it is written: even with the most urgent deadline, walk away for an hour or so. Better still leave it overnight or over a weekend. Then come back with a fresh eye and re-read your work. At this point you will always see something that could have been said better!

Get some feedback

Always ask a colleague to read it for content. Specify that you want comments on content or some colleagues will merely try to improve your grammar and miss the big points. Ask them specifically to look for:

- material that just looks wrong (e.g. statistics for circumcisions that exceed the number of male births in your locality)
- important issues that have been missed (e.g. abortion clinics as well as maternity units in a study of conception).

If possible, though this is often difficult, ask someone like the intended reader to review it for clarity.

Don't get defensive when people point out errors, inconsistencies, etc. Be grateful.

Consider the distribution list carefully

Send it to your intended readership, but also think 'Who else should see this?' This is particularly important for correspondence.

Do a mental check of people in your own organization and in other agencies. Other organizations won't distribute it internally to everyone you think should see it, so mail them directly. In general anyone who will be affected by what you write should see it.

Offer to meet the individual or group you have sent it to

Offering your time shows your commitment to the cause, as well as the opportunity to lobby, and clarify any issues.

Summary

These rules may seem daunting, but as with so much in life they become much easier with practice. Writing well can be one of easiest ways of improving your personal effectiveness. Moreover, reading well can be a good way of writing well—improving your ability and experience in both spheres is an enjoyable art form in itself.

Further resources

Albert T (1996). *Publish and prosper. BMJ,* **313(7070):** Classified Supp.

Albert T (2000). *A–Z of medical writing.* BMJ Books, London.

Albert T (2000). *Winning the publications game,* (2nd edn). Radcliffe Medical Press, Oxford.

Asher R (1986). *Richard Asher talking sense.* Churchill Livingstone, London.

Bryson B (1987). *Troublesome words,* (2nd edn). Penguin, Harmondsworth.

Burchfield RW (ed.) (1999). *Fowler's Modern English usage,* (revised 3rd edn). Clarendon Press, Oxford.

Economist style guide. Profile Books, 1999. www.economist.com (accessed 15 February 2001).

Effective written communications. www.timalbert.co.uk (accessed 15 February 2001).

Strunk W and White EB (1979). *The elements of style,* (3rd edn). Allyn and Bacon, Boston.

Tufte E (1983). *Visual display of quantitative information.* Graphics Press, Connecticut.

Tufte E (1990). *Envisioning information.* Graphics Press, Connecticut.

Tufte E (1997). *Visual explanations.* Graphics Press, Connecticut.

Writing a report: position, problem, possibilities, proposal.

7.4 **Working with the media**

Alan Maryon Davis

Objectives

After reading this chapter you will be able to:

• develop a strategy for working with the media both as an individual practitioner and as a representative of your department

• review and strengthen your strategy if you already have one in place.

This chapter addresses the basics of working with the print and broadcast media. More provocative engagement with the media is described elsewhere in this handbook (see chapter 3.5).

Working with confidence

As health professionals, we tend to be rather wary of working with the media. Like fire, publicity can be a great source of light—but it can also be erratic and risky. Besides, it often takes an awful lot of matches just to get it started. Yet, the media's influence and reach are invaluable to us. We need to engage large numbers of people and convey information, change attitudes, and trigger actions for health improvement. We must therefore learn how to make the most of this potential with a few basic skills and a coherent approach.

We talk of 'the media' as a single entity. In reality of course it is very plural—not only in terms of its various modalities, like print, radio, or television, but also because it comprises a diverse collection of individual journalists and programme makers, all trying to attract readers, listeners, or viewers. Fortunately for us, health issues make good copy, and media professionals need us as much as we need them. This makes our task a little easier.

Be clear about what you're trying to achieve

As with all forms of communication, your starting point must be:

• what am I trying to say?

• who am I trying to say it to?

• how best can I get it across to them?

To which should be added:

• what support or follow-up should I provide?

• what parallel approaches should I adopt?

• how will I know if I've succeeded?

Simple, clear messages, tailored to your target group, delivered through an appropriate media mix, is the recipe for success. If you can back that up with support—for example by providing a helpline or an information leaflet—and ensure that health services are ready to respond to increased demand, your intervention is likely to be even more effective.

Make use of available help

Use your organization's press officer or communications manager. They can advise you on how to *frame* your messages and which media are best for reaching the target group (see chapter 3.5). More importantly, if you *don't* use your organization's press officer, not only will you not be availing yourself of quality advice, your messages may be out of step with your organization's current policy. Always be clear, to the press and to others, on whose behalf you are speaking. Even if you claim you are speaking as an individual, it may be thought more newsworthy by journalists if they forget this.

Your organization's press officer will usually have a working relationship with key journalists and producers, and perhaps a budget which can be used to set up a press conference or pay for an 'advertorial' in the local paper. If you don't have this level of support, try to link in with a partner organization that does.

Cultivate the media

Be familiar with their output and look for opportunities. Talk to, and if possible, meet with health reporters and producers. Explain what you're trying to do—and what you can do for them. Try to be available if they need instant public health advice or information. By and large they want to get it right.

Writing a press release

Unlike a paid-for advertisement or advertorial, a press release doesn't guarantee your story will be covered. Newsdesks are buried under mountains of press releases. How can you make yours stand out?

Ten important guidelines:

1. Keep it short and simple—preferably one side of A4 maximum.
2. Devise a 'catchy' headline based on the main angle of the story.
3. Use short sentences and only a few key statistics.
4. The introductory paragraph should summarize the whole story in a few lines—what, why, who, where, when, and how.
5. The second paragraph fleshes out the detail—fuller background can be given in a 'notes for editors' section at the end.

6. The third paragraph can give a direct quote from the spokesperson and a plug for any action you want taken.

7. Editors are more inclined to use the story if they can lift text directly from the press release.

8. Always give a contact name with daytime and evening phone numbers.

9. Follow up with a phone call offering information booklets, photographs, or photo opportunities.

10. Consider putting on a formal press conference with a panel of speakers and convivial hospitality.

It should be possible to cut a press release at any word count and for it still to make sense.

Responding to press enquiries

If you are rung up by a journalist
make a note of their name and their publication or programme

• be open, fair, and honest. Don't try to bluster and pretend you know what you don't

• if they ask a question you are not sure about, say you'll check it out and call them back—and make sure you do

• avoid saying 'no comment'. Explain why you can't answer that particular question—perhaps because of confidentiality or because the matter is *sub judice*

• avoid making 'off the record' comments—they have a habit of finding their way onto the record.

Working on radio or television

Approach each programme separately via the producer or researcher. Whether you call them or they call you, you are likely to find yourself being assessed not only on the merit of your story but also on how well you put it across. If you seem to be saying the right things in the right way, you may be invited to take part.

Before committing yourself to being interviewed, try to find out:

• what is the programme's format and style?

• what sort of audience does it have?

• how are they pitching the item?—what is the topical hook?

• in what capacity are you appearing?—personal or representative?

• is it a one-to-one interview, or a studio discussion? If so, with whom, and what's *their* angle?

• is it live or pre-recorded?

- how long will your item be? (you need to know how to pace yourself)
- what are the likely questions?
- will it be in the studio, or will they come to you? (you may need to obtain permission for the recording to take place).

When deciding what your messages should be:

- decide on a few key messages and get them clear in your head—you can use brief notes for radio, but not for TV. Make sure they're jargon-free
- one or two real examples may add colour—but avoid using names unless you have been given permission to do so
- quote statistics very broadly—rather than '34.7%' say 'about a third' or 'about one in three'
- get your points across *early*—you never quite know when the item will be over
- a light touch of humour *may* help, but only if appropriate. If in doubt, don't
- make sure that any resource you're promoting, such as a leaflet or a service, is in plentiful supply and someone is primed to provide it.

Radio interviews or phone-ins

Radio is a cosy, intimate medium—so just talk naturally with the interviewer. Remember that the listeners are usually doing something else at the same time, so be upbeat, friendly, and plain-speaking.

If you find yourself taking part in a phone-in, here are a few more points to bear in mind:

- agree the ground you want to cover with the anchor-person so that callers are kept to the subject
- write each caller's name down so you can personalize your answers
- talk directly to the caller as if you were giving one-to-one advice
- don't ramble on too long with each call—keep moving on to the next.

Television interviews

Dress simply and plainly. No glinting jewellery or jarring patterns. Avoid white, bright red, green, or blue, which can 'flare' on the screen. Go for gentle, muted colours instead.

When you are in front of the camera:

- sit up—don't slouch—look alert and engaging
- if your mouth is dry, have a sip from the water on the table
- maintain eye contact with the interviewer, otherwise you'll look shifty
- don't fidget.

Feedback

Ask someone to listen to or watch the programme to give you some honest feedback. If possible, record it so you can learn how to do better next time.

Media training

As with most things, you learn best by doing. But you can help to avoid the pitfalls by having media training. Check to see if your organization can arrange this.

Further resources

Gabbay J and Porter J (ed.) (1995). *Communication skills.* Faculty of Public Health Medicine, London.

Karpf A (1988). *Doctoring the media: the reporting of health and medicine.* Routledge, London.

7.5 **Communicating risk**

Nick Steel and Charles Guest

> *'Learn what people already believe, tailor the communication to this knowledge and to the decisions people face, and then subject the resulting message to careful evaluation'.* [1]

Objectives

By reading this chapter you will be able to use an understanding of risk perception to communicate about risk more effectively.

Why is this an important public health issue?

Policy makers, scientists, clinicians, and the public do not always share a common understanding of risks to public health in many areas. Examples are the safety of food or medicines, control of infectious diseases, risks from pollutants or natural hazards, or the dangers of a poor diet. Public perceptions of the risks can be very different from 'expert' perceptions. However, there are some predictable patterns. Risk communication is relevant to all staff dealing with potential public health risks. There is an increasing moral and legal requirement for the public sector and private industry to inform populations about the health hazards to which they might be exposed.

Definitions

Risk is the probability that a particular adverse event occurs during a stated period of time, or results from a particular challenge.[2] It can never be reduced to zero.

Absolute risk is the probability of an event in a population, as contrasted with *relative risk*, which is the ratio of the risk of an event among the exposed to the risk among the unexposed.

Attributable risk is the rate of an event in exposed individuals that can be attributed to the exposure. Some people find the number needed to harm (NNH) more comprehensible than the attributable risk. The NNH is the number of people exposed that would result in one *additional* person being harmed over and above the background risk in the general population.

Risk assessment is the qualitative and quantitative assessment of the likelihood of adverse effects that may result from exposure to specified health hazards (or from the absence of beneficial influences). It has two components, risk estimation and risk evaluation.

Risk estimation relies on scientific activity and judgement. Statistics about past harmful events can be used to predict both the size and likelihood of future harmful events, including estimates of uncertainty. It involves identifying the health problem and the hazard responsible, and quantifying exposure in a specified population.

Risk evaluation relies on social and political judgement. It is the process of determining the importance of the identified hazards and estimated risks, from the point of view of those individuals or communities who face the risk. It includes the study of risk perception and the trade-off between perceived risks and benefits. The term 'outrage' has been used to describe the things that the public are worried about that experts traditionally ignore.[3]

Risk communication is the way in which information about risk is communicated to various audiences. It is a two-way process that needs to be considered at all stages of risk management (Figure 7.5.1).

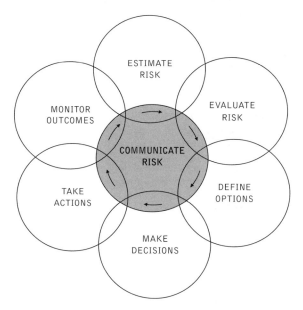

Figure 7.5.1 The risk management cycle[4].

Tasks for effective risk communication

Identify and involve relevant stakeholders

The first step is to identify all those within the organization who will be involved, in order to:

- agree a line to take to avoid sending contradictory messages
- identify who will lead the communication process
- involve public affairs or press office if available
- consider legal advice
- consider the time-scale.

Involving external stakeholders early will improve trust and generate useful information. Accept and involve the public, media, professional groups, experts, special interest groups, the local community, patients, politicians, manufacturers, environmentalists, and health officials as partners in risk communication.

Clarify objectives

Who are you trying to communicate with? Do you want to warn, reassure, or inform? You are unlikely to resolve all conflict over a controversial issue, but may clarify disagreements, minimize conflict, and improve decision making. Extra care is needed when you wish to both reassure (the risk is tolerable) and at the same time to warn (but if, in the unlikely event that the situation changes, the following emergency action will be necessary). If behaviour change is desired, consider the wider influences on behaviour.

Anticipate potential pitfalls

Check the source of your information. Is it consistent with other knowledge? Is it peer reviewed? Expert over-confidence is a common cause of failure in risk communication. It can be countered by explicitly seeking to uncover uncertainties, and by seeking different views to expose assumptions about your scientific evidence. Listen to the language and signs of concern of all persons involved. Pilot messages before releas.

> *'One should no more release an untested communication than an untested product'.*[5]

Resist the temptation to offer bland reassurance where there is real uncertainty. If the news is bad, share the burden with other stakeholders. Distinguish between scientific knowledge and value judgment, and recognize that emotion is an appropriate force for policy change.

Consider the target audience's risk perceptions

Analyse the different perspectives of, for example, politicians, the media, and scientists. What relative weights should be given to the results from different domains, such as the health and environment sectors? Produce written materials and other information sources if needed.

Monitor and review each communication routinely

Keep records of decisions taken and the resulting outcomes, and identify learning points.

What are the competencies needed to achieve these tasks?

Effective risk communication requires:

* commitment to openness and acceptance of the need to share uncertainty
* familiarity with risk language
* understanding of risk perception
* recognition of the benefit of continual learning from experience.

Commitment to openness

Early, ongoing, open, and honest interaction is a prerequisite to effective and ethical risk communication.[6] Uncertainties should be openly addressed, if only because subsequent events may show that a risk prediction was flawed, or result in a contradictory message. These will reduce trust, which is easy to lose but hard to gain. If we do not trust the source, we will not trust the message. People find it difficult to judge between experts when they disagree.

Risk language

The range of risk magnitudes that we face is so wide that the extremes can be hard to grasp. A logarithmic scale can span this wide range and provide a basis for describing risk. Such a scale can be anchored to the size of human communities, or use the analogy of a 1 metre 'risk stick' in a certain distance (Table 7.5.1). A potential problem of using risk comparisons is that people tend to over-estimate the risk of death from dramatic causes such as lightning, and underestimate the risk from common problems such as stroke.

Risk perception

Risk perception involves people's beliefs and feelings within their social and cultural context. A particular risk or hazard means different things to different people, and different things in different contexts. An understanding of risk perception underpins all effective risk communication.

Table 7.5.1 Risk scales.

Risk	Risk magnitude	Unit in which one adverse event would be expected ('community risk scale')	Distance containing one 'risk stick' 1 m long ('distance analogue risk scale')	Example (based on number of deaths in Britain per year)
1 in 1	10	Person	1 m	
1 in 10	9	Family	10 m	
1 in 100	8	Street	100 m	Any cause
1 in 1000	7	Village	1 km	Any cause, age 40
1 in 10,000	6	Small town	10 km	Road accident
1 in 100,000	5	Large town	100 km	Murder
1 in 1,000,000	4	City	1000 km	Oral contraceptives
1 in 10,000,000	3	Province or country	10, 000 km	Lightning
1 in 100,000,000	2	Large country	100,000 km	Measles
1 in 1,000,000,000	1	Continent	1,000,000 km	
1 in 10,000,000,000	0	World	10,000,000 km	

(Source: Calman and Royston[7])

(i) Framing

The way information about risk is framed affects the choices that will be made (see chapter 3.5). For example, both patients and doctors prefer treatment with a 90% *survival* rate to treatment with a 10% *mortality* rate, although the measures are equivalent.[8]

(ii) Absolute and relative risk

It is important to distinguish between absolute and relative risk. The anxiety generated in the UK over the doubling of the relative risk of venous thrombosis with third generation oral contraceptives compared with second generation ones obscured the message that the absolute risk was minimal.[9] Estimated reduction in relative risk gives a more favourable impression of the benefits of medical treatment than reduction in absolute risk.

(iii) Acceptability

It cannot be assumed that a risk is acceptable just because it is smaller than another risk that people already take. The qualitative aspect is more important than the quantitative aspect in risk perception. Risks are usually considered less acceptable if they:

• are involuntary (e.g. genetically modified food or pollution) rather than voluntary (e.g. skiing or smoking)

• arise from a novel or man-made source

• cause hidden damage, perhaps through onset of illness many years after exposure

• pose a danger to small children or pregnant women

• are poorly understood by science

• damage identifiable rather than anonymous victims

• are close—concern diminishes with distance

• threaten a form of illness arousing particular dread (e.g. death from cancer rather than a sudden heart attack).[10]

Working with the media

Journalists are constrained by the nature of their work to convey complex information about health risks simply, unambiguously, and dramatically. Public health practitioners need to acknowledge the uncertainty of many health risks.

> *'In a fight between 'terribly dangerous' and 'perfectly safe', the winner will be 'terribly dangerous'. But 'modestly dangerous' is a contender. Activists can afford to exaggerate, but industry and government cannot. Move to the middle of the seesaw'.*[3]

The following are indicators of potential media interest:

• questions of blame

• secrets and 'cover-ups'

Box 7.5.1 **Communicating the BSE–CJD epidemic in the UK and Australia**

(Adapted from Banwell and Guest[11])

United Kingdom

The Ministry of Agriculture was perceived to be secretive, and was criticized for denying the possibility of a link between BSE in cattle and vCJD in humans. The Minister for Agriculture denied risks of human infection from BSE, but later a group of 'eminent scientists' reported that they had stopped eating British beef. Articles in the press contained estimations of wildly differing numbers of people who may have contracted vCJD.

Australia

The government provided easy access to information via the media and a telephone information line to prevent the release of contradictory information and to acknowledge that there were risks involved, although small. Co-ordinated media liaison between government agencies helped to promote balanced reporting by the Australian media. It is not possible to say whether the government's media strategy would have been as effective if BSE had been discovered in Australia.

Key points:

Avoid secrecy, the denial of risk, and contradictory messages. Acknowledge uncertainty promptly.

- conflict (between experts or experts versus public)
- links to sex or crime
- human interest through identifiable heroes or villains
- links with existing high-profile issues or personalities
- strong visual impact
- signal value, or suggestion that the story is a sign of further problems.[10]

Continual learning from experience

Routine and honest review of experiences and dissemination of learning points improves future risk communication.

Examples of success and failure in risk communication

Success

The recovery of UK immunization rates with MMR (mumps, measles, rubella) vaccine after a high-profile scare that MMR immunization might be related to Crohn's disease and autism in the UK. Key points were the building of trust through the provision of high quality information, and the open acknowledgement of uncertainty. This approach allowed most people to see that the likely benefits of immunization far outweighed the potential disadvantages.

Failure

The complex saga of Bovine Spongiform Encephalopathy (BSE) in cattle and its possible links with a variant of the human disease Creutzfeldt-Jakob Disease (vCJD) has aroused considerable public concern (Box 7.5.1).

How will you know if your communication about risk has been successful?

Success means reaching a shared understanding of risk with the relevant target audience. This can be assessed in terms of how close you have come to fully meeting your objectives about the purpose of the communication. Absence of outrage is usually the desirable outcome, and, as usual, this attracts little attention or gratitude!

Further resources

Bennett P and Calman K (ed.) (1999). *Risk communication and public health*. Oxford University Press, Oxford.

Bernstein PL (1996). *Against the gods: the remarkable story of risk*. John Wiley and Son, Inc., New York.

Dickson D (1997). UK policy learns about risk the hard way. *Nature*, **385**, 8–9.

Golding D, Krimsky S, and Plough A (1992). Evaluating risk communication: narrative vs. technical presentations of information about radon. *Risk Analysis*, **12**, 27–35.

Henderson M (1990). *The BMA guide to living with risk*. BMA, London.

Keeney RL and von Winterfeldt D (1986). Improving risk communication. *Risk Analysis*, **6**, 417–24.

Mason JO, Ogden HG, Berreth DA, and Martin LY (1986). Interpreting risks to the public. *Am J Prev Med*, **2**, 133–9.

Petersen A and Lupton D (1996). *The new public health: health and self in the age of risk*. Sage Publications, London.

Slovic P (1987). Perception of risk. *Science*, **236**, 280–5.

Smith AFM (1996). Mad cows and ecstasy: chance and choice in an evidence-based society. *J R Statist Soc*, **159**, 367–83.

Risk and the inadequacy of science. *Nature*, 1997, **385**, 1.

References

1. Morgan MG (1993). Risk analysis and management. *Scientific American*, July, 24–30.
2. Royal Society Study Group (1992). *Risk: analysis, perception and management*. Royal Society, London.
3. Sandman PM (1993). *Responding to community outrage: strategies for effective risk communication*. American Industrial Hygiene Association; Fairfax VA.
4. The presidential/congressional commission on risk assessment and risk management (1997). *Framework for environmental health risk management*, Final report Vol. 1. Government Printing Office, Washington DC.
5. Morgan MG, Fischhoff B, Bostrom A, Lave L, and Atman C (1992). Communicating risk to the public. *Environmental Science and Technology*, **26**, 2048–56.
6. National Research Council (1989). *Improving risk communication*. National Academy Press, Washington DC.
7. Calman KC and Royston GH (1997). Risk language and dialects. *BMJ*, **315**, 939–42.
8. McNeil BJ, Pauker SG, Sox HC, and Tversky A (1982). On the elicitation of preferences for alternative therapies. *New Eng J Med*, **306**, 1259–62.
9. Calman KC (1996). Cancer: science and society and the communication of risk. *BMJ*, **313**, 799–802.
10. UK Department of Health (1997). *Communicating about risks to public health: pointers to good practice*. Department of Health, London.
11. Banwell C and Guest CS (1998). Carnivores, cannibals, consumption and unnatural boundaries: the BSE–CJD epidemic in the Australian press. In *Mad cows and modernity: cross-disciplinary reflections on the crisis of Creutzfeldt-Jakob disease*, (ed. I McCalman, B Penny, and M Cook), pp. 3–36. National Academies Forum, Canberra.

Falsehood flies and truth comes limping after it; so that when men come to be undeceived, it is too late, the jest is over and the tale has had its effect.

Jonathan Swift 1667–1745

7.6 Developing public health strategies: the consultant's role

Charles Guest

Objectives

This chapter introduces the steps for developing a public health strategy. It should help you to play a constructive role as a public health consultant (see definition below), working closely with government officials, policy advisers, and other stakeholders in the creation of a major strategy.

You will consider:

- the definition of a public health problem and the development of a strategy as a response to it
- the need to create and clarify objectives
- the need to collect and analyse relevant information
- the development of proposals and options, with appropriate balance between brevity and comprehensive detail
- the importance of a detailed study of options, which should include the case against, as well as for, the options favoured by the consultant
- consultation, one activity for improving a draft of the strategy.

Implementation and evaluation of the strategy are addressed only briefly.

Definitions

In this chapter, the word '*consultant*' is used in a general sense to indicate a provider of independent professional advice or services, on a contractual basis. An independent consultant working alongside government agencies will have a quite distinct role from that played by employees of those agencies (public servants). Also, distinguish the role played by medical specialists as salaried officers of a health service (e.g. consultants in public health medicine).

A *public health strategy* is an organized programme for public health activity at a local, regional, or national level. In this chapter, '*strategy*' consists of the development and documentation of a specific agenda in public health (see chapter 6.3). '*Policy*', a more general term, refers to a course of action, expedient or prudent, that may be less adequately documented than a specific public health strategy (see chapter 3.2).

Development of a strategy should include many of the same evidence-based steps that apply to the development of guidelines (chapter 6.10). This chapter assumes some familiarity with the latter process and addresses additional steps and departures from the more circumscribed activity of developing guidelines.

Why is this an important public health activity?

Strategies represent tangible public health activities that often have large associated budgets. Most people are affected by a number of public health strategies. At some time, most practitioners will participate in the development or implementation of a public health strategy.

Methods, stages, and tasks of developing a public health strategy

Initial clarification

Whether or not to develop a major public health strategy is usually a decision taken at a high level in a government department after politicians, special interest groups, or journalists have moved an issue onto the national agenda. People in the public health field may have participated in that process, or their influence may have been slight. As the consultant, you should appreciate the circumstances that produced the requirement for a strategy, such as changes in:

+ government
+ population health status
+ health services
+ perspectives in sectors other than health (e.g. environment or transport)
+ financing
+ economic and performance pressures
+ alliances.

A potential for improvement in at least some of these variables may justify the development of a strategy. If you are contributing to early decisions about the possible development of a public health strategy, your advice should:

+ provide structure to promote systematic thought and action about a major problem that has been poorly understood
+ gather the minimum necessary information, with appropriate analysis
+ indicate a range of options for public health action
+ communicate results of this work to the client in a timely and understandable way.

Other stages may then follow:

Defining the scope of the public health problem

A more formal definition will usually be required, in consultation with a reference group of senior officials and stakeholders, referred to in this chapter as the steering committee. A review of the relevant epidemiology and potentially effective interventions is usually required, with reference to the current position. Public opinion survey data may be available: they should be considered early in the strategy process. (Alternatively, surveys may be planned as a research activity, noted below.)

Establishing the policy framework

This includes identification of guiding principles (including, but not restricted to, 'government policy') and appropriate key partners, and then, according to the circumstances, contributing to the:

* establishment of priorities
* definition of roles and responsibilities
* planning of research and development
* scope of intervention—tools for the strategy, e.g. guidelines, governance, standards, regulation, legislation, grants, subsidies, tax credits
* development of a workplan for some or all of these tasks (implementation)
* planning of the evaluation (measurable achievements and other outcomes).

Consultation

You may play a role in the conduct of consultations, of possible relevance at several phases in the development of a strategy. These may serve to obtain critical information and to foster a receptive attitude among stakeholders to the development of a strategy. The methodology for consultation should be developed to include views from a wide range of individuals and organizations by such methods as focus groups, interviews, and written submissions.

Drafting the strategy

This will be then be informed by:

* views of the government (the client) and the steering committee
* results of the consultations
* review of the literature
* your own observations.

The draft strategy is then usually subject to further consultation and revision before approval at senior levels.

Managing the strategy's development

Assemble essential resources

Influence with policy makers, peers, and the public, for any activity in public health, has to be earned, and cannot be granted by fiat. You will have earned at least some influence if you play a major role in the development of the strategy. If you do not also have them, ensure that your contract[1] enables you to obtain the necessary:

- legal authority
- convening power
- information
- scientific and technical expertise (e.g. for community health assessments, epidemiology, health education campaigns, or detailed policy analysis (see below))
- advocacy, lobbying and public relations skills.

The development of many strategies requires simultaneous attention to inputs and process:[2]

Inputs

(i) Management

Good management is essential for the development of a strategy, including:

- competent leadership and senior management
- effective communication of objectives and priorities by the executive to all staff
- openness that seeks positive external linkages
- performance guidelines that adequately define success and failure, with due reference to integrity and ethical standards.

(ii) Staff

Appropriately qualified and motivated staff may need to be recruited and retained. Time must be allowed for this. Training may be relevant to the development of staff in major national policy activity, but you may not have time for this during the more constrained schedule for developing a new strategy.

(iii) Information technology

Is your equipment adequate? For example, do you have enough storage and processing power and software to perform tasks efficiently in the field?

Process assessment

The public health consultant needs to identify rapidly and use networks, within government (within and between portfolios) and outside it. The views of those likely to be affected should be sought actively and carefully incorporated in the development of the strategy.

Detailed analysis should establish:

- the successes and failures of previous and related programmes
- possible consequences, intended and unintended, of options for the strategy
- the institution's capacity to implement the strategy, including the support at middle and lower levels necessary for the achievement of objectives.

Outputs

An immediate output of a strategy's development is represented by its publication. The published strategy may be accompanied by other background or technical reports.

The publication should specify:

- the problem to be addressed, with adequate analysis
- the scientific basis on which the strategy was developed
- who will do what, when.

Desirable features include:

- creative approaches to options and their implications
- coherence with other programmes and strategies
- practicality
- cogent advocacy of the preferred options.

A background report[3] could specify:

- how the need for the strategy was identified
- how the strategy was developed
- how strategy development has been funded, and the resources available for implementation
- who was responsible for development of the strategy
- who was consulted
- possible—as well as probable—outcomes of the strategy
- cost-effectiveness of solutions identified
- the time-frame for evaluation.

Dissemination and implementation require much greater attention than previously accorded to many major strategies. Approaches now include:

* summaries on the internet and elsewhere
* mass media
* professional and consumer organizations
* incentives.

Engaging people in the importance of a strategy

The whole spectrum of public interests, government, and management must be engaged if a public health strategy is to achieve its goals. You should promote the development of goals that all health and other sectors can share.

As with any collaborative venture:

* seek the early involvement of partners
* identify reasons (additional to the public health concerns) for others, including representatives of industry or the private sector, to become actively involved
* expect and listen to a wide range of opinions about the development of the strategy
* obtain influential endorsements.

Potential pitfalls

Under-estimating complexity

Public health strategies may cross conventional governmental portfolios, or require new inter-governmental relations. Consider institutional constraints early. Avoid too large a task with too few resources.

Inadequate communication

For example, lack of awareness and understanding of the strategy among the target population, or failure to legitimate the approach among professionals of all affected sectors, may lead to people ignoring or undermining the new approach.

'We have the Minister's full support'

Continued support from within government should not be assumed, even if the development of a public health strategy was the minister's initiative. Choosing not to decide about possible government projects is sometimes the preferred option for politicians and their advisers. They will sometimes go to extremes to avoid association with an initiative that could fail.

The development of a strategy distorts the political process, while the real questions remain undebated

Perhaps the worst pitfall, from the citizen's perspective. Technical issues should not be allowed to obscure political questions, while the public health consultant cannot and should not assume the responsibilities of the elected representative.

Particular problems for the independent consultant

Avoid:

* arrogance
* self-censorship (tell clients what they need to know, not what you think they want to hear)
* creating problems rather than solving them
* neglect of current clients while chasing new ones.[4]

What are the key determinants of success?

* political support
* committed, adequate financial resources
* collaboration across sectors
* community participation.

How will you know when/if you have been successful?

Development of the strategy

Desirable qualities of the process and outputs of the strategy include:

* comprehensiveness
* timeliness
* responsiveness (e.g. evidence of adequate consultation with interested parties)
* clarity
* practicality
* relevance
* fairness (e.g. recommendations are balanced and equitable, as well as objective)
* cost-effectiveness (comparative costs to various solutions should be provided).

Subsequent evaluation

* were the objectives of the strategy met?
* did the original objectives remain in place?
* what has actually been implemented?[5]
* has the public health problem itself changed?
* what relevance does the strategy now have?
* what were the outcomes? Were they anticipated or not?

Your role as consultant

- was your analysis of the problem accurate?
- if the strategy was developed according to your plans, did you predict the outcome?

Also assess your efficiency, e.g. the timeliness of preparation and real costs of your input to the strategy. The measurement of effectiveness assumes a causal link between your role as a consultant and the outcome of the strategy. This will probably remain a matter only for speculation, but see chapter 4.3.

Conclusion

Like any project in public health, a strategy requires:

- collaboration that may be broad, while retaining sufficient focus for effectiveness
- adaptability to local and regional needs
- careful attention to the allocation and use of resources, including government and other infrastructure.

Further resources

Walt G (1994). *Health policy*. Zed Books and Witwatersrand University Press, London.

References

1. Lasker RD and the Committee on Medicine and Public Health (1997). *Medicine and public health: the power of collaboration*. New York Academy of Medicine, New York.
2. Uhr J and Mackay K (ed.) (1996). *Evaluating policy advice: learning from Commonwealth experience*. Federalism Research Centre, Australian National University and Commonwealth Department of Finance, Canberra.
3. National Health and Medical Research Council (Australia) (1999). *A guide to the development, implementation and evaluation of clinical practice guidelines*. NHMRC, Canberra.
4. Nelson B and Economy P (1997). *Consulting for dummies*. IDG Publications, Foster City CA.
5. Rist RC (1994). Influencing the policy process with qualitative research. In *Handbook of qualitative research*, (ed. NK Denzin and YS Lincoln), pp. 545–57. Sage Publications, Thousand Oaks.

7.7 Assessing and improving your own professional practice

Caron Grainger

Overview

Improving your professional practice is both a duty, and an important method of maintaining your own feeling of self-worth. Professionals have a responsibility to continuously monitor and improve their own practice *and* to make it as easy as possible for others to do the same. This second obligation (i.e. towards our fellow professionals) distinguishes corporate/clinical governance from earlier methods of professional quality improvement.

Objectives

This chapter should:

- emphasize the importance of objectively demonstrating competence and commitment to professional development (both for yourself and others)
- enable you to understand the role of performance review in improving performance
- enable you to understand the principles of setting, and recording, a personal development plan (PDP) or equivalent
- enable you to understand the principles of mentorship
- help you appreciate the importance of individuals and leaders in creating public health 'learning organizations'.

Why assessing and improving your professional practice matters

Identifying, and communicating the need for change, and helping the change happen is the essence of public health action. The most fundamental process of change is simply that of genuine learning: learning by individuals, by teams, and by organizations. Assessing and improving your professional practice is important in *all* professions. However, it is *particularly* important in public health practice for at least three reasons:

- many people do not understand the broad range of work of public health professionals. It is important to be able to communicate quickly to many different people how, as a public health professional, you can add value to the clarification of an issue or the solution of a problem (or both)

- the challenges that face public health professionals can change quickly; hence the need to realign existing skills and develop new ones as the need arises

- professional competence is an increasingly important part of professional regulation that both regulatory agencies and the public expect and require. Maintaining and improving competence is easier if this is an integral part of your *own* work. It can be difficult to convince others to do something that you don't seem be prepared (or able) to do.

The importance of insight, reflection, and unlearning

Before you can improve your own practice, you need to be able to assess it; hence the importance of insight. Perhaps the most difficult part of developing insight is appreciating what you don't already know, sometimes called the unconscious incompetence. Mentors and buddies are essential in helping you discover what you don't know that you don't know. However, as the Johari window (Figure. 7.7.1) illustrates, developing personal insight with the help of others cannot guarantee success because there will always be areas unknown to others as well as yourself (box 4). The task is to minimize this area. Similarly in Figure. 7.7.2, the objective is to identify the critical areas contained within your area of conscious incompetence.

Insight will help discover not only what is not known, but what is thought to be correct that is wrong: this will lead to necessary unlearning—the unlearning of previous beliefs.

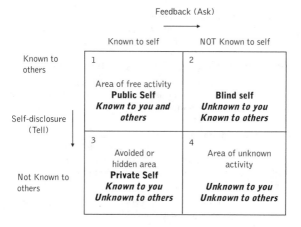

Figure 7.7.1 The Johari window (after Joseph Luft-Kurtz and Harry Ingham).

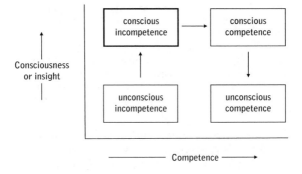

Figure 7.7.2 Developing competence and insight.

Lastly, insight and reflection are important to know how you can, as a public health professional, contribute to a public health organization. Every public health professional has a different set of competencies. Every competent public health professional will know a little about a lot (breadth) and a lot about a little (depth). It is important to know:

• what this picture of breadth and depth looks like at any particular time for you

• how this matches the needs of the public health organization(s) in which you work

• how your professional competencies need to be developed in order to match the present and future demands of teams and organizations of which you may be a part.

Terms used in improving your professional practice

All detailed areas attract phrases, acronyms, and jargon. It is important to know when these terms mean something very particular. Perhaps the most common words and processes to be confused are assessment and appraisal:

• *appraisal:* a non-threatening, confidential dialogue exploring and agreeing on objectives to be attained, or progress in attaining agreed objectives, and the individual development needs of the appraisee, enabling them to get the most from their experience in order to develop specific competencies

• *assessment:* a formal, one-way process, assessing performance against pre-set competencies, standards, or objectives.

Appraisal and assessment may be related (Table 7.7.1). For instance, appraisal might reveal that one career direction is better suited to the individual than another. This may influence the targets, milestones, criteria, and standards that are set for subsequent assessments. Similarly, the formal findings of an assessment process could well be discussed during appraisal. Confidentiality is an important feature of appraisal. However, there will be situations where it would be difficult to ignore the findings of an appraisal (considering, for example, the competence of an individual, appraised information may be needed in an assessment process). It is critical that any such information elicited and subsequently used elsewhere (e.g. at an assessment process) is done with the appraisee's consent. If this is not done, the trust is broken.

Table 7.7.1 Assessment and appraisal.

Summative assessment 'Assessment'	Formative assessment 'Appraisal'
Summates/assesses progress so far	Reflects on progress to indicate future direction—leads to formation and learning
Measures targets met; grades; marks	Checks and sets goals and values, and builds, but rarely attracts marks/grades
Looks back against generic standards—data capture, tick box	Looks backwards and forwards with respect to person—involves planning and motivation to develop the individual
Process concentrates on information about the person's objective progress (skills, knowledge, competencies)	Process includes (a) feedback on general performance, and (b) help with personal development and career progression
Mainly one way process of checking milestones and benchmarking	A two-way, informal, subjective, iterative, negotiated process using quality feedback
An explicit, external, formal process of measurement at critical points, measuring progress against explicit standards	A confidential and personal process that should be supporting and non-threatening
Asks: can I/you reach that standard?	Asks: how am I/are you doing now/in the past and how do I/do you do better in future?

Many meetings include elements of both processes. Because assessment and appraisal have different objectives and consequences, however, it is important to be clear at any one time exactly which process is underway:

• **performance review:** a formal process, usually between employee and line manager, of assessing performance against agreed objectives, identifying training and development needs, and setting objectives for the next work period. It encompasses elements of both appraisal and assessment

* **learning need:** the gap between your current and your desired or optimal level of competence required to undertake a task
* **continuing professional development** (CPD): a purposeful, systematic activity by individuals, teams, and organizations to maintain and expand their knowledge, skills, and attributes required to fulfil their potential to do their job competently
* **personal development plan** (PDP): a recorded method of identifying gaps in professional knowledge, skills, or attributes and planning how to address these deficits, often performed with another professional e.g. boss, mentor, colleague. The aim should be to identify and record training needs for individual development and to support the individual's development in relation to the role they play in meeting the organization's present or future requirements. (Alternative terms include personal learning plan, learning agreement/contract).

Developing a personal development plan

A personal development plan, or equivalent, is a blueprint for continuing professional development. Essential elements include:

* it should be recorded (on paper, electronically) such that it can be objectively retrieved and reviewed
* it should be systematic (i.e. logically structured, and addressing all necessary competencies)
* it should be agreed (initially with a mentor or buddy), or failing that, a consensus on what is not agreed should be recorded.

Ultimately every public health professional should be able to demonstrate that they have mechanisms for developing insight into their professional competence, clarifying their professional role, and identifying their learning needs, and how they are being, or planned to be, met. This involves:

* a systematic and agreed plan of what these needs are, and how these needs may be met
* a process whereby progress is monitored explicitly and plans adapted accordingly
* an open record of this complete process
* a willingness to share this record with others.

This process requires critical awareness, an appreciation of the context in which knowledge and skills will be applied, an understanding of a practitioner's personal learning style, and reflection. Many individuals find it helpful to review their learning needs, and identify means of meeting them, with another practitioner (e.g. boss or mentor) who provides an external, balanced view of both strengths and weaknesses.

Developing a PDP requires:

(a) identifying learning needs

(b) prioritizing learning needs

(c) recording learning needs and objectives

(d) organizing the right sort of learning to meet these needs (and getting the necessary resources)

(e) evaluating the outcome of learning.

(a) Identifying your learning needs

Group your learning needs into four broad areas:

• to fulfil the duties of your *current* role (involves careful analysis of job description and person specification)

• to meet the requirements of a change in duties or role e.g. a new job (it is vitally important that public health practitioners maintain the right balance between depth and breadth)

• general keeping up-to-date

• specialist interest or personal development needs (developing depth).

(b) Establish which of these needs are most important and most urgent, by considering:

• the organization's needs vs. your department's needs vs. your personal needs

• how big the learning need is

• how urgent the need

• whether resources are available

• the commitment of the organization to support the department and the commitment of the department to support the individual in meeting the need.

(c) Recording learning needs and objectives

This may sound bureaucratic and tedious but it is both important and useful. A need identified today may be forgotten tomorrow. If a need is validly identified by a colleague or manager and then formally recorded, it is more likely that the resources can be found to address it.

Having identified learning needs and potential outcome indicators, it is possible to set a learning objective according to SMART criteria:

• Specific

• Measurable

- Achievable
- Realistic/Relevant
- Timed.

(d) Organizing the right sort of learning and locating resources for learning

Opportunities for learning are many: on-the-job vs. formal training, active learning vs. observation learning, theoretical vs. practical learning. Not only do different people learn in different ways, but, within the same person, different sorts of knowledge, skills, and attitudes are learnt in different ways. Furthermore, these learning styles can also change over time.

In practice, there are two main settings for learning (external or internal), each with two dimensions, planned and unplanned. Various learning opportunities arise in each of these four categories (Table 7.7.2). Identifying opportunities in each category is a first step to finding the resources for learning.

Table 7.7.2 Categories of learning opportunities.

Example: learning how to chair meetings better (see chapter 7.2)		
	External **'Off-the-job'**	**Internal** **'On-the-job'**
Planned	e.g. Attend a one-day course on improving chairing skills	e.g. Have someone assess your chairing skills at the beginning and end of a meeting
Unplanned	e.g. Noting styles of chairing on a TV documentary	e.g. Observe chairing skills in others

(e) Evaluating the outcome of learning

As part of setting learning objectives it is important to recognize how you will evaluate the impact of your learning. Evaluation criteria can be either:

- *qualitative* e.g. your perception of change, your insight as a result of learning; or
- *quantitative* e.g. the use of an objective assessment tool, such as an examination, or external assessment of performance.

It is worth noting the difference between output, i.e. the knowledge or skill that has been acquired, and outcome, or how you are applying this knowledge and skill to greater effect. A simple way of assessing outcome is to ask whether what you have learned has resulted in change in practice.

Example: An example of a well thought out learning objective would be:

To improve chairing skills (specific) over a six-month period (timed, realistic) to ensure that all meetings have a clearly defined agenda, adequate time for discussion involving all parties, and clearly agreed decisions/actions which are appropriately recorded (achievable, measurable).

Learning portfolios

These can help to demonstrate and distinguish learning achieved and learning needed. A good portfolio will comprise:

• evidence of learning
• reflection and commentary on the learning, including how learning has been applied to your everyday practice.

Your portfolio should eventually build into an inventory of your skills and achievements, together with future aspirations. Items to include in a learning portfolio are shown in the Box 7.7.1.

Box 7.7.1 **Items to consider including in a learning portfolio**

• examination certificates, registration certificates, etc.
• CV
• summary of posts to date, and learning from those posts
• appraisal forms
• objectives of current post
• (adverse) incidents and reflection upon them
• audit projects
• teaching experience
• research experience and aspirations, publications
• career intentions
• personal development plan
• anything else that you feel is relevant, which demonstrates learning from an event.

The process of conducting a performance review

Any system of performance review should be focused on motivating staff through unbiased, objective feedback in *both* directions between manager and staff member. Successful performance review is a cyclical activity, which takes a joint problem-solving approach, reviewing personal, career, and organizational goals through:

• assessing performance against agreed objectives and standards of competence

- a two-way appraisal reviewing and reflecting upon personal, educational, and job-related achievements and training or development needs

- recognition of the contribution of an individual towards organizational goals, including the collaborative setting of standards for future work in context of the local business plan.

It is important to recognize that good performance review includes consideration of the wider development needs of an individual outside the immediate job, for example, developing them for a new job, or within their wider professional activities. Similarly, there must be recognition that duties and responsibilities, and the environment in which we work, and therefore learning needs, change over time. These elements should all be considered as parts of performance review.

Mentors

A mentor (literally 'wise one') can be a useful source of support in identifying and planning personal development for public health professionals. A good mentor will help you consider your roles and responsibilities 'in the round', i.e. the balance of work and home, development needed in the current job and for future jobs, and will play a variety of roles (Box 7.7.2).

Box 7.7.2 **Roles in mentoring**

- sounding board
- joint problem solver
- ratifier
- mirror
- coach
- repository
- referee
- flaw finder
- connector and networker
- empathizer
- guide.

Key issues for managing a mentoring relationship include:

- agree a mentoring contract i.e. how long the relationship will last for, how often the meetings will be held, confidentiality, boundaries

- give thought to who you approach as a mentor. Whilst they are not necessarily friends, they must be a trusted and respected individual you can relate to easily

- look for someone who can translate his or her personal experience into generic 'how to's'

- your learning needs will vary over time. One individual may not be able to provide all the help you need, but should be able to direct you to others as appropriate. Similarly, consider whether one individual should be used on an ongoing basis, or should be picked for particular skills to help resolve a short-term training need, or a mixture of the two

- mentors are usually senior to you and usually work in a different organization. If mentors come from the same organization, however, this can be sensitive, particularly if they are your boss's boss and you are seen to be going above your boss's head!

Departments and organizations

After the individual, another level of analysis is the organization you work for. The individual influences the organization and the organization influences the individual. Public health has always worked (and is always likely to work) in a rapidly-changing environment. It is therefore imperative that individuals and leaders do all they can to make the unit a learning organization: an organization where reflection, learning, and improvement are integrated into every activity.

Summary

- develop insight into what your strengths and weaknesses are (possibly with the help of other trusted colleagues)

- distinguish and map your breadth skills and your depth skills

- understand how these strengths and weaknesses relate to the contribution expected from you by the public health organization(s) you work with

- identify a plan to close the gap between what you have and what you need

- ensure you have a vision for the sort of skills you may need in a rapidly changing public health environment

- record whenever possible, very simply, this whole process, in order to demonstrate to others your insight, your progress, and your commitment to improving your professional practice and that of your team and organization.

Further resources

Schön DA46 (1983). *The reflective practitioner*. Temple Smith, London.
The whole of this handbook addresses the improvement of public health practice. In particular, see chapters 7.1, 8.1, and 8.5.

Keep your eyes on the stars, and your feet on the ground.

Theodore Roosevelt, 1858–1919

Part 8
Organizational development

Introduction

'*Give us grace to accept with serenity the things that cannot be changed, courage to change the things which should be changed, and the wisdom to distinguish the one from the other*[†].'

We live with too much change in too short a time. Some changes are deliberate, planned, and purposeful, some appear random and chaotic, and others are merely fashions. To survive requires a careful examination of ourselves, dealt with in part 7. Part 8 is about examination of our surroundings: the organizations and relationships that are integral to the public health practitioner's role.

Many approaches are required to cope in a changing environment, to develop public health as a constant learning activity. Being prepared to study the process of change from perspectives that include psychology and management need not lead to an eclectic free-for-all.

This part contains two chapters about people: working with others engaged in the public health endeavour (teams), and working with those we purport to serve—'consumers'; and three chapters on development techniques: project planning, business planning, and assessing good public health action.

Assessing our effectiveness is a critical element for collaboration in public health. Working with consumers should now be considered essential for all of us. We are all consumers.

CSG

[†] *Reinhold Niebuhr (1892–1971).*

8.1 Working in teams

Annabelle Mark

Introduction

Very few endeavours today are achieved effectively and efficiently without the use of teams at some stage. This is particularly important in areas such as public health which are, by their very nature, often bureaucratic, political, and multi-disciplinary.

Objectives

By reading this chapter you will know:

- what a team is
- how to make it work
- what the problems can be in team working and ways of avoiding or overcoming them
- how to recognize success.

Definition

- teams are groups of people working together towards *common goals*
- they are more effective than groups because 'the whole is greater than the sum of its parts'
- teams provide a sense of belonging, a source of help and support; a sense of shared purpose.

Why is this an important public health issue?

No individual in public health knows all the answers, or can represent all the issues and opinions—so teams help bring these together and achieve effective outcomes. In summary, teams are more likely than individuals to be effective functional units.

What are the defined tasks?

There are important tasks that any team member must take seriously if the team is going to work effectively:

- understanding individual roles and behaviour
- sharing the development process
- identifying problems
- improving team activity and effectiveness.

When joining a team, ask yourself what you will gain:

• I will look important = *status*
• I will feel important = *self-esteem*
• I like to mix with others = *affiliation*
• I like to have influence = *power*
• I achieve my goals faster with others = *goal achievement*.

Different team members seek different things from teams. It is important to acknowledge and to identify what motivates individual team members.

Once you have assembled your team you need to think about how it works. Remember that teams thrive on variety. Teams of clever people or people with similar personalities are often *not* as effective as might be imagined. Mutually respecting heterogeneity is preferable to competitive homogeneity.

Key competencies

An essential competency in participating in any team is recognizing the different behaviours of team members and using them to the team's advantage in achieving its objectives.

Example: the development of hierarchies

Hierarchies develop in any group (although genuine teams are often characterized by their lack of formal hierarchy). We can see this by looking at the pattern of interruption—more interrupting often equates to desire for more influence. Professionals do this constantly: doctors interrupt more than nurses, men tend to interrupt more than women. Observing interruptions can often indicate how hierarchies within a team are changing.

Effective team working depends on every person:

• knowing what the team is here to do
• taking full advantage of how the team can help each person to do it
• minimizing the ways in which the team may hinder any individual contributing fully.

Sharing this information regularly within the team helps members think about their own behaviour. This information needs to be compared with individual needs for status, self-esteem, affiliation, power, and goal achievement identified above.

Developing the team

This requires an explicit sharing and development of:

• *norms* or 'the usual methods we adopt here'
• an understanding of the *roles* of team-members.

Role of team members

Roles can be categorized:

- *functional roles*—what I do as a doctor, nurse, accountant, or community representative (often *professionally* defined)

- *team roles*—how I like to behave and contribute, by for example leading the team or collecting information, or contributing ideas (often *personally* defined).

While most people know their functional role, identifying your team role is critical to success.

Belbin[1] described eight essential team roles which should be allocated within the team:

1. Co-ordinator = chairing role.
2. Resource Investigator = external liaison.
3. Shaper = goal setter.
4. Implementer = translates ideas to action plans.
5. Plant = the ideas person.
6. Monitor Evaluator = analyst of ideas and action.
7. Team Worker = develops team spirit.
8. Completer Finisher = minds details and targets.

(The Belbin Self-Perception Inventory[1] will assist in identifying these roles for each team member.)

Team members can have more than one preferred team role, but all roles must be covered by members, *even if the team is smaller than eight in number.*

Knowing which are the least favoured roles shows where a weakness in the team may appear—ask team members which roles they most and least wish to fulfil.

How do teams in public health work?

Teams in public health involve many professions and sometimes members of the community. The way each one works will vary according to the *task* and *time-scale*. They are usually one of three types:

- a crisis team
- a project team
- a planning team.

Examples

- a *crisis* team will need to move fast to achieve its task, so some unhelpful behaviours may be reinforced, for example failing to listen to others (see chapter 4.8).

- a *project* team will have specific goals and time-scales, but may need help in developing ideas and a shared view, especially if members rely only on their representative or professional roles to guide them (e.g. re-engineering the emergency admissions system for a busy hospital)

- a *planning* team will have more time. This is not always an advantage—especially when individuals lose the motivation and pressure to contribute (e.g. strategy groups—see chapters 6.3 and 7.6).

Remember, the less time the team has to do something, the more it will focus on the task, rather than the team. To avoid poor team-working, good team leadership is essential. Good leaders share mutual trust and respect with their followers—leaders are thus best chosen by the team but can change according to the task or roles required.

Potential pitfalls in teams

Language

Agreeing on a common language is about culture. Specialists must not exclude others by their technical perspective and use of jargon.

Stereotyping

Get each member of the team to express their attitudes to other roles like doctors or managers or the public. The group then shares this information to see how they see others and how others see them. This activity is an essential part of team building. Time spent on such activities is rarely wasted; it breaks down barriers and increases trust.

There are many other soluble barriers to good team working:

- poor listening
- domination by individuals or subgroups
- negative (destructive) criticism
- hidden conflicts
- divisive arguments
- absenteeism.

Effective team building requires good personal interaction to build trust and openness.

Engaging people in team building

Like individuals, teams have recognizable development paths and life-cycles, and, like life, some stages of this development can be uncomfortable.

Stages of development

The most frequently used model[2] to describe the team development process consists of these phases:

- *forming* = the testing phase—information gathering

- *storming* = infighting and demotivation—barrier recognition
- *norming* = sharing ideas and tasks—developing shared interdependence
- *performing* = achieving together—group maturity and task progress.

These stages represent a circular process which may stop, get stuck, or begin again, when there are changes in:

- team membership
- task
- environment
- team norms or roles.

Avoidance of any of these stages damages the development of trust and team effectiveness.

To summarize, team-building involves:

- setting shared goals
- shared understanding of each other's roles and personalities
- understanding of the team process.

Conflict, conformity, and team work

Conflict between *personalities* can have very negative effects, but conflict over *ideas* enhances team development. Conflict therefore has both a negative and positive role in groups. Conflict in teams usually appears as either disputes about what to do (objectives), or who should do it (boundaries).

Public health professionals may find themselves in conflict with others because their concern is with the health of the community as a whole, rather than specific individuals within it (objectives). (Similarly, in other areas, many nurses can find their clinical role sometimes conflicts with that of the doctor (boundaries).)

Conflict can also indicate communication failures—don't assume everyone understands your role, even if it seems obvious. If in doubt, check by asking for feedback.

Is conformity better?

In team terms, a *lack* of conflict can cause 'groupthink'[3]; the group becomes more important than the tasks it has to perform. This can have disastrous results, because the team risks developing any or all of the following characteristics:

- a sense of invulnerability
- unquestioning belief in its own morality
- pressures to conform, suppressing opposition
- rationalizations of the unacceptable to achieve consensus

- an illusion of unanimity
- self-censorship of any deviation from the group.

Some tensions are both healthy and productive, especially where teams are unreceptive to ideas that come from elsewhere.

How do you recognize poor team working?

There are ten warning signs of poor team working[4] (this list can be used as formal exercise within a team):

1. People are often late or miss meetings.
2. Positions are entrenched by professional roles ('it's not my job').
3. Too much time is spent going over the same ground.
4. Individuals are doing complete projects in their own right.
5. Too much work is changed or has to be redone.
6. Some people seem to have their own hidden agenda.
7. People accept tasks but never get them done on time.
8. Deadlines are OK, but there are too few detailed plans.
9. Teams seem to produce long reports but are short on real output.
10. Priorities keep being changed as problems arise.

(List adapted with permission of the publisher, Kogan Page.)

Agreement to more than three of these statements suggests there may be a significant problem. Agreement to more than five indicates that you have a serious problem causing stress to team members.

Characteristics of effective teams

Effective teams know how to . . .

- make decisions
- develop new ideas and ways of achieving specific objectives

. . . by using and developing all available skills and resources.

(a) Make decisions

Decision making in a team should include:

- presentation of the problem
- seeking information
- not accepting the first solution
- looking for alternatives
- avoidance of conflict-reducing techniques such as majority voting
- encouragement of difference and risk-taking
- establishing agreement/consensus.

(b) Develop new ideas and ways of achieving specific objectives

.Developing creativity can be essential to effective team working. An effective way of developing creativity is to brainstorm. This method separates idea generation from critical examination, as this latter part will inhibit spontaneity and creativity.

Brief guide to *effective* brainstorming

A team member notes ideas on a board that everyone can see:

- members contribute ideas for a fixed period e.g. ten minutes
- each new idea is displayed separately and clearly
- do *not* criticize or make any evaluations at this point
- once the time limit is up, proceed to evaluation, keeping the best for further work.

Brainstorming allows group members to participate fully in the creative process, because no critical barriers are allowed to develop. In any creative exercise, the team leader should:

- avoid competing with the team
- be a good listener
- not allow others to be put on the defensive
- keep the energy level high
- use every member
- avoid manipulating the team.

Summary

Successful teams comprise members who:

- share norms and goals
- understand their environment
- appreciate each other's different roles
- welcome innovation and new ideas
- value each other
- are exciting to work with
- constantly review and renew
- *achieve their objectives.*

References

1. Belbin RM (1996). *Management teams—why they succeed or fail.* Butterworth Heinemann, London. www.belbin.com (accessed 1 September 2000).
2. Tuckman BC (1965). Development sequence in small groups. *Psychological Bulletin*, 63(6), 384–99.

3. Janis JL (1982). *Groupthink*, (2nd edn). Houghton Mifflin, Boston MA.
4. Davis J, Milburn P, Murphy T, and Woodhouse M (1992). *Successful team building*. Kogan Page, London.

No one individual is perfect, but teams can be.

8.2 Involving 'consumers'

Vikki Entwistle and Bec Hanley

Objectives

After reading this chapter, you will:

- understand why consumer involvement can help achieve public health goals
- be aware of a range of forms of consumer involvement
- be able to start planning appropriate consumer involvement in diverse public health tasks.

Definitions

In this chapter, we use the term '*consumers*' to refer to people who are more likely to be at the receiving end than the delivery end of public health or health care interventions. These include members of the general public or of specific local communities or ethnic groups, health service users, potential health service users, carers, self-help groups, consumer advocates, and organizations that represent the interests of health service users or people with particular health problems.

We use the term '*involvement*' to cover a range of ways that people who work in organizations that have responsibility for the health of a defined population can use to ensure that their work benefits from consumers' input. We are talking about doing things *with* people rather than doing things *to* people. Different forms of involvement are discussed below.

Why is consumer involvement important for public health?

There are two basic reasons for involving consumers in public health activities:

(a) consumer involvement can improve the quality of public health activities, for example by:

- ensuring that public health needs are appropriately identified and prioritized
- ensuring that public health interventions are acceptable and appropriate to the people who are supposed to benefit from them
- encouraging support for public health goals

(b) consumer involvement might be an explicit public health or policy objective.

(a) Consumer involvement can improve the quality of public health activities

Professional education and training can equip public health workers with important knowledge and skills. They do not, however, provide all the insights that are needed to carry out all public health projects in the best possible way. Consider the questions in Box 8.2.1.

Box 8.2.1 **Do you really know...**

- what it is like to live with asthma, depression, diabetes (or any other health problem or disability)?

- what it is like to be addicted to alcohol or an illegal drug? what it is like to try and then to fail to give up smoking?

- what it is like to care for a severely disabled child, a spouse with cancer, or a parent with Alzheimer's disease?

- what it feels like to be on the 'receiving end' of services in your local family planning clinic, orthopaedic outpatients clinic, or general surgical ward?

People who engage in behaviours risky to health, who live with particular health problems or disabilities, or who have experience of particular health care interventions or services often have insights into these behaviours, problems, and services that health care professionals and health service managers do not have. They see things from different perspectives.

Some public health projects are developed on the basis of public health workers' assumptions about what the intended beneficiaries need, want, and will respond to. Your projects are more likely to be effective if you actively try to find out how they themselves see their needs and concerns and if, where possible, you work with them to achieve jointly agreed goals.

Greater awareness of consumers' views and concerns might affect:

- how you assess health needs

- what you define as a public health problem

- how you define and measure or articulate a public health problem

- what interventions you think should be used to address the problem

- how you judge the effectiveness and appropriateness of interventions.

In addition, active consumer involvement might enhance the effectiveness of what you do. For example, it might ensure that any interventions you use are appropriate and credible. It might help mobilize support for your goals.

Box 8.2.2 **Three examples of consumer involvement**

Evaluating infertility treatments

A group of health care professionals planned to review research evidence about the effects on pregnancy rates of giving drug and surgical treatments to infertile couples. After discussing their work with consumers, they shifted their emphasis. They started to look at the effects of a broader range of interventions, including information-giving and counselling, for couples who wanted a baby and were seeking help. The group also considered a variety of outcomes, including anxiety, relationships, and having a baby, as well as pregnancy rates.

Developing consumer health information materials

A team preparing an information leaflet about screening for prostate cancer ran focus group discussions with men over 40 from various backgrounds. Most of the men thought that cancer screening programmes were generally a good thing. They thought there should be a national screening programme for prostate cancer. Once the team was aware of these views, they could address them directly. In the leaflet, they contrasted screening programmes for breast cancer and prostate cancer before summarizing the research evidence about screening for and treating prostate cancer.

Planning services for people with back pain

Public health staff in one health authority held a citizen's jury to hear local people's views about whether the authority should redirect money spent on physiotherapy for people with back pain to fund osteopathy and chiropractic. After hearing evidence from experts, jurors called for an integrated system, with osteopaths, chiropractors, and physiotherapists working together and sharing expertise.

Box 8.2.2 gives three examples of how consumer involvement has made a difference.

(b) Consumer involvement as a policy objective

Public health activities are often politically motivated and may have political implications. In several countries, government policy requires that consumers are involved in certain public health and health care activities. There have been lay members on research ethics committees for many years now, but consumer involvement policies are now being extended to research funding programmes, professional regulatory bodies, and government advisory groups.

What is consumer involvement?

Examples are given in Box 8.2.3.

Box 8.2.3 **Consumer involvement can take various forms**

A team that needs to carry out a health needs assessment exercise among a minority ethnic community might invite a respected member of that community to join them. They might also train and employ other members of the community to carry out interviews. These forms of involvement might help ensure that the project is seen positively by the community, that appropriate questions are asked in a culturally sensitive way, and that the views of the local people are appropriately understood.

A multi-agency working group that is trying to reduce teenage pregnancy rates might commission focus group discussions with young teenagers to find out what factors might influence the teenagers' use of contraception and the types of contraceptive services they would feel most able to use. Insights from these discussions might inform any interventions that the working group plans.

Researchers planning a clinical trial might meet with members of a patient-based organization that provides information and support to people with a particular condition. The meetings might help the researchers understand the problems that people with that condition face and the hopes and concerns they have about the intervention being studied. They might thus help ensure that the researchers select appropriate outcome measures for their trial and that their approaches to recruitment and data collection are as acceptable as possible to the people who are asked to participate. At a later stage, meetings to discuss the trial results might help ensure that the findings are appropriately interpreted and their implications are fully thought through.

Before you start

For any given situation and task, some forms of consumer involvement will be more appropriate than others. But there are no hard and fast rules about which forms of involvement are 'best'. We suggest you think about four interlinked questions:

(a) what do you want to achieve?

(b) what constraints are you operating under?

(c) which consumer(s) might/should you involve?

(d) how might/should you engage them?

(a) What do you want to achieve?

Whatever the task you are considering, think about what you hope to achieve from consumer involvement. For example, you might want to:

- understand the views and concerns of a group of people in order to improve the relevance and quality of interventions intended for their benefit
- work more closely with community members to help them ensure they have access to the health services they most value
- ensure that a decision about the reconfiguration of health services has political legitimacy.

(b) What constraints are you operating under?

- how much time and what resources do you have at your disposal?
- how negotiable are your aims and approaches? (How will you be able to respond if some of the consumers you involve say they would prefer to see things done differently?)
- are there any confidentiality policies that might prevent consumers from participating in discussions?

(c) Which consumer(s) might/should you involve?

A variety of people have insights, expertise and opinions that you might (or might not!) want to influence your work. Some of these are listed in Box 8.2.4.

Box 8.2.4 **Whose views might be important?**

People who have experience of particular circumstances

- people living in a particular geographical area or community
- people of a particular age, sex, or sexual orientation
- people from a particular ethnic or religious group
- people who engage in 'risky' behaviours (e.g. smokers, injecting drug users)
- potential users of specific services (e.g. older people, pregnant women)
- people who have, or have had, a particular health problem
- people who use, or who have used, a particular health service
- carers and family members of people with health problems.

Consumer representatives

+ leaders of local, ethnic, or religious groups
+ people who work or volunteer in organizations that serve or represent health care consumers:
    – organizations with generic health interests (e.g. consumer councils, community health forums)
    – organizations with specific health interests (e.g. breast cancer support groups).

The different types of consumer obviously vary in their expertise and skills. Even within types there is a wide variety of individuals!

Consumer representatives are usually more able to work with health professionals and health service managers around committee tables than arbitrarily chosen individuals with experience of living in particular circumstances. Some consumer representatives have particular skills, such as research appraisal or the production of information materials. However, they are not usually appropriate substitutes for testing the responses of ordinary people to information materials or other interventions.

Box 8.2.5 **How might you engage with consumer views?**

+ read consumer publications or academic studies of consumer views
+ hold focus group discussions
+ consult with key individuals in consumer or community organizations (who might then consult with their members before feeding back to you)
+ hold open meetings
+ run citizens juries or lay consensus conferences
+ conduct surveys (using self-completion questionnaires, telephone or face-to-face interviews)
+ include consumers as members of project teams, working groups, or committees
+ invite consumers to comment on drafts of project plans, research proposals, advertising ideas, information leaflets
+ ask consumers to lead or undertake projects themselves.

(d) How might/should you engage them?

Box 8.2.5 lists some of the ways that can be used to identify consumer views, consult, or involve consumers.

The approaches vary among other things in terms of:

- the extent to which they allow consumers to directly influence agendas and activities
- the expertise and skills that they require consumers to have
- time and resource implications.

What counts as good practice in consumer involvement?

Many of the principles of good practice for consumer involvement apply to any consultation exercise or team effort. We suggest that the following points are particularly important:

Offer a clear invitation

When asking consumers to get involved, be ready to tell them:

- about the project or activity you are asking them to contribute to
- why you have asked them to help
- what you are (and what you are not) expecting of them in terms of expertise, time, effort
- what support you propose to give to enable them to contribute effectively (briefings, training, child care arrangements, expenses, fees)
- what (if anything) you hope that they (or their communities) will get out of it.

Accept that people may choose not to become involved.

Remove practical barriers to involvement

Make sure that:

- meeting places are accessible. (e.g. that the venue is served by public transport and that people in wheelchairs can get around the building)
- communication media are appropriate (e.g. do you need to provide facilities for people with hearing or sight impairments?)
- participants' travel and child care expenses are covered.

Take active steps to enable people to contribute

- provide clear briefings about the aims and context of the task
- offer training if necessary
- avoid unnecessary jargon and explain necessary jargon

...and if you are inviting consumers to join a committee:

Consumers often feel isolated and intimidated in professionally dominated committees or working groups. They might feel more comfortable if you:

* invite more than one consumer
* encourage the chairperson to visit them on their own territory
* ensure that the chairperson enables the consumers to have their say
* provide training or awareness-raising exercises to encourage committee members to get to know each other and respect each other's views.

Be flexible

The consumers whose views you seek might suggest that you do things differently. If you are not prepared to take their ideas seriously, then your efforts to involve them will be wasted. However, this does not mean that the 'best' consumer involvement requires that you do whatever any individual consumer or group of consumers asks you to.

Two possible distractors

(a) The issue of representativeness

The claim that the consumers who tend to participate in public health projects are rarely typical is often raised as an objection to consumer involvement. This objection, however, often misses the point. An articulate consumer advocate might not look like the average person of the group you are interested in but might well be able to contribute important insights from a consumer perspective and might also be able to present a range of consumer views for consideration.

(b) The injunction to 'involve consumers at all stages'

This widely-used recommendation reflects the point that the benefits of consumer involvement are more likely to materialize if consumer views are considered at all (particularly early) stages of projects than if consumers are just brought in to comment on almost-completed tasks. It does not have to mean expecting consumers to take on every task in a project.

Pitfalls

The most common type of consumer involvement trap is based on the principle that some types of consumer are simply not suited for some tasks. These traps are easily avoided with a bit of common sense.

We suggest that you steer clear of:

- asking a special interest group to provide *the* consumer perspective on a general priority-setting task. (Consumer involvement at its best does not simply reflect the 'who shouts loudest gets' phenomenon)
- putting undue responsibilities on 'ordinary' people with experience of living in particular situations. For example, a 13-year-old mother is likely to flounder if asked to participate unsupported as a member of a high level committee that is formulating policies to try to reduce teenage pregnancy rates.

What constitutes success in consumer involvement?

Because consumer involvement can be undertaken with a variety of aims, it may be judged by a variety of criteria. Opinions will differ as to which are the most important.

You can ask:

- did consumer involvement (positively) influence what you did?
- did it seem to make a (positive) difference to the outcome?
- was the process itself valuable?
- did people enjoy the process?
- did people learn from it?

Finally, as you learn from your experiences of consumer involvement, do share your insights with others. Many people are grappling with the practicalities of involving consumers to benefit public health and progress in this area will be faster if we can learn from each other.

Further resources

Bastian H (1998). Speaking up for ourselves: the evolution of consumer advocacy in health care. *Int J Tech Assess Hlth Care*, **14**, 3–23.

Consumers in NHS Research Support Unit offers (free) publications, advice, seminars, conferences, etc. on involving consumers in health research. Contact details: conres@hfht.org or www.hfht.org/ConsumersinNHSResearch.

Consumers in Research in the NHS (1999). *Involvement works: second report of Consumers in Research in the NHS*. NHS Executive, Leeds.

Entwistle VA, Renfrew M, Yearley S, Forrester J, and Lamont L (1998). Incorporating lay perspectives: advantages for research. *BMJ*, **316**, 463–6.

Jakubowska D and Crossley P (1999). Developing skills in consulting with the public. *BMJ*, **319**, S2.

Kelson M (1997). *User involvement: a guide to developing effective user involvement strategies in the NHS*. College of Health, London.

NHS Executive, Institute of Health Service Management, and the NHS Confederation (1998). *In the public interest: developing a strategy for public participation in the NHS*. Bridge Consultancy, Cambridge.

Oliver S, Entwistle V, and Hodnett E (1998). Roles for lay people in the implementation of health care research. In *Getting research findings into practice*, (ed. A Haines and A Donald), pp. 43–51. BMJ Books, London.

Arnstein's hierachy of involvement: informing; consulting; collaborating; conferring control.

8.3 **Project management**

Gabriel Scally

Objectives

By reading this chapter you should understand the general principles of project management and what it might contribute to your effectiveness as a public health professional.

Definition

Project management is the skill of successfully balancing time, quality, and resources in order to produce a particular change or product.

Why is this an important public health skill?

There are many factors connected to contemporary public health practice that make the set of skills and approaches used in project management very useful.[1] The time-scales of delivery of public health work, whether it be a health impact assessment or an acute service review in the health service, do not allow the luxury of a prolonged, sequential approach to undertaking tasks. Indeed the computer jargon phrase 'multi-tasking' can be said to apply to much of public health work. Similarly, the complexity of relationships between all those involved has grown, as partnership working across organizational boundaries is central to the achievement of public health goals.[2]

The planning skills that have been part of public health practice for many years are still important, but an emphasis on 'delivery' has accompanied the introduction of general management into health systems worldwide. The ability to see a project all the way through to successful completion is as important as the initial research and professional opinion about what needs to be done.

What is a project?

Consider projects as one-off tasks with a definite outcome or product. The task will never have been done before and there is not usually an opportunity to try again and perhaps get better each time. They therefore carry a higher than usual risk of failure; using a project management approach is an attempt to reduce those risks and achieve a successful outcome. Project management is used very frequently in the construction industry and in the world of information technology. In both these sectors time-scales are short, the price of failure can be extremely high, the processes are highly complex, often involving many different participants, and, crucially, it may not be possible to have a second chance.

In public health, tasks such as the production of a complex report, the development of a health strategy, or the reorganization of a hospital or community service all lend themselves to project management.

What is involved in getting started?

Building commitment

Sometimes the decision to proceed with a project is obvious to all concerned. It may be however that different contributors have different perspectives on what needs to be done, or even if it needs to be done at all. It is usually impossible to get widespread commitment to a project without those whose involvement in it is essential being aware of the work or resources required of them. It is therefore necessary to try to develop a shared vision of the goals of the project. This can then be built on to construct a clear and unambiguous definition of the task. Of particular interest to participants, or their managers, will be the resources that the project will consume and the time-scales predicted for the various stages. The engagement of proposed participants or supporters can be achieved by consultation on a written proposal or by means of a developmental workshop where they can be actively engaged in creating the vision and defining the goals. The importance of community involvement, and even leadership, is stressed in much of public health work, and gaining trust and respect amongst community leaders may take time.

Feasibility

The issue of feasibility is a central feature at this point. A review of the steadily growing literature on the effectiveness of interventions may provide clear evidence as to whether what is being suggested is likely to be beneficial or not. The absence of a strong evidence base does not necessarily invalidate a proposed course of action, but it may indicate that a pilot stage might be appropriate. It might also argue for the project to take the form of a research study, with implications for the design, funding, and objective of what is being proposed.

Build the team

There are many situations where an individual may work on a complex task unaided, but increasingly public health professionals work in teams. Of all the serious constraints to successfully negotiating the 'start-up' phase, the difficulty of identifying and building the team that is necessary to achieve overall success may be the most serious. Almost inevitably, high-performing individuals will have a host of tasks awaiting their attention and this may make it difficult to gain their commitment. The nature of multi-agency or cross-directorate working means that individuals may never have worked together before, and may have loyalties to their own organization or professional group which need to coped with. Team building is a particular skill which is important in any work setting but particularly so in project work (see chapter 8.1).

What are the key components in planning the project?

If and when the go-ahead for a project is given, the process of detailed planning begins. A crucial part of the planning process is to use every opportunity to gain commitment from all those important to the success of the project. Effective communication is therefore vital. The essence of the planning phase is to break down the project into a series of tasks that can be allocated an appropriate amount of resource in terms of time or money. The allocation of time will of course depend on the nature of the project and the input, but should be quantified, whether it is in hours, days, or weeks. The sequence of these tasks is identified and detailed time-scales given to each task so that they are scheduled to flow one from another. The usual way of illustrating this is using a Gantt chart; that is a bar chart, or timeline, of greater or lesser complexity. The interrelation between the sub-tasks determines the timing and allows the identification of milestones.

Quality control

Those most engaged in the work of the project might well be too deeply involved to be able to provide objective analysis of the quality of what is being done. This is overcome by a checking of the quality by an identified individual or group at predetermined points along the schedule. This may be by someone who is the main 'customer' or by external advisers.

Identification of risk

Risk may take many forms, for example the policy may change from on high during the course of the project, new research may discredit an intervention, or an important contributor may leave for a new job. The important thing is to identify potential risks and what impact they might have on the project. Then, if they are deemed to be significant, an assessment can be made of what can be done to avoid the risk or lessen its potential impact if it does come about.

Approvals

It may be necessary to get further approvals before implementation commences. A major project will consume substantial resources and may well be critical to the work of several organizations, so getting high-level approval may well be a wise course.

How is the project executed?

The most important person in the course of a project is the project manager. This individual has to have the confidence of her or his seniors and be able to command a response from the individual team members when the time is right for them to make their contribution. The choice of project manager is therefore vital. The tasks during this phase include the monitoring of progress against the plan, dealing with conflicts and delays, and defining and agreeing any deviations from the plan. The project manager should be highly visible during all this activity, particularly if many organizations are involved and there may be variability in the levels of commitment.

Controlling progress in a complex project will rarely be easy, as things will inevitably go off-schedule or be seen to be more difficult than envisaged at the planning stage. The ability to think creatively to overcome problems will be an important skill for the team to exercise. Should the obstacles become insuperable, a decision making process will need to be constructed in order to redefine the project, perhaps by making it less ambitious, or perhaps even to agree its abandonment.

How will you know if you have been successful?

If the task definition has been a precise and collectively owned one then it should be obvious when the end point has been achieved. The most rewarding part of any successful project is completing it and standing back to admire the results whilst accepting all the praise that is given. However, it is easy to lose the attention of team members as minds inevitably drift into thinking about what their next assignment is or how they will cope with the backlog of work that has built up in their absence. Getting the last little effort in order to finish the project may take a disproportionate amount of effort on behalf of the project manager, but achieving completion is important if the project is not to drag on needlessly. Similarly you should try to have a definite finishing point at which the product, whatever that might be, is handed over and accepted by those who gave it the go-ahead. Planning the party for the team is a way of drawing things to a close as well as letting off steam.

Some projects may have to be repeated in the future, even if not in exactly the same form, so it is useful to conduct a brief evaluation of how the project went. A particular public health report may have to be produced annually for example, and the next person who is assigned responsibility may be very grateful for details of what exactly went wrong during the proof-reading stage. It is also a useful contribution to staff appraisal, as they may have been working outside their usual line management structure for the duration of the project. The identification of skills developed during the course of the project may identify some that are transferable to other areas of work. The documentation of successes and failures may seem like a pointless task when the main body of work is already over, but if the organization is to get better at doing what it does, then evaluation is vital.

Further resources

The project management system, PRINCE2, is the UK government standard for use in information system projects. 'PRINCE' is an acronym that is derived from PRojects IN Controlled Environments. Although developed for IT applications, its use has spread to a wide range of public sector bodies and it is used to manage projects in many different areas of work, including public health. Details of the PRINCE2 method are available from www.ccta.gov.uk/prince/index.htm (accessed 4 September 2000). One of the major advantages of PRINCE2 is that there is no licence charge for its use. As public health projects are often components of structured programmes, an overarching programme management approach may also be valuable and the same website contains details of programme management publications.

Central Computer and Telecommunications Agency (1998). *Managing successful projects with PRINCE2*. The Stationary Office, Norwich.

Turner RJ (1993). *The handbook of project-based management*. McGraw-Hill, Maidenhead.

References

1. McKinlay JB and Marceau LD (2000). To boldly go . . . *Am J Public Health*, **90**, 25–32.
2. UK Department of Health (1999). *Saving lives: our healthier nation*. Cm 4386. The Stationery Office, London.

A vision without a task is a dream; a task without a vision is drudgery.

8.4 **Operational and business planning**

Paul Watson and Peter Wightman

What is business planning?

Any organization (including public health organizations) has corporate plans. These describe what an organization as a whole will do over a specific time period. The focus is on the greater good, balancing different priorities. Corporate plans are made at two levels:

• *strategic planning*: this process outlines the overall direction for a service area or organization over a long time-scale, usually a minimum of five years (see chapter 6.3)

• *business planning* is one of the two ways in which corporate plans are put into action. Business plans usually cover a single financial year and are the main process for allocating resources within an organization.

Objectives

This chapter will help you:

• understand the fundamentals of *business* planning

• understand the steps in using the business planning to commission services

• develop an effective business case.

Why is business planning important in public health?

Failure to engage in an effective manner with your organization's planning process will severely limit your ability to effect change. For example you may have spent months or even years on developing a funding bid only to see it fail by missing a bidding deadline or being unaware of a key planning meeting. Public health practitioners need to be as central to the decision making of the organization as possible. The business planning of any organization concentrates on:

• securing agreement about the main *priorities* for an organization

• allocating its *resources* (see chapter 2.6)

• outlining how *strategies* will be implemented (see chapters 6.3 and 7.6).

Using the business planning process to commission services

The corporate process could be run by a purchaser with its service providers or within a provider with its budget holders.

Step 1: Clarify the strategic direction—and ensure that the business planning relates to this

- what is the longer-term strategy of your organization?
- is it realistic and credible e.g. is it (likely to be) owned by constituencies (such as those from whom you may be commissioning services?)
- is the way in which you plan to implement the strategic plan (through business planning) consistent with other priorities (e.g. national priorities, priorities of local partner agencies . . .)?

Step 2: Identify pre-existing commitments and priorities outside your immediate control ('must dos')

The first call on any resources involves pre-existing agreements (e.g. commitments from previous years) and the 'must dos'. Must dos include:

- inevitable service pressures (e.g. a continuing rise in emergency admissions)
- national political imperatives such as the achievement of waiting time targets.

Defining 'must dos' is a key element of negotiations both between and within organizations.

Step 3: Preliminary work with service providers/budget holders

There are three stages here:

- aim to make a forecast early in the planning cycle regarding the funding that will be available (perhaps a minimum and maximum) and ensure the service providers/budget holders know these details
- establish if any funding is left for discretionary developments after commitments (see below)
- invite service providers to prepare their own individual business cases (ensure these are likely to be realistic—hence the importance of providers knowing the resource limitations and avoiding wasted effort if resources are limited). You, as a commissioner of services, should provide an indication of your organization's priorities.

Step 4: Prioritization of discretionary developments

* priority-setting work takes place before and after funding is announced
* a local, inclusive, and open process is needed
* aim to involve key local constituencies in the emerging plan (e.g. public watchdog organizations)
* once funding is announced, Board takes decision on priorities for consultation.

Step 5: Consultation

* it is essential to run a public consultation process if there are likely to be high-profile changes to the quantity or configuration of services available.

Step 6: Implementation

* finalize service delivery agreements with the providers: financial resources and the process of quality assessment on your part; activity levels, indicators of quality, change objectives, and deliverables on their part.

Developing a business case

When promoting a particular development you will need to prepare a *business case*. This outlines what you would like to develop and how. Remember, whatever you are proposing, you will be competing with other people with their own business cases. The focus should be:

* planning the details of the way forward from the perspective of an individual service ...
* usually within a known and agreed wider strategy and ...
* presenting the case to funders.

The six steps are therefore:

Step 1: Is there a strategy?

* ideally the business case is written in the context of an agreed strategy.

Step 2: Reality check

* It is important to assess if the case stands a realistic chance of success to avoid wasted effort:
* is it financially feasible? (What is likely to be the upper limit of resources available?)
* is it politically feasible?

Step 3: Inclusive process

A standard structure for a business case:

- strategic context
- objectives
- costs: capital and revenue
- staffing
- timetable: what will be achieved by when
- wider impact (e.g. implications for support services of a new consultant appointment)
- success criteria: enable evaluation
- source of funding: national bids, local authority, charities
- risk assessment (e.g. recruitment, sources of funding)

Appraisal of other options will be required if major investment is involved.

Step 4: Prepare the case

If you forget to prepare, prepare to be forgotten.

Principles for preparing the case:

- define the problem to which you consider your case to be (part of) the solution. Carefully chosen data that are properly referenced, appraised, and presented can be very powerful at this stage
- genuinely consider the different options, particularly across professional boundaries (e.g. a health visitor versus a community development worker)
- be inclusive: involve all interested parties. Backing from key opinion leaders is essential
- be clear which parts of the process are the responsibility of the funder and which are the responsibility of the provider.

Step 5: Convincing decision makers

Use the *formal channels*. Ensure you meet the required deadlines in the required manner. Make specific links to the organization's strategy or identified priorities. Ideally you (or someone you know very well) should present the case directly instead of relying on others presenting the case for you.

Use the *informal channels*: explain the case to key decision makers (clinical and managerial) and the key support officers who are involved with, and administer, the corporate process. Ensure clinical champions are involved early in the process, not forgetting to use *their* informal networks to present the case. Senior, direct sponsorship is highly desirable (by the Chief Executive or a Director). Avoid the over-use of informal networks.

In presenting the case *your message* should be clear about what the health problem is and how the proposal addresses this.

Step 6: Implementation

If the case is successful but less funding is available than desired, you may need to renegotiate priorities. If you have developed a realistic and mutually respecting relationship with the providers, this need not be difficult. You will need to ensure careful management of change in implementation: never lose sight of the key objective(s) and maintain a close focus on the key success criteria.

Key determinants of success

* genuine initiatives always cost more and take longer to implement than you think—add 50% to your initial estimates!
* know all the deadlines—months of hard work can be wasted by missing a deadline
* always base your day-to-day activities on the formal processes—however, also use informal networks to build up a constituency for your case
* it is possible to bring about change that defies the spirit of the times or existing political priorities. However, this takes much longer and needs far more work—be selective when you go against the flow!
* *always* be on the look out for opportunities that can further your cause—luck is often about spotting and exploiting opportunities. Be ready and prepared to take advantage of any fortuitous changes in policy, people, or resources
* pay attention to shifts in the regulatory framework and political priorities; this will often be the making or breaking of your case.

Box 8.4.1 **Case study 1**

Securing funding for diabetes services in a UK Health Authority responsible for commissioning health care

How were funds secured through the corporate planning process even without this problem having national priority? The successful business case included:

* *senior sponsorship*: two health authority directors and the trust medical director personally supported the case
* *inclusive development*: the strategy was developed through a process of interviews and group discussion of multi-disciplinary groups, and also a GP questionnaire
* *clear message*: four key parts to the message: (i) comparison showed lower levels of medical and nurse staffing; (ii) there

were specific service problems illustrated by the complaints of patients and the written concerns of GPs; (iii) benchmark comparisons showed many service shortfalls; (iv) international trends for increasing incidence

- *pragmatism*: shortage of public funding meant the start was delayed. However, firm commitment was gained to meet the full year effect the following year (i.e. a prior commitment).

  It can be easier to get people to agree to something if it can be deferred

- *realistic*: three-year investment plan costed at an affordable level.

Lesson There is no magic bullet to ensure that business planning is successful. However, there are many approaches and techniques that are likely to increase the chance of success. Combining approaches and techniques often helps.

Box 8.4.2 **Case study 2**

The service and financial framework in the UK NHS

Since 1991 the UK National Health Service (NHS) has been funded through a series of service agreements between purchasers and service providers. This process put hospitals and community services in competition with each other and encouraged a 'bidding up' mentality, with each provider trying to secure the largest slice of purchasers' funds possible. This often meant that both purchasers and providers overspent against available resources as the system became over-extended. Since 1998, each Health Authority has had to produce a Service and Financial Framework for its district. This includes an early, open declaration of cash limits for individual NHS organizations within the district. This helps give providers a sense of what its business plan can realistically contain and means that it is made clear that individual organizations can only increase their budget at the expense of another organization within the local NHS. This helps avoid an over-bidding culture in what is strictly a cash-limited system.

Lesson Be open, honest, and realistic, and warn colleagues that compromise may be necessary.

Further resources

Chapters 6.3, 6.4, 6.5, and 7.2, this handbook.
Handy C (1976). *Understanding organisations*. Penguin, Harmondsworth.
de Geus A (1997). *The living company*. Nicholas Brearley Publishing, London.

8.5 **Criteria to assess effective public health action**

Chris Spencer-Jones

Objective

This chapter should help you to understand and measure your progress towards creative and sustainable public health practice. It is intended to address the absence of criteria and standards against which to audit public health work.[1]

Definition

'Effective public health action' is defined as the work that achieves the desired public health outcome. This must include some improvement in measurable health outcome, or a clear indication of likely possible benefit in terms of process. When commissioning public health work, it may be an impact on a problem, or a change in environment that is sought.

Understanding success criteria in public health will help with evaluation of the work we do. It will help us to shift our efforts to where they are most beneficial. Always ask yourself and your colleagues: 'If this endeavour were to be successful, how would we know?'

Deconstruct to reconstruct

Right task, right person, right time

It is your responsibility to ensure that any work you do is likely to improve health. Your relationship with the objectives of the organization is two-way. You need to *shape* them in the longer term as well as *meeting* them in the shorter term.

You need to ensure that the right task is being performed (in the right way) by the right person at the right time. Use the check-lists in Tables 8.5.1–8.5.3.

Table 8.5.1 Right Task?

Consider	Essential	Desirable
Opportunity cost	The work is likely to bring health benefits	There are health benefits available that can and will be measured
Management support	The work is supported explicitly by the public health department you are associated with	The organization you work for requests a plan, agrees on the plan, and supervises the plan

Work programme	The task fits into a portfolio of work that offers job satisfaction	At completion you will meet both personal and organizational objectives
Allies	The people affected by the work expressed willingness to support the work	The people affected by the work are part of the commissioning process
Whether it can be done	There is an end-point that can be identified	The task is to change something specific—not the world!

Table 8.5.2 Right Person?

Consider	Essential	Desirable
Your engagement	You were asked to become involved because you have competencies essential to progress the issue	You were consulted about the nature of the work from an early stage and are able to comment upon your contribution
Skill-mix	The work can only be done if you possess the required skills or can develop them effectively on the job	The task requires public health skills in proportion to the time you are requested to invest
Politics	Your involvement in this work strengthens your links with the people who make decisions affecting health	Your contribution is likely to be appreciated

Table 8.5.3 Right Time?

Consider	Essential	Desirable
Timing	Your involvement is welcomed by key individuals	You don't have to push the door wide—somebody is holding it open for you
Timetable	Something is going to happen within an explicit time-scale and this piece of work will influence events	A timetable is agreed at the start—that takes account of relevant external constraints

Table 8.5.3 (continued)

Consider	Essential	Desirable
Timing of engagement	There is time to consider the value of your contribution	You can weigh up the benefits of involvement in the context of your own and your department's overall work programme
Product	The outcome of the work is anticipated by an audience	The product is of wide interest—perhaps it is publishable

The politics of effecting change is not something be avoided in public health. Part of the work of public health practitioners is to change people's understanding, attitudes, opinions, and actions in a way that improves health. In one description, 'public health is where the action isn't'—meaning that public health practitioners need to constantly activate neglected areas.

Organization for excellent execution

Wherever you are working, the capable practitioner will work effectively in a wide diversity of environments, with a wide variety of people and organizations, always holding the public health objectives in mind, before any other objectives. This requires turning problems into tasks that are possible, that will create outcomes that are beneficial and definable.

Table 8.5.4 Criteria for excellent execution.

Steps	Essential	Desirable
Problem into tasks (see chapter 2.2)	Definable blocks of achievable work	Every person relevant identified
Project planning (see chapter 8.3)	A structured project plan endorsed by your department	Project plan endorsed by your organization
Engagement	Identify people who share common objectives	Share project planning with possible partners in action
Consultation	Project plan shared with key players following approval	Project plan agreed with key players in advance
Communication	Ensure everybody in your organization who acts in the same field is aware of developments	Define a network of key players and interested parties and keep them informed

Project monitoring	Regular reports on progress to your department	Supervision by trusted colleague or mentor
Time-keeping	Complexity of task matches timetable	Other relevant timetables identified
Record-keeping	Details of all work undertaken kept separately	Annual report on activity of individuals

Achieving positive change requires careful forethought and preparation. Whenever a piece of work seems set to extend beyond a few weeks or take more than a few hours it is useful to define the work in terms of a project. When we are 'consulted', a less formal approach will suffice. A project should have a project plan, and be managed accordingly (see chapter 8.3).

Effective public health action is creative and proactive. Many of us work in a reactive environment, with pressures that bend us towards consultancy and away from defined projects. Whatever the circumstances, we have to make the best of them, carrying a positive message and remaining firmly focused on our public health objectives.

What went wrong?

Even with careful commissioning, precise and careful planning, and deployment of adequate personal skills, a piece of work may be less than successful. The major pitfalls and preventive tips are noted (Table 8.5.5).

Table 8.5.5 Preventive action against pitfalls.

Pitfall	Prevention
Underestimation of complexity	Achieving change is complex. Detail the stages required to make change happen and the complexity soon emerges
Taking too much on oneself	Remember: in public health the highest standard is to involve others fully, not to do well only what you can do. We will have optimal impact when we work to gain the understanding and commitment of others
Expectations too high	A clear project plan with agreed aims, objectives, and methods overcomes this if circulated to all key people. It will tell them something useful is going to happen— even if it will not do all they seek
Lack of focus	Talk over what you are trying to achieve with somebody else. If it still isn't clear then start from scratch. If it was somebody else's project then go back to them for clarity. If it still isn't clear then downgrade this work quietly, quickly

Table 8.5.5 (continued)

Pitfall	Prevention
Undermining	Let facts, reason, and logic solve this one. Remain resolute!
Impossible	Look through the files and find out how many people have been involved in the recent past. If more than two other people have had a go already then assume you will do no better. Fresh soil is generally more fertile, though it may look harder to dig over!
Hurry and fudge	Difficult tasks can be done quickly, but complex tasks cannot. Differentiate and spell out complexity through a project plan. It is worth thinking carefully in order to prevent taking on a complex task with inadequate time or resources
The boss mucks it up	It is his or her prerogative. Take it well and find a way of entering the event into the vocabulary of the department. It helps if you understand your boss! Do you always get it right? Use humour

All these pitfalls cause us strain and stress. They are all common and we need to have the humility to take responsibility for our contribution. When we feel stress we need to identify the source and apply a remedy. In particular when we are away from our known competencies it is best to consider ourselves more as a trainee than as a practitioner, taking cautious steps and with a degree of supervision.

If things are not working well you need help:

• tell somebody it's not working—but not just anybody. Tell somebody who is in a position to help

• start asking people about their success stories. Ask them for tips

• identify which criteria you are failing on, which competencies you are light on

• consider whether you would benefit from supervision (or different supervision!)

• is it you? If you think everybody around you is OK then it probably isn't you, but if everybody else looks bad, well what about you? Consider paying a professional listener to listen to your story.

Formal public health audit, with other members of your department or within a looser affiliation, is helpful. Together with self-reflective learning it is the best way to increase your effectiveness.[2]

Competencies

To undertake successful public health action you need most, if not all of the currently defined public health competencies. In particular you need to be able to:

- deconstruct and reconstruct an issue
- plan in detail
- work with others—and make them work with your agenda
- win over other people
- reflect on your own work with honesty.

Key determinants of success

What really matters is that we make ourselves useful. Ideally, indispensable. We have to take part in agendas that are shaped by and matter to the communities we serve. We must have a sense of responsibility for the work that we do; a sense not only that it matters but also a certainty that it will achieve health benefits.

Key determinants:

- right task, right time
- planning and execution of plans avoiding pitfalls
- patience
- prioritization
- partnership working
- participation in the execution of one's own plans
- explicit goals
- reflection incorporated in action.

How will we know when we have succeeded?

Public health outcomes are diverse. They can be 'hard', such as community action to address deprivation. They can be 'soft', such as clarifying what may need to be done to make specific improvements. They may be highly organized, such as instigation of a preventive programme. They may be *ad hoc*, such as clarifying evidence on effectiveness. They may be concerned with the wider public health agenda, such as advocacy on behalf of excluded communities. They may be concerned with the bio-medical model, such as health service reviews. We know when we have been successful when we take time to look (Table 8.5.6).

Table 8.5.6 Our sucess criteria.

People indicators of success	*Activity* indicators of success
Commissioners increasingly ask for work that seeks to achieve public health goals	Information and ideas developed by you and your colleagues are adopted by other people or agencies
Partners from other agencies build public health into their work programmes	Measurable health gains are linked to your initiatives

Table 8.5.6 (continued)

People indicators of success	*Activity* indicators of success
Our colleagues and seniors feed back that we are working well, through a formal process of review	Acceptance by peer-reviewed journals of reports of your work. Positive column inches in the media, successful input to radio or television

It is helpful to hold regular reviews, discussing issues using an agreed, structured approach. The preparation and implementation of a public health annual report provides a good opportunity for reflection on successes and failures.

Further resources

Wright K, Rowitz L, Merkle A, Reid WM, Robinson G, Herzog W, Weber D, Carmichael D, Balderson TR, and Baker E (2000). Competency development in public health leadership. *Am J Public Health*, **90**(8), 1202–7.

References

1. Richardson A, Jackson C, and Sykes W (1992). *Audit guidelines in public health medicine: an introduction.* Nuffield Institute for Health Services Studies, University of Leeds, Leeds.
2. Jacobs R and Gabbay J (1994). *An action research report on audit in public health departments.* Faculty of Public Health Medicine of the Royal College of Physicians of the United Kingdom, London.

I long to achieve a great and noble task, but it is my chief duty to accomplish humble tasks as though they were great and noble. The world is moved along, not only by the mighty shoves of its heroes, but also by the aggregate of the tiny pushes of each honest worker.

Helen Keller

Part 9
Case studies

Introduction

Academia often provides poor preparation for action. In theory knowledge is power but it would be more appropriate to say that knowledge was potential energy, and the conversion of that potential energy into power requires know-how—the practical ability to get things done.

The principle of the modern professional in action is that a university education provides the practitioner with the tools needed to be effective. However, there is a great difference between knowing about something and doing something, particularly when doing, as is the case in public health, is a complex action involving many people and agencies. In preparing this handbook, we have concentrated less on the underlying academic disciplines of public health—for example anthropology, sociology, psychology, epidemiology, political science, and statistics—and more on practical topics such as becoming a more effective professional or making better decisions.

However, being an effective public health practitioner requires much more than acquiring the individual skills described in earlier sections of the book and then hoping they hang together when action is required. In the middle of a major public health task, it is impossible to distinguish whether one's effectiveness (or lack of it) is due to one's professional development or the strength of the organization in which one works. To learn how to be effective in public health it is necessary to look at other public health practitioners or organizations that have been effective (or, at least as useful), and ineffective. The wonderful case-book compiled by Benjamin Paul,[1] which could have been sub-titled 'Great public health failures', demonstrates just how useful failures are as a means of learning.

In this part of the handbook we have therefore concentrated on a small set of case studies, necessarily highly selective, which illustrate the skills and competencies described elsewhere in the book in concert and in action. In future, we hope to develop this collection of case studies into an electronic public health case-book, designed to promote debate about how to improve public health practice. Your engagement in this process could begin with thoughtful completion of the evaluation form.

How does it feel to be a rolling stone?

Most books are about knowing; fewer books are about doing, and we have certainly tried to make this a book about doing rather than knowing. Many people considering a career in public health wonder what it feels like to be a public health professional as compared to being, for example, an orthopaedic surgeon, a pathologist, or a nurse in coronary care. How does it feel, in Bob Dylan's immortal words, to be a rolling stone? Feeling is as important as doing for the public health practitioner, particularly when life seems frustrating and the bold rhetoric of the new age of public health seems oddly at variance with the grisly reality of working in an organization facing budget cuts and tackling short-term objectives determined by a pressurized chief executive and a risk-averse Board.

The cases presented in this final section take the most important public health lenses through which practitioners analyse and act, namely: by assessment and analysis (disease clusters), by setting (within a particular community, within a less industrialized country), by population subgroups (disability in older people), by determinants/risks/exposures (genetics, tobacco), by diseases (diabetes, depression), and by consequences (injuries).

We close this handbook with a challenge; that practitioners should:

- share not only what they have achieved, but also how they have achieved it
- share not only their successes, but also their failures.

The evaluation form provides a mechanism for you to respond to this challenge.

Although one is often exhorted not to reinvent the wheel, in reality it is often necessary to do exactly that. More importantly, let us at least avoid reinventing the flat tyre.

Reference

1. Paul BJ (1955). *Health, culture and community: case studies of public reactions to health programs*. Russell Sage Foundation, New York.

JAMG

9.1 Investigating a disease cluster

Jill Meara and Amanda Burls

Objectives

The following chapter will:

- provide a structured approach for responding to reports of disease clusters
- show how to calculate how often an observed cluster would occur by chance
- warn practitioners how apparently significant disease clusters are created artefactually
- emphasize the need for a communication strategy.

Definition

This chapter is about responding to reports of disease clusters in the community (*post hoc* clusters). A disease cluster is defined as an aggregation of relatively uncommon events in space and/or time that are believed or perceived to be greater than could be expected by chance.[1] (Different methods apply if you are investigating the health impact of a known exposure.)

Why are disease clusters important?

Diseases clusters are important to public health teams because:

- they may indicate a common risk factor; their investigation may provide evidence about environmental causes of disease
- whilst the overwhelming majority of reported 'clusters' are simply due to chance, they can cause considerable alarm
- media interest means that public health practitioners must be able to respond coherently to enquiries.

Competencies

In order to deal effectively with disease clusters the following basic public health skills are necessary:

- communication
- epidemiology
- statistics
- knowledge of local resources
- networking with experts.

Cluster investigation—six key steps

There are six key steps in the investigation and management of a suspected disease cluster:

(a) responding to initial report

(b) initial enquiry

(c) local liaison

(d) regional and national information

(e) published literature

(f) involving the public.

(a) Responding to initial report

'I am telephoning from *The Times*. What are you are doing about the cluster of childhood leukaemia in your local school?'

You are unaware of any concern at the school. Request details of the alleged cluster and his informant and tell the journalist you will get back to them later that day. Assuming that there is no one more informed or more competent to pass the call to, begin collecting data for the initial enquiry. *Always call back if you promise to.*

(b) Initial enquiry

The aim of the initial enquiry is to verify the information received, to develop a case-definition, and to obtain data about cases and environmental exposures in the relevant area and one or more comparison communities. National data can be useful for comparisons. It is best to corroborate information from a variety of sources.

(c) Local liaison

A number of local people may need to be informed about the problem or may have information:

- clinicians in primary and secondary care
- people (communicable disease specialists) who run relevant local demographic or disease databases (e.g. the child health register) or surveillance systems
- environmental health department
- other contacts, including the voluntary sector and local authority (e.g. social services and education)
- keep public relations staff informed—they may be able to help.

(d) Regional and national information

Get in touch with relevant organizations on the first day. Examples of such organizations are:

National:
- UK childhood cancer registry; national statistics (for denominator information, congenital abnormalities).

Regional:

- communicable disease epidemiologists
- cancer registries.
- public health observatories

Other:

- National experts e.g. Environment Agency, universities, UK National Radiological Protection Board
- Small Area Health Statistics Unit, Imperial College
- published cluster studies on the same topic (see below).

Arrange for preliminary data to be sent as soon as possible.

(e) Published literature

Search for information about:

- causes of the disease in question
- health effects of hypothesized environmental factors
- relationships between environmental factors and the disease.

(f) Involving the public

Involve the public from the outset, and involve them well. Good communication with the public is the key element that distinguishes a well-handled enquiry from a poorly-handled enquiry—there is no point conducting an excellent study and obtaining compelling scientific evidence if the public do not trust or believe your results. Different people see the risk of different threats in different ways. Assume nothing about other people's perception of threat and risk (see chapter 7.5.):

- listen sympathetically to their concerns (people are often reassured by simple information well communicated (e.g. the life-time risk of cancer is about 1 in 3)—avoid condescension
- however apparently trivial the problem, make clear you are *concerned* and that something is being done—obviously, be prepared to explain what and why
- be *honest* at all times—be prepared to admit lack of information and uncertainty
- interpret the evidence—*explain* the limitations of scientific methods
- *invite key worried people* to discuss the matter personally or in small meetings—public meetings are often unrepresentative and people may not be able to express their concerns (including you)
- patient *confidentiality* is paramount—even when people have been identified in the media, do not release identifiable information.

Developing a case-definition

Every cluster is different. However, some general principles apply:

- *disease*: only include the disease or diseases known to be related. Be sure your choice has a rational basis. If the 'cluster' involves a specific cancer, you may also wish to look at all-cancer rates. Choose the most relevant ICD codes *before* you look at the data

- *time*: use a time period relevant to, but not wholly defined by, the original reported cases. Use whole months or years. Cover a number of years with the same quinquennials as the comparator data. (The case-definition should include how you will deal with cases who have migrated in or out. This will depend on the aetiological hypothesis)

- *geographical boundaries*: a line drawn simply to enclose the house locations or other putative exposure points related to the cases will not suffice. Where possible, use routine units of evaluation that have not been constructed to fit the data. Postcode and electoral ward boundaries can be used.

Calculating whether a cluster may be due to chance

Use the Poisson distribution, which assumes independence of events, to calculate the probability of the specific number of events observed (*obs*) given the expected number of events (*exp*):

$$\text{pr}(\text{Obs} = obs | \text{Exp} = exp) = (exp^{obs}\, e^{-exp})/obs!$$

Example: Calculate the probability of seeing 1 case of a disease where the expected number was 1.789

$$\text{pr}(\text{Obs} = 1 | \text{Exp} = 1.789)$$
$$= (1.789^1 e^{-1.789})/1!$$
$$= 1.789 e^{-1.789}$$
$$= 0.2990$$

Tip: spreadsheets (e.g. the Poisson function in Excel) allow you to do these calculations painlessly—even with large numbers.

How likely is it that we would see at least as many cases as observed, simply due to chance? To do this subtract the probabilities of seeing each number of cases less than the number observed from the total probability of 1.

Example: Calculate the probability of seeing 3 or more cases of a disease when only 1.789 are expected by chance.

$$\text{pr}(\text{Obs} \geq 3 | \text{Exp} = 1.789)$$
$$= 1 - \text{pr}(\text{Obs} = 0 | \text{Exp} = 1.789) - \text{pr}(\text{Obs} = 1 | \text{Exp} = 1.789)$$
$$- \text{pr}(\text{Obs} = 2 | \text{Exp} = 1.789) = 1 - 0.1671 - 0.2990 - 0.2674$$
$$= 0.2664 \text{ (one-sided)}$$

The *relative risk* is the observed number of cases divided by the expected number.

Should the cluster be investigated further?

Few cluster investigations have been scientifically worthwhile. Most are under-powered and should not have been undertaken. Criteria that suggest that it is scientifically worthwhile investigating a cluster further are shown in Box 9.1.1.

Box 9.1.1 **Criteria to assess importance of suspected cluster**

1. There are at least five cases and the relative risk is very high (20 or more).

2. The disease is one for which a unique, detectable class of agents has been responsible in the past, or the pathophysiological mechanism is understood.

3. This agent is persistent in the environment and can be measured.

4. The agent is persistent or leaves a physiological marker in the bodies of people exposed to it but is rare in the normal population, so it can be used as an index of exposure.

5. People who live in the same neighbourhood have different levels of exposure to the possible cause so that effect of exposure can be assessed.

6. The plausible route of exposure is such that subjects would be able to accurately assess their own relevant exposure on a questionnaire or it could be reconstructed from records.

7. It is feasible to carry out a multi-community study of several similarly exposed and some unexposed communities.

8. The cluster represents an as-yet-uninvestigated, endemic space cluster, rather than a space-time cluster. Suggesting a stable, persistent problem and perhaps a persistent agent in the environment.

Working with the press

This is where you can make big mistakes. However, it also gives you the chance to minimise fear (if appropriate), inform, and elicit help (if necessary).

- be honest—admit what you do not know
- be concerned and sympathetic
- be positive where information is available—'overall the cancer rate is no higher than the national average'

- outline the steps you, or others, are taking, e.g. mention if you are:
  - developing a case-definition
  - searching the records for cases
  - organizing meetings
  - calling on 'national experts'
- beware of committing yourself to a specific type of investigation at an early stage—it may not prove appropriate and changes in plan can be interpreted as lack of interest or incompetence
- you may be asked 'what are the immediate implications for the local community?'—prepare an answer.

Many of the questions put by the press are standard and predictable (except in times of stress). Role play is a useful method of becoming more competent in this area if you get little exposure to the real thing. Listening to others dealing with the media and analysing it carefully with others can be an effective way of improving your skills (see chapter 7.4).

Pitfalls

There are three important pitfalls about which you should be aware:

(a) 'chasing chimeras'

(b) multiple hypotheses and vested interests

(c) inter-organization co-operation.

(a) Chasing chimeras

The biggest danger in any cluster investigation is 'generating' an apparently significant cluster when cases really occurred by chance. Not surprisingly, this can cause anxiety, waste time, and lead to inappropriate courses of action. It is common and occurs for several reasons:

- random events do not occur regularly—clusters identified *post hoc* can be simply due to chance
- it is easier to identify cases in the area of concern than in a comparison population
- national data for comparison may be incomplete or out-of-date
- boundaries (e.g. the time period, age, case-definition, and geographical area) are unconsciously set *post hoc* in a way that maximizes the number of cases in the 'cluster'. (This is known as 'Texas sharp shooting'—the target is drawn to fit the bullet holes!)

(b) Multiple hypotheses and vested interests

The media and public will be bombarded by information from external sources. Ranging from the extremely helpful (e.g. the

Meningitis Trust), to the downright eccentric. Be wary of people with vested interests e.g. local politicians, lawyers, commerce, pressure groups. Stick to the case and population definition and the major hypotheses—do not allow these definitions or hypotheses to drift. If they need to change, do it explicitly with consensus, and communicate the facts widely.

(c) Inter-organization co-operation

Organizations with expertise in the environmental aspects of cluster analysis may not give timely help or may not be keen to participate if the press is involved. Avoid criticizing other statutory organizations, as this may undermine public confidence. Recognize the constraints on other organizations.

Strengths and weaknesses of this approach

- the initial work on case-definition, case-finding, consulting data sources, and talking to contacts *is* an investigation and should be reported in positive terms
- setting up a case-control study which has no power to detect an effect wastes time and may be unethical
- maintaining that a cluster is likely to be due to chance when the public is worried is not always easy.

Evaluation

A successful investigation:

- has good written records
- has a clear case and population definition
- carefully considers the quality and quantity of data available about the 'cluster' and the reference population
- uses networks and others' expertise
- communicates effectively and helps the audience understand the scientific issues (e.g. how apparent clusters can arise by chance)
- avoids embarking on studies which do not have the power to produce meaningful answers
- identifies ongoing studies or recommendations for future research that might provide answers
- develops recommendations about protective measures and future disease surveillance (see chapter 1.2)
- is clear about current uncertainties and what action should be taken if more cases occur or more information becomes available.

Further resources

Centers for Disease Control (1990). Guidelines for investigating clusters of health events. *MMWR (Morbidity and Mortality Weekly Report)*, **39**, 1–23. www.cdc.gov/epo/mmwr/preview/mmwrhtml/00001797.htm (accessed 29 August 2000).

Elliott P, Cuzick J, English D, and Stern R (ed.) (1992). *Geographical and environmental epidemiology: methods for small-area studies.* Oxford University Press, Oxford.

Handbook and guide to the investigation of clusters of diseases. Leukaemia Research Fund, University of Leeds, Leeds, 1997.

Hertz-Picciotto I (1998). Environmental epidemiology. In *Modern epidemiology*, (ed. KJ Rothman and S Greenland), (2nd edn), pp. 555–84. Lippincott-Raven, Philadelphia.

Neutra RR (1990). Counterpoint from a Cluster Buster. *Am J Epidemiol*, **132**, 4–8.

References

1. National Conference on Clustering of Health Events. *Am J Epidem*, 1990, **132:1 (Suppl)**, S1–S202. In *Dictionary of epidemiology*, (ed. JM Last), (4th edn). Oxford University Press, Oxford, 2001.

9.2 **Public health in poorer countries**

Nick Banatvala

Objective

The objective of this chapter is to give the reader a basic understanding of the major public health issues among the poor populations of the world, and approaches to tackling them. The chapter is based on the approach of the UK Government's Department for International Development drawing extensively from its policy papers.[1,2]

Definition

More than a quarter of the developing world's people still live in poverty as measured by the human poverty index (a composite measure including life expectancy, basic education, and access to public and private resources).[3] One-third of the developing world's people (1.3 billion) live on incomes of less than $1 a day.[3] The chapter looks at the broader determinants of health and the links to other sectors.

Why is this an important public health issue?

Not only is health a long-recognized human right, improving health is associated with a decrease in poverty by securing better livelihoods. This is so at both a micro (family) level—less time caring for the sick means more time to earn and learn, and at a macro level—less sickness leads to regional and national economic growth.

Communicable diseases are the most important reason for the existence of the 'poor–rich' gap (world's poorest 20% to richest 20%), accounting for 77% of deaths and 79% of DALYs.* Non-communicable diseases account for less than one-fifth and accidents for one-tenth of the gap.[7] While a narrowing in the gap would occur with communicable disease control, the gap would widen with an overall decline in non-communicable diseases.[4]

There is huge variation in health between the poor and the rich globally and within developing countries. The poorest 20% of the world's population are ten times more likely to die before they are aged 14 years than the richest 20% and the greatest burden of ill-health is in sub-Saharan Africa.[3] If all children in developing countries had the same life chances, 11 million fewer children would die each year.[2] In Guinea, for example, there is a ten-fold variation in the percentage of richest and poorest fifths benefiting from public subsidy for health.[5] A spend of $12 per person per year on essential health care is sufficient to make a real difference to the suffering of poor people if resources were used effectively (Table 9.2.1).

Table 9.2.1 Estimated cost of a minimum essential package of health services in a low-income (*per capita* income = $350) country (Adapted from World Bank[6]).

Package	Package elements	Cost/person/year (US$, 1990)
Public health package	Expanded Programme on Immunization (EPI-plus), school health (including deworming), micronutrient supplementation, health education, information on health, nutrition, and family planning, tobacco and alcohol control programmes, disease monitoring and surveillance, vector control, AIDS prevention	$4.2
Minimum essential clinical services	Directly Observed Treatment, Short-course (DOTS) tuberculosis treatment ($0.6); management of the sick child ($1.6); prenatal and delivery care ($3.8); family planning and sexually transmitted diseases (STD) treatment ($1.1); limited care for other ailments ($0.7)	$7.8
Total		$12

Currently, many developing countries spend less than $5 per person per year and these funds are often not distributed equitably within the countries.

What are the approaches to subdividing a programme of work around this issue into defined tasks?

To tackle this massive agenda, clear targets are required to provide milestones against which progress towards the goal of eliminating poverty can be measured. These are based on recent UN Conventions and Resolutions. These International Development Targets (IDTs)* are given in the section 'Key determinants of success' below.

IDTs will only be achieved if there is the political will to address international development in both poorer and richer countries.

Objectives to eliminate poverty

Four primary objectives can be considered when poverty elimination is your objective in poorer countries:

- policies and actions which promote sustainable livelihoods (pro-poor policies, development of efficient and well-regulated markets, access of poor people to land, resources, and markets, prevention and resolution of conflicts, etc.)
- better education, health, and opportunities for poor people
- empowerment of women through gender equality[3,7]
- protection and better management of the natural and physical environment (sustainable management of physical and natural resources, efficient use of productive capacity, protection of the global environment).

Key areas to intervene

In order to achieve these objectives, there are key areas where intervention is likely to be more effective. Most of them relate to a primary aim of poverty elimination: the support of local and self-sustaining economic growth:

- water and food
- education
- essential health care
- population growth
- basic infrastructure
- income and employment opportunities
- good governance, corruption, and the rule of law
- gender inequalities
- rights of the child
- disasters and emergencies (see chapter 4.9).

The four key areas for *health gain* are:

- infant and child mortality
- maternal mortality
- reproductive health
- HIV incidence and prevalence.

HIV is a massive threat to global development and threatens to overturn many decades of development investment. The epidemic is affecting *both rich and poor* countries, economically, socially, politically, and culturally. However, poorer countries have pitifully few resources to address such a devastating problem.

What are the tasks needed to address these objectives and key areas?

There are four key responses that, taken together and vigorously pursued at national and international levels, would impact on the health and wealth of poor populations (Table 9.2.2).

Table 9.2.2 Response and action to improve the health of the poor.

Priority Response	Specific priorities	Examples of actions
1. Addressing the priority problems of the poorest billion, strengthening access to care, services and products	• Making pregnancy safer and improving reproductive and sexual services	Developing appropriate local policies and strategies, empowering communities, improving access to essential obstetric care including abortion services, promoting availability of contraceptives, generating school-based programmes
	• Reducing child mortality and improving child health	Introducing Programmes for the Integrated Management of Childhood Illnesses (e.g. immunisation, malaria, diarrhoea and acute respiratory illness management) access to safe water and sanitation, female education.
	• Communicable diseases	Malaria, tuberculosis, STDs* (including HIV/AIDS); Eradication of polio, onchocerciasis, guinea worm and lymphatic filariasis
	• Injuries and non-communicable diseases	WHO Tobacco-Free Initiative; Understanding the impact of mental illness
2. Investment in strong, efficient and effective health systems (public, private and informal)	• Supporting coherent systems rather than fracturing effort	Developing institutional and financially sustainable health systems, promotion of intersectoral actions towards health improvement, utilising public subsidies to assure equal access to health services for equal need
3. Creating conducive social, political and physical environments that enable poor people		Increasing safe shelters, road and vehicle safety; Minimising environmental hazards, violence, pollution and waste

Table 9.2.2 (continued)

Priority Response	Specific priorities	Examples of actions
4. A more effective global response to HIV/AIDS	◆ Raising the profile	Advocacy at local, national and international level
	◆ Enabling environment for HIV prevention and control	Improving gender equity; Programmes to reduce stigmata and discrimination
	◆ Caring for people living with HIV/AIDS	Improving access of poor to HIV care and support
	◆ Improving knowledge and technology	Vaccine and viricides development; Understanding social and behaviour issues such as risk behaviour

No one single player is able to transfer the above policies into action. Those involved in developing strategies to implement international policy need to:

(a) work in partnership
(b) use both multilateral and bilateral initiatives effectively
(c) ensure local ownership of initiatives
(d) encourage donors to match political commitment with funding and debt relief.

(a) Work in partnership with poor countries, private and voluntary sectors, research community, multilateral development organizations, and government departments. Examples include the partnerships developed in the WHO's Roll Back Malaria programme, the work to eradicate polio and river blindness. Many of the programmes developed by Oxfam, CARE, CONCERN, and other international development organizations have focused on generating programmes sustained by in-country government, private organizations, or local NGOs.*

(b) Use both multilateral and bilateral initiatives effectively. Examples include strengthening the technical and operational arms of UN agencies such as WHO, UNICEF (UN Children Emergency Fund), and UNIFEM (UN Development Fund for Women) and working directly on projects with governments and other partners in poor countries. The World Bank, the African Development Bank and the IMF are key partners for development work, with the former for example contributing in areas as diverse as understanding the costs of gender inequality for growth and development, and the effects of, and treatment strategies for, multi-drug resistant TB.

(c) Ensuring local ownership of initiatives and local capacity development, and where an evidence base exists basing activities on this. The sustainable livelihoods approaches encourage a holistic approach rather than collapsing the focus onto a few factors (e.g. economic issues, communicable disease, food security). The principles of sustainable livelihoods are that activities should be people-centred, responsive and participatory, multi-level, conducted in partnership, sustainable, and dynamic.[8]

(d) Encourage donors to match political commitment with a real increase in funding and an effective response to debt relief.

Potential pitfalls

The agenda above is more likely to succeed if a number of fundamental principles are adhered to. Success is unlikely where there is failure to:

- address the causes rather than just the symptoms of ill-health
- remove barriers that prevent the poor accessing services
- assure standards, accountability, and responsiveness to health service users
- strengthen the state in policy making, regulation, and providing services
- encourage the private sector to deliver appropriate services to poor people
- recognize that the UN system needs support in order to provide the necessary leadership for health
- believe that the IDTs will be easy to meet.

Fallacies

International public health policy is as prone to dogma as any area of domestic public health.

Fallacy 1: Models concentrating on one particular discipline are most effective in tackling the public health problems in developing countries

Approaches to international health have changed over time, with biomedical, economic, and institutional approaches each promulgated at varying times. Present consensus is that poverty reduction should be at the core of international health policy.

Fallacy 2: Either vertical or horizontal public health programmes are always better

Vertical programmes have been successful in areas such as immunization and useful in introducing new concepts (e.g. Directly Observed

Therapy, Short course for TB; (DOTS)). In the longer term, however, sustainable services need health systems that integrate into national health systems rather than focusing on a few specific interventions and services.

Fallacy 3: The cost of action and attaining the IDTs cannot be met

The targets are not easy but can be met through international co-operation (the harnessing of private and public sectors, global alliances including governments, NGOs, philanthropists), increased funding for programme activity as well as research and development, and employing principles of sustainable livelihoods.

Fallacy 4: Models of health care delivery developed in Western settings can be effectively transferred to other situations

Enthusiasm for health sector reform based in new management trends in Europe (decentralization, managerial autonomy, contracting, and internal market mechanisms) has been dampened by a realization that reforms must be closely tailored to local circumstances.

Fallacy 5: Cost-recovery systems are an effective approach to providing long-term delivery of health services

Cost-recovery systems (self-sustaining systems financed by the local community) have rapidly fallen out of favour, with concern on equity consequences with poorer patients excluded and subsidies benefiting the non-poor. In any event, revenue yields have often been minimal.

Fallacy 6: In developing countries there is no place for anything other than public funded and run services

The private sector in terms of services delivery, support of health systems, research and development, as a policy maker and donor are to be encouraged and valued. Indeed in some of the most desperate countries such as Afghanistan, private health care will form a greater component of overall health delivery than government-funded health care. The private sector cannot therefore be ignored.

Fallacy 7: There are too many players in international health, with policies muddled through the competing agendas of UN agencies, NGOs and others

While there has been a proliferation in agencies responding to global health needs over the last 20 or so years, the challenge is to co-ordinate these actors. Compared with the number of agencies in developed countries (c.f. partners in any one of the UK district's HImPs*) the number of agencies in development projects in resource-poor countries are often few. It is fair to say however that high-profile relief events (Rwanda 1994, Kosovo 1999) often result in a number of competing agencies searching for financial and media opportunities. Governments and other institutional donors have a responsibility to distribute funds to agencies with proven track records in the field of work and geographic region.

Fallacy 8: The real threat to development is globalization

Globalization is far from detrimental—there are plenty of opportunities, if harnessed appropriately, that come from a global community: economic, trade agreements and an international response to debt relief, communication and rapid transfer of information, maximizing finance and capital flows, and investment, competition, and private sector.

Fallacy 9: Funding development activities is more effective than the funding of relief

Disaster preparedness and prevention are an essential component of development assistance. Disasters, natural and man-made, including war, are more common in poor *countries*. The 'relief-development continuum' (cycles of relief and development), with agencies co-operating in different areas of expertise, and 'developmental relief' (development models being used in chronic relief efforts often seen in complex emergencies) are both increasingly accepted approaches.

Examples of successes, failures, and lessons learnt

Readers interested in specific geographic or sector initiatives are best referred to either a health database search or contacting donor and implementers in these areas (see chapter 3.6). Almost all donors and implementing agencies will produce annual reports which often identify recent programmes. Examples include those produced by the UK Department for International Development (DFID), Oxfam, and Médecins sans Frontières.[9–11]

What are the key determinants of success?

Measures of success are the international development targets (IDTs). The overarching target is a reduction by one-half in the proportion of people living in extreme poverty by the year 2015. In addition to this economic target there are targets for human development, and environmental sustainability and regeneration (Box 9.2.1).

Box 9.2.1 **International Development Targets**

Economic well-being

- a reduction by one-half in the proportion of people living in extreme poverty by the year 2015.

Human development

- reduction by two-thirds the rate of infant and child mortality by the year 2015
- reduction by three-quarters the rate of maternal mortality by the year 2015
- attain universal access to reproductive health services before the year 2015
- achieve a 25% reduction in HIV infection rates among 15–24-year-olds in worse affected countries by the year 2005, and globally by the year 2010.

Environmental sustainability and regeneration

- the implementation of national strategies for sustainable development in all countries by the year 2005, so as to ensure that current trends in the loss of environmental resources are effectively reversed at both global and national levels by the year 2015.

How will we know if we have been successful?

(a) continually check the IDTs as outlined above

(b) monitor core indicators of health that are most appropriate in the locality, e.g.:

- infant mortality rate
- under-five mortality rate
- maternal mortality rate
- births attended by skilled health personnel
- contraceptive use prevalence rate
- HIV prevalence in 15–24-year-old pregnant women.

Acknowledgement

This chapter is based principally on recent policy documents emanating from the UK Department for International Development (DFID) for the benefit of developing countries. The views are not necessarily those of DFID.

Further resources

Banatvala B and Zwi AB (2000). Conflict and health: public health and humanitarian interventions: developing the evidence base. *BMJ*, **321**, 101–5.

www.cdc.gov (accessed 29 August 2000).

www.dfid.gov.uk (accessed 29 August 2000).

www.msf.org (accessed 29 August 2000).

www.oxfam.org.uk/publications.html (accessed 29 August 2000) and www.oxfam.org.uk/development.htm (accessed 29 August 2000).

www.undp.org (accessed 29 August 2000) and their human development reports: www.undp.org/hdro (accessed 29 August 2000).

www.usaid.gov (accessed 29 August 2000).

www.who.int (accessed 29 August 2000).

www.worldbank.org (accessed 29 August 2000) and its reports: www.worldbank.org/wdr (accessed 29 August 2000).

References

1. *Eliminating world poverty: a challenge for the twenty-first century*. HMSO, London, 1997.

2. UK Department for International Development (1999). *International development strategy, better health for poor people: target strategy paper*, (consultation document). UK Department for International Development, London.

3. United Nations Development Programme (1997). *Human Development Report 1997*. Oxford University Press, Oxford.

4. Gwatkin DR, Guillot M, and Heuveline P (1999). The burden of disease among the global poor. *Lancet*, **354**, 586–9.

5. United Nations Development Programme (2000). *Human Development Report 2000*. Oxford University Press, Oxford.

6. World Bank (1993). *World development report 1993: investing in health*. Oxford University Press, 1993.

7. UK Department for International Development (2000). *International development strategy paper, poverty eradication and the empowerment of women people: target strategy paper*, (consultation document). UK Department for International Development, London.

8. www.livelihoods.org (accessed 29 August 2000).

9. UK Department for International Development (2000). *Department report 2000*. The Stationary Office, London.

10. Oxfam (1999). *Annual review 1998–9*. Oxfam, London.

11. Médecins sans Frontières (1999). *1999: year in review*. MSF, Brussels.

9.3 Empowering community health: women in Samoa

Pamela Thomas

Introduction

Empowering communities to take responsibility for health-promoting initiatives is an important way of ensuring widespread and sustained improvements in health, most particularly in poorer countries. A review of successful and sustainable community-based primary health care systems in developing countries indicates some common strategies and processes. An example is provided by the Women's Health Committees in Western Samoa, which in 1929 were hailed as 'the most brilliant illustration of the possibilities of preventive medicine amongst native peoples'.[1] Sixty years before a global policy for primary health care was enshrined in the Alma Ata Declaration of 1978, Western Samoa had an extensive rural network of community-based health care which fulfilled all the criteria for primary health care outlined in the Declaration. Today, Samoa has almost 100% child and maternal immunization, very low maternal mortality, and an infant mortality rate of 12 per 1000 live births—comparable to that of many industrial nations.

Empowerment is neither a single nor a simple intervention. Improvement will not be maintained unless the strategy is constantly revisited, reviewed, and renewed.

Key prerequisites for community empowerment for health

A number of prerequisites are required if communities are to become actively and successfully involved in public health. The most important appear to be:

- *establishing* community involvement:
  (a) a supportive administrative and health department philosophy
  (b) knowledge and analysis of the health, social, and political context, including the establishment of clear health priorities
  (c) establishing community health systems in ways that conform to accepted social norms and values

- *maintaining* community involvement:
  (a) tactics for maintaining community involvement
  (b) monitoring and evaluation.

These are exemplified by the establishment of the Samoan Women's Health Committees.

Establishing community involvement

(a) A supportive administrative philosophy

Successful community empowerment and involvement in health care requires an underlying philosophy which, like that of the Alma Ata Declaration, is based on:

- equality of access to health-related information and affordable health services
- helping communities fulfil their local health needs
- the rights of individuals and communities to plan and implement health care initiatives
- providing communities with the knowledge and capacity to make and act on health-related decisions
- accepting and supporting community decisions
- a firm belief in, and practical support for, community health
- making fullest use of local and national resources.

Community health initiatives established solely as a means of cutting health costs are almost never successful. Implementing such changes nearly always involve an increase in health (care) costs. The importance is that the added benefit has great value in long-term community investment.

> ## Box 9.3.1 **Diverse groups with common goals**
>
> In the early twentieth century, New Zealand was known for its socialist policy and commitment to equal access to public and preventive health. Two community-based self-help health systems had already been established—a Maori Nursing Service, in which trained Maori nurses worked with Maori communities to involve them in health, hygiene, and child care, and the Plunket Society, an association based on neighbourhood groups, the idea of mutual assistance, self-help, and education for the care of mothers and infants. In 1923, the New Zealand administration in Western Samoa, alarmed at the very high infant mortality rate and deteriorating health status of the people,[†] considered adapting these two models to suit Samoan health needs and social structure. As always, genuine community improvement involves diverse groups working towards common and shared goals.

....

† Following the 1918 influenza pandemic and successive epidemics of measles, whooping cough, and typhoid, it was thought that the populations of Samoa and other Pacific Island countries would die out.

(b) Knowledge and analysis of the health, social, and political context

Any community health initiatives must be based not only on firm knowledge of the major health problems and what is required to address them, but also on what is feasible for a community to successfully undertake, given the social, political, economic, and geographical context. The major steps are:

- a review of health status by age, gender, and rank[‡]
- an analysis of lifestyle, infant rearing practices, and living conditions
- consultations on village perceptions of health and illness
- an assessment of major village health concerns
- a review of village social structure, including authority structures and gender roles
- an analysis of village capacity to undertake health-related initiatives that were most likely to be effective
- clear knowledge of the capacity of government or non-government health services to support a community health initiative.

Box 9.3.2 **Priorities, needs, and feasibility**

In Samoa, a review was undertaken by local and international experts to consider health priorities, local needs, and what was feasible given local conditions. The priority health problems were found to be high levels of infant mortality, often related to lack of hygiene and poor weaning practices, and infectious diseases, also related to poor sanitation and lack of hygiene. It was decided that the health focus should be on community and household hygiene, and infant and child nutrition as: (a) these were preventive health measures that required no expensive outside inputs and were within the capacity of the community to implement and (b) they are the basic principles of public health and social reform. The decision conformed strongly to an over whelming and longstanding community concern about the death of so many infants and young children and a feeling of powerlessness to deal with the problem.

---

‡ Gender, rank, and occupation were considered particularly important, as during the influenza pandemic a very high proportion of those who died were men of high rank and/or church pastors. An occupational hazard was obesity.

This is of course an ideal list of steps. In reality, not all will be practically or financially feasible. However, if the potential exists (e.g. good local data), it should be used.

(c) Introducing the concept of community involvement in health: conforming to social norms and values

The successful introduction of the concept of community involvement in health requires time and careful planning. In particular, sensitivity to local social norms and values is paramount. However, it is important to remember that empowerment of some groups within communities may directly challenge those norms, which others may perceive as oppressive and contrary to true empowerment. Key concerns are:

- careful consideration and conformity to social and political values and local etiquette
- ensuring women, as well as men, have a voice and are involved
- support for local values regarding rank and authority
- speaking and listening to the appropriate people first—getting permission when necessary
- being able to offer something considered to be of value—knowledge, status, opportunities
- positioning major health problems and local needs within a local framework of knowledge
- providing an opportunity to be involved in something prestigious and exciting
- acknowledging and trying to meet perceived needs.

Maintaining effective community involvement in health

Many successfully established community-based health initiatives eventually fail because there is lack of adequate follow-up, support, monitoring, and evaluation. This is often related to reduced resources allocated to community health, lack of appropriately trained personnel, a change of health policy away from community and preventive health to more centralized, curative systems—often exacerbated by the policies and practices of development assistance agencies—and the perceived loss of prestige or authority of the community group. If there are no perceived benefits to the community, whether health related or not, the initiative will collapse. Occasionally this will require a trade-off between early perceived benefits to sustain long-term local commitment.

Box 9.3.3 **Working within the system I**

In Samoa, the introduction of the concept of community involvement in health was undertaken in strict accordance with indigenous etiquette and the ceremonial requirements of a hierarchically-ranked society based on a system of chiefly titles. The ability to work within this system and to reinforce traditional rank and authority was essential. A team of health and administrative personnel together with a group of high-ranking Samoan chiefs and orators formed a traditional travelling party and, carrying lavish gifts of food and fine mats, in accordance with tradition, formally visited village councils to discuss the health of the people.[2] By stressing the need for Samoan assistance, local pride and dignity were maintained and it was agreed that village women should take responsibility for health. The highly visible support of the highest ranking Europeans in the country—the chief medical officer, a woman doctor,[§] and the New Zealand administrator, gave the new undertaking not only very high status but legitimacy.[3] News of this obviously prestigious undertaking spread quickly and there were soon demands for Women's Health Committees from villages all over the country.

(a) Tactics for maintaining community involvement

Community development may be easier to *initiate* (in a first flush of enthusiasm from all) than it is to *maintain*. In order to sustain meaningful community involvement, there are important tactics to consider adopting:

- regular visits and follow-up by well-trained health personnel and occasional visits by high status personnel
- building on successes even if they are small
- giving praise where it is due
- ongoing support and encouragement for local ideas and initiatives
- clear lines of communication between community health group and health service personnel, building on pre-existing channels of communication
- regular distribution of equipment and preventive and educational materials
- regular feedback of information on local and national health status
- opportunities for the use of local authority in health issues

....

§ It was a remarkable coincidence that at a time when there were few women medical graduates, there were two women doctors in Samoa. Both had a deep interest in community health.

Box 9.3.4 **Working within the system II**

In Samoa, the Women's Health Committees were considered highly prestigious organizations to which all women wanted to belong. The Department of Health trained a number of high-ranking young Samoan women as maternal child health nurses who visited the Women's Health Committees each month. They were supported by visits from the Department of Health personnel and women doctors. Day-to-day health care and large-scale village health initiatives were left to the Committee to devise and organize. Committee executives were given first aid training and provided with medical kits. They held weekly meetings with all women and ensured all women and children attended the clinics when the nurse or doctor visited. Other areas of community service included maintenance of a supply of fresh drinking water, the provision of clean bathing facilities, the use of food safes, the construction of fly-proof latrines, keeping pigs out of the village, and in time the construction of a special Committee house which served as a meeting house and village hospital. Through a direct link to government and through the use of their own authority, the executive of the committees put in place village health regulations to which all families had to conform. Committee prestige was further enhanced by the visits of health teams with slide shows and movies** and by regular reports on the excellent work they were doing.

• provide variety in approaches and in health education
• involve communities in developing national health policy (emphasizing that any endeavour is a learning exercise that can be shared more widely).

(b) Changing contexts and the need for monitoring and evaluation

In most societies, health status, health problems and social situations change, requiring community-based systems that are able to adapt to new contexts. This is a challenge and requires:

• empowering communities to respond to changing health problems in different ways
• regular surveillance of health status by age, gender, and location by the community

....

** The Rockefeller Foundation was active in preventive health in the Pacific at the time and provided two magic lanterns, a film projector, and six sets of slides on nutrition, hookworm, filariasis, and the danger of flies. These were shown in committees throughout the country and were 'seen by a great majority of the Natives' (*Wellington Post*, 22 May 1925).

- regular surveillance of social and economic data and gender roles by the community
- health policies which support community involvement in health
- regular reassessment of community activities in health
- continued support for community health initiatives.

Box 9.3.5 **Empowering community groups**

As the Samoa example shows, the empowerment of communities to take responsibility for health can have unexpected results. The introduction of the Women's Health Committees not only brought about changes in health but considerable changes in women's authority, their daily activities, their perceptions of women's roles, and ways in which women interacted with one another. For the first time they participated in a single group that cut across traditional groupings which were divided by age, rank, and status. The Committee became the largest organized group in the village, with considerable political and economic power. It had greater access to labour than the church or village council. It became responsible for a wide range of health-related activities. They raised money for, and built increasingly large and impressive committees houses, health centres, and district hospitals. They provided regular inspections of village sanitation, built village latrines, provided piped water. They later engaged in small business and agricultural projects and became the leading fund raising organization in the village—sometimes to the detriment of their strictly health-related activities. By the 1940s the Women's Health Committees had become so well integrated into village life that they were considered to be a traditional Samoan organization to which women had always belonged. Ironically, although based on an ideology of equality, the success of the Committees was based on the legitimate use of traditional authority.

Today's challenge for community empowerment in health

In Samoa today, the situation continues to change, demanding new approaches to community health. Traditional authority, including that vested in the leaders of the Women's Committees, has weakened. With improved education and better transport, many younger women, including those with children—the Committees' traditional labour force—have paid jobs or have migrated. Twenty-five years of declining assistance for public and preventive health, together with persistent shortages of transport, insufficient nurses with appropriate public health training, and a widespread lack of equipment and maintenance of rural health facilities, have added to the decline of Committee importance and attendance. At a time when non-communicable diseases are now reaching epidemic proportions and effective, community-based preventive health care is urgently needed, the Women's Health Committees in their current form are no longer likely to provide a 'brilliant illustration of the possibilities of preventive medicine'.

It is important to consider which features of this case study from Western Samoa are transferable to other contexts: none will be generalizable everywhere but all will be relevant somewhere (see Further resources).

Further resources

Development Studies Network, Research School of Social Sciences, Australian National University, Canberra, Australia. devnet.anu.edu.au (accessed 29 August 2000).

Feuerstein MT (1993). *Turning the tide*. Macmillan, London.

Feuerstein MT (1997). *Poverty and health: reaping a richer harvest*. TALC, Macmillan, London.

Johnston M and Rifkin S (ed.) (1987). *Health care together: training exercises for health workers in community based programmes*. TALC, Macmillan Press, London.

Morley D, John E, Rhode JE, and Williams G (1983). *Practising Health for All*. Oxford University Press, Oxford.

Rifkin SB (1985). *Health planning and community participation: case studies in South-east Asia*. Croom Helm, London.

References

1. Lambert S (1929). *Medical conditions in the South Pacific*. The Australian Medical Publishing Company, Sydney.
2. Christie M (1926). Child welfare work in Western Samoa. *Appendices to the Journals of the House of Representatives*. New Zealand National Archives, Wellington.
3. Flood Keyes (Roberts) R (1927). Report on the Women's Health committees. *Appendices to the Journals of the House of Representatives*. New Zealand National Archives, Wellington.

9.4 Disability and ageing: a public health issue

David Melzer and Jack Guralnik

Objectives

In this case study we hope to show how epidemiology has contributed to a complex area of public health activity.

The chapter illustrates:

- the issues concerning measurement of disability
- the effect of social roles and environmental factors on health status
- the problems in interpreting international differences that relate to the measurement of burden of disease.

The chapter aims to provide:

- clear definitions and explanations concerning an important public health area
- some background to the importance and availability of measurement tools
- information on local and international terminology
- informed comment on the future challenges to be addressed.

Development of concepts of disability in older people

Much of contemporary public health is discussed in terms of specific medical diagnoses. Ironically, this model of discrete and well-defined disease works poorly for the largest population group with morbidity in industrialized countries, namely older people. Many older people have more than one disease, and in any event, disease status does not correlate well with everyday functioning.

Disability as impairment

Early attempts to assess disability emphasized physical impairment. For example, in workers' compensation legal cases in the first half of the last century, the loss of a hand was considered '60%' disability, by English medical review boards.[1] This model made:

- physical impairment the only criterion of disability
- doctors the overall judges of disability.

Inevitably, this approach led to sharp contradictions. For example, loss of a big toe can have devastating effects on an athlete, but less so on her coach.

Disability as loss of expected functioning

Gradually, a conception of disability developed that is based on everyday functioning, dependent on a person's normal roles, expectations, and environment. Disability in this model is the result of a gap between physical or mental capability on the one hand and the demands of the environment on the other. In this wider vision of disability it is clear that the impact of physical impairment can be highly variable. Mental health problems are also accepted as being disabling, not just physical lesions.

Disability thus has more to do with the impact of disease severity in a specified environment, and is much better suited to assessing at least the rehabilitation, support, and long-term care needs of ageing societies. Disability summarizes the overall impact of coexisting disease and environmental limitations in a way that disease classifications cannot.

Measuring disability

After definition, the next step in the public health approach to disability has been to develop measures for assessing disability. Disability is now usually assessed by asking the person themselves (or an informant) about inability or difficulty carrying out 'everyday activities of daily living', such as eating, bathing, and dressing. This can be supplemented by questions about 'instrumental activities of daily living', such as answering a phone, taking a message, or arranging payment of bills—activities that mostly require intact cognitive function.

Exploring the causes of disability in older populations

The overall analytic agenda on disability has covered most of the aspects of the public health approach to analysing a health problem. Early attempts aimed at identifying the scale of disability prevalence in the older population. Cross-sectional studies were undertaken, and the accepted pattern of rising rates of disability with age, and higher rates in women than men, soon emerged.

The next step was to identify the causes of disability—with much work concentrating on personal factors, but also geographic (place) factors and time trends. The need to identify pre-existing risk and to measure incidence of disability soon became pressing, and longitudinal studies emerged.

In longitudinal studies, the concept of recovery from disability had to be combined with the usual view that disability in old age is progressive—one of the surprises to emerge from epidemiological studies was the identification of large numbers of older people who recover between baseline and follow-up stages of longitudinal studies.

Disability and risk factors

Some specific risk factors for disability have emerged from this epidemiological work.[2] Consequently, it is now clear that disability is not an inevitable part of ageing—a substantial proportion is attributable to potentially avoidable risk factors. There is now strong epidemiological evidence that inactivity, cigarette smoking, obesity, depression, and alcohol and drug misuse are important risk factors for loss of mobility and functional decline in old age.

In the traditional notion that disability is mainly linked to age, the differences seen between socio-economic groups could also not be explained. In fact, people who had an elementary education only are roughly twice as likely to be disabled at older ages compared to those who received a college education in the USA, with very similar findings by occupational social class in the UK.[3] Clearly, your age, the number of times the earth goes round the sun with you on board, is not the only determining factor in disability.

Influencing policy and health care

Despite the evidence of potentially avoidable disability in old age, governments and international bodies have continued to see disability as an immutable burden. The strong association between disability and hospital and nursing home costs has led to a demand for better data on trends in disability. In the 1980s, evidence emerged, especially from the USA, of modest declines in disability prevalence.[4]

Public health practitioners have responded by establishing long-term studies of health status and have also developed a battery of sophisticated measures of health status that combine mortality and disability information, to help estimate the overall burden of different risks or diseases. Examples of these measures include 'disability free life expectancy'[5] and disability-adjusted life-years (DALYs*)[6] as summaries of population health status, and clinical outcome measures such as the RAND SF36 questionnaire, which incorporates questions about disability.

Challenges ahead

Having travelled this distance, troubling problems remain. One of the authors (JG) was involved in a study of disability in rural Italy, and was surprised to find considerably higher rates of disability in older Italians than in older Americans. Analysis of the data showed that the Italian sample's excess disability was mostly due to inability to bath without help. Visiting the homes in question revealed high-sided cast iron baths, which required quite a climb to get into. Disability is about the gap between physiological ability and environmental demand. This comprehensiveness makes it useful in assessing individual people, but problematic in comparing health status between populations, especially where culture and environment differ.

While clinicians and epidemiologists have concentrated efforts on identifying risk factors, quite another approach has emerged from the Disability Rights movement. The demand for public policy and public space that does not disable people is a very important part of the future agenda on disability and ageing. This illustrates how public health is everybody's business, identifying avoidable personal risks, forcing policy change, and modifying the environment to reduce disability.

Conclusion

Disability was once regarded as an inevitable consequence of ageing, and disease or physical impairment assessed by doctors was seen as its cause. The public health approach has clarified the concept, developed survey measures to assess its prevalence and incidence, and identified a series of risk factors, many of them potentially avoidable. While the media focus on the prospects of finding a biological panacea for ageing, the public health approach of identifying risks and modifying environments (together with improved health care) may already be delivering improvements in functioning in old age.

Further resources

Ebrahim S and Kalache A (1996). *Epidemiology in old age*. BMJ Publishing Group, London.

Guralnik JM, Fried LP, and Salive ME (1996). Disability as a public health outcome in the aging population. *Annu Rev Public Health*, **17**, 25–46.

Hickey T, Speers M, and Prohaska T (1997). *Public health and aging*. Johns Hopkins University Press, Baltimore.

References

1. Mor V (1984). *A modern lexicon of disability. Public policy toward disabled workers: cross national analyses of economic impacts*. Cornell University Press, Ithaca NY.

2. Stuck AE, Walthert JM, Nikolaus T, Bula CJ, Hohmann C, and Beck JC (1999). Risk factors for functional status decline in community-living elderly people: a systematic literature review. *Soc Sci Med*, **48**, 445–69.

3. Melzer D, McWilliams B, Brayne C, and Johnson T (2000). Socioeconomic status and the expectation of disability in old age: estimates for England. *J Epidemiol Community Health*, **54**, 286–92.

4. Manton KG, Corder L, and Stallard E (1997). Chronic disability trends in elderly United States populations: 1982–1994. *Proc Natl Acad Sci USA*, **94**, 2593–8.

5. Robine JM and Ritchie K (1991). Healthy life expectancy: evaluation of global indicator of change in population health. *BMJ*, **302**, 457–60.

6. Murray C and Lopez AD (1996). *The global burden of disease*. Harvard School of Public Health, Boston MA.

9.5 **Genetics in disease prevention**

Ron Zimmern

Objectives

By the end of this chapter you will:

• understand the principal associations between genetics and disease

• be able to discuss their implications concerning disease prevention both for

  • the health of the public

  • public health practice.

Introduction

All human variation and all disease processes are, with few exceptions, determined both by environmental and by genetic factors. These often interact, and individuals with a particular set of genes may either be more or less likely, if exposed, to be at risk of developing a particular disease. These effects may be measured by showing that the relative risk of exposure to the environmental factor is significantly greater (or lesser) for the subgroup with the abnormal gene, than the risk in those without.

Genetic variation exists in all populations. Clinically relevant polymorphisms, as these genetic changes are known, will be identified and associated with different diseases over the next few decades. While classical epidemiology presupposes that the genetic features of populations under study are homogenous, and compares groups of people exposed to with those not exposed to the environmental factor under study, the new genetic paradigm will seek to compare two genetically different populations under similar environmental conditions for disease outcomes.

It is the appreciation that gene and environment interact that will allow greater effectiveness and efficiency in the use of preventive and public health strategies. Preventive strategies which rely on an understanding of genetics are not about genetic manipulation, nor do they embrace eugenic processes such as attempts to prevent couples from exercising their own choice to reproduce, or to put pressure on them to abort affected foetuses. Public health interventions will continue to be directed at environmental or behavioural factors, but greater genetic knowledge will allow interventions to be focused on those subgroups of individuals whose genes make them particularly susceptible, rather than on the general population.

The extent to which genes contribute to disease form a continuum, but it is useful in practice to distinguish three types of situation. First, where the presence of the genetic abnormality reasonably accurately predicts whether the individual has or will develop the disease. These are usually caused by a single gene defect and transmitted from generation to generation in a Mendelian fashion, and are conventionally referred to as genetic diseases (Box 9.5.1). Second, where, in complex common disorders such as breast or colorectal cancer, Alzheimer's disease, or hypertension, rare genetic subgroups which behave like conventional genetic diseases can be defined (Box 9.5.2).

Box 9.5.1 **Examples of conventional genetic diseases**

- Duchenne muscular dystrophy
- cystic fibrosis
- Huntingdon's disease
- phenylketonuria
- adult polycystic disease of the kidney
- neurofibromatosis.

Box 9.5.2 **Examples of rare, genetic subtypes of common complex diseases**

- familial polyposis coli
- familial hypercholesterolaemia in coronary disease
- BRCA1 and BRCA2 in breast cancer
- PS1 and PS2 in Alzheimer's disease.

Third, where the presence of known genetic abnormalities alters the risk of disease in an individual, but does not predict it with any degree of certainty. These changes, often referred to as polymorphisms, are found much more frequently than the gene mutations in conventional genetic disorders, but their penetrance, or probability of developing the disease in question given the presence of the abnormality, will be much less. Knowledge of the status of genetic polymorphisms will be akin to knowledge about biological markers such as cholesterol levels, or blood pressure, in individuals. They define a risk, or probability, of developing (in this example) heart disease or stroke, but whether the disease actually develops or not will be the consequence of unidentified, multitudinous interactions between the genetic abnormality in question, other genes, and environmental factors.

Public health skills

Public health practitioners should appreciate the growing influence of the genetic contribution to disease, and the potential of using that knowledge for more efficient and effective disease prevention. Consider:

(i) if involved in research:

- be aware of the genetic heterogeneity of population groups
- question proposals for large-scale epidemiological studies which do not measure relevant genetic factors
- think not just in terms of the greater risk of disease posed by an environmental exposure, but also of the genetic factors that might determine why some exposed individuals develop the disease and others do not.

(ii) in relation to conventional genetic diseases appreciate that:

- their total burden is quite considerable, even though each disorder is comparatively rare
- many service issues remain to be addressed, including those of service quality, of neo-natal and ante-natal screening programmes, of the organization of laboratory genetic services, of the development of new genetic tests, and of commissioning and funding.

(iii) in relation to the rare, genetic sub-types of common complex diseases:

- seek to establish a minimum level of knowledge about the clinical epidemiology of the genetic determinant (Box 9.5.3)
- be aware of familial aggregation in these subgroups, and the importance of family history as a means of assessing risk
- question the utility of making the genetic diagnosis and ask if there are proxy criteria, such as clinical manifestations that might lead to the genetic diagnosis without the use of molecular genetic tests
- be aware, not only of the relative risk of possessing the genetic defect, but its absolute risk over a defined period of time
- question how individual patients in these subgroups should be managed in order to prevent the disease from developing or to improve survival (Box 9.5.4)

Box 9.5.3 **Epidemiological characteristics of a genetic determinant**

- the gene and its chromosomal location
- its known allelic variants
- their prevalence in the population at risk
- the relative and attributable risk of the variant in the diseased population
- the positive predictive value, or penetrance, of the variant
- the population attributable risk and population attributable fraction
- the potential for molecular genetic tests
- the sensitivity, specificity, and predictive value of the test
- the nature of any known interaction with other genes or with environmental exposures.

Box 9.5.4 **Intervention strategies for prevention or reducing mortality**

Early detection	colonoscopy for colorectal cancer (HNPCC)
	mammography for breast cancer (BRCA1 and BRCA2)
Chemoprophylaxis	tamoxifen for breast cancer (BRCA1 and BRCA2)
	statins for familial hypercholesterolaemia (FH)
Removal of target organs	oophorectomy for ovarian cancer (BRCA1)
	mastectomy for breast cancer (BRCA1 and BRCA2).

(iv) in relation to low penetrant susceptibility genetic influences on common complex disorders:

- realize that the examples of susceptibility genes of clinical relevance are as yet few, but that in the next decade these are likely to multiply
- endorse the principle that, in most situations, the use of genetic tests for detection and diagnosis should be avoided where there are no effective preventive or therapeutic interventions

- appreciate that there are significant ethical implications in relation to privacy and confidentiality and to employment and insurance

- assess the positive predictive value of carrying a genetic polymorphism, appreciating that it is similar to the concept of penetrance as used by geneticists

- understand that there will also be many examples where the possession of the abnormal gene is protective of disease in the context of specific environmental factors

- be aware that much research will be needed before these concepts result in interventions which will change significantly the incidence and prevalence of common diseases

- understand that high penetrance genes which matter in complex, common disorders are rare and are unlikely to contribute to a significant population risk, but will be of crucial importance to the individual and the family

- be aware that the more common polymorphisms, responsible for susceptibility, have yet to be identified, but that their penetrance and population prevalence will together determine the population attributable fraction, an indicator of the significance of their contribution to the burden of disease.

(v) in general:

- be sensitive to the ethical, legal, and social issues surrounding all aspects of genetics and genetic testing

- be aware of the importance of taking into account the views of the public, which, if mishandled, may hinder the translation of basic research into technologies that will benefit the patient in the clinic and the public health.

Conclusion

Public health perspectives are broad, and encompass not only scientific, epidemiological, and medical, but also sociological and other perspectives. This wide approach is essential to the formulation of public policy, particularly in the context of genetics, where its impact over the next two decades on the organization of clinical services and on society is likely to be considerable. Practitioners of public health must contribute to this endeavour, remaining aware of the growing importance of genetic mechanisms in disease, and of the potential to utilize the new genetic knowledge for the benefit of both individuals and society.

Further resources

Collins FS (1999). Shattuck lecture: medical and social consequences of the Human Genome Project. *N Engl J Med*, **341**, 28–37.

Coughlin SJ (1999). The intersection of genetics, public health and preventive medicine. *Am J Prev Med*, **16**, 89–90.

Khoury MJ (1997). Genetic epidemiology and the future of disease prevention and public health. *Epidemiology Reviews*, **19**, 175–80.

Khoury MJ and Thomson E (ed.) (2000). Genetics and public health in the twenty-first century. Oxford University Press, Oxford.

Khoury MJ, Beatty TH, and Cohen BH (1993). *Fundamentals of genetic epidemiology*. Oxford University Press, New York.

Zimmern RL (1999). Genetics. In *Perspectives in public health*, (ed. S Griffiths and DJ Hunter), pp. 131–40. Radcliffe Medical Press, Oxford.

Zimmern RL (1999). Human Genome Project: a false dawn? *BMJ*, **319**, 1282.

Zimmern R and Cook C (2000). Genetics and health: policy issues for genetic science and their implications for health and health services. The Stationery Office, London.

9.6 **Action against smoking**

Muir Gray

Objectives

At the end of this chapter, the reader will be able to check their strategy or programme for tobacco control against a template. It assumes that the reader is working with a defined population and is only indirectly able to influence national policy making, being directly responsible for promoting the health of their population through a public health department.

Programme objectives

Every programme must have objectives. For smoking and tobacco control, two objectives are important:

- to stop children from starting smoking
- to help people who want to stop smoking.

These two objectives are helpful as they are morally unassailable. It is, of course, possible to set a wide range of objectives which pit the public health practitioner directly against the tobacco industry, but these can cause unnecessary problems for the practitioner. For example, if an objective such as 'to campaign for tighter controls on tobacco advertising and sponsorship' is adopted as a high-level objective, the practitioner may be criticized by some member of their Board who believes that this is not the function of the public health department. If however, this objective is a sub-objective to the two main objectives of stopping children starting and helping smokers quit, then it becomes acceptable because conflict with industry is seen as a means to an end and not an end in itself.

For each of the main objectives, therefore, it is possible to list a second level of objectives, some of which are common to both. The second level objectives of a tobacco control programme are typically:

- to ensure that everyone is aware of the risks to health caused by tobacco
- to create a smoke-free environment for young people
- to protect young people from the influence of advertising and sponsorship
- to help young people understand the motives and techniques of advertising and sponsorship
- to help young people say 'no' to cigarettes
- to ensure that all health professionals give appropriate advice to smokers whenever possible

- to make easily available pharmacological agents which help people stop smoking and stay stopped
- to campaign for higher taxes on tobacco
- to campaign for tighter controls on advertising and sponsorship.

Choosing criteria

For each objective the practitioner should identify criteria that could be used to measure progress, or the lack of it. Criteria should be:

- *valid*—they should measure a variable that gives an accurate estimate of progress towards the objective
- *reliable*—they should give the same result when collected by different people
- *feasible*—it should be possible to measure them.

The most valid measure of progress towards stopping young people starting is, of course, smoking prevalence among younger people, but that may not be very feasible to measure on a regular basis, and proxy measures may have to be chosen. For example, national rates of smoking may have to be used with periodic sampling in the local population. Alternatively, use national data and calculate the locally-attributable data.[1,2]

Public health can, however, be unfairly criticized if it takes smoking prevalence as the outcome measure for which it wishes to be held responsible. National decisions such as those which influence the price of cigarettes have a major influence on smoking prevalence. Thus it would be possible for a public health practitioner to run a very effective tobacco control programme based on the second level objectives set out above but for smoking prevalence among young people to rise because the relative price of cigarettes was falling.

Thus, a more valid measure of the effectiveness of a public health programme at local level would be levels of knowledge about smoking and health among young people or adherence to regulations about advertising near schools.

It is all too easy for public health professionals to be criticized because they have not brought about a rapid reduction in lung cancer or smoking prevalence as the power to do so is not within their hands alone.

Do not equate feasibility with ease; it is sometimes an effective public health intervention to choose a measure that requires a considerable amount of effort. For example, to involve all schools in a study of advertising near schools, measuring the distance to the nearest advertisement and photographing advertisements on hoardings or outside shops near schools. It is not a simple thing to organize but the measurement becomes an intervention.

Helping young people stop starting

In developing this sub-programme, it is useful to think of three main elements:

(a) the context
(b) direct action
(c) indirect action.

(a) The context

It is important to appraise the context, as it partly relates to the context of young people's culture and the way they view risk, the language they use to describe risk, and the future; the fact that cigarette smoking increases the likelihood of having a myocardial infarction at the age of 55 is of little relevance to someone who regards the age of 56 as being a human condition of very low value. Neither can it be assumed that parents rank cigarette smoking among their highest worries in modern society; some parents may be more concerned about other drugs.

An analysis of context is therefore important as the first stage of the programme.

(b) Direct action

The direct actions that a public health department can take include:

- integration of information about smoking into the general school curricula

- specific educational programmes designed to help people understand advertising and giving them insight into the social pressures to smoke because young people start to smoke for social reasons but continue because of pharmacological dependence

- monitoring sales to young people and taking action to discourage this

- monitoring advertising near schools and taking action if there is abuse.

Box 9.6.1 **Incentives in California**

Pierce et al.[3,4] in California ran a successful campaign very cost-effectively. Schools would be awarded prizes of music concert tickets if children, chosen at random from participating schools, had undetectable levels of tobacco through breath testing. This proved they had not smoked, *and, more importantly, had not been in the company of any peers who had smoked*. Advantages:

- cheap to monitor (only one person needs testing)

- incentives tailored to age-group

- action taken *within* the group (peer pressure brought by one child on another to stop smoking).

(c) Indirect action

The public health practitioner should keep their national political representatives informed of the evidence concerning young people which helps them to resist ever starting the habit—lobbying is an important part of public health (see chapter 4.10).

Helping smokers quit

Again, consider the same three dimensions:

(a) The context

Social attitudes towards smoking are changing in developed countries although there are great variations from one country to another, with Australia and California probably being in the lead in terms of creating an environment in which non-smoking is the norm in all social classes. In other countries such as the UK the culture varies from social class to social class, with changes taking place on the promotion of a smoke-free culture while making concessions to people who cannot stop smoking; this is an important part of their public health programme.

(b) Direct action

Direct action by public health practitioners includes:

- public education about risks, as not everyone is fully informed
- the encouragement of clinicians to identify smokers and give them advice to stop and support if they do
- the provision of nicotine replacement therapy and public advertisement of its availability
- high-profile events such as 'stop smoking days'; it is often best if these are co-ordinated nationally because national media coverage can be very supportive.

(c) Indirect action

Practitioners can campaign for:

- tax increases
- control on advertising
- more explicit labelling
- support for litigation.

Evidence-based public health action on smoking

This is one aspect of public health in which an evidence-based approach is relatively easy. Not only do we have good information about the effects of smoking on health; through the Cochrane Library there is an increasing evidence base for the effectiveness of different interventions, including policy changes. The Cochrane Database of Systematic Reviews[5] contains reviews that are continuously updated.

Big issues in public health

Tobacco control is a big public health issue, on the same scale as AIDS. This is especially important in developing countries as the tobacco industry switches its attention to countries where public health is less well organized. Deaths in China could rise to 2 million a year by the year 2025.[6]

However, it is also a big issue because of its ethical implications. In 2000 a jury in Miami ordered five tobacco companies to pay $145 billion compensation to half a million smokers made ill by cigarettes, the key factor not being the harm but the techniques that the tobacco companies had used to conceal information about the harmful effects of smoking and their use of substances to increase the probability of dependence. Welcome though this decision was, there were doubts expressed, articulated by a writer in *The Guardian* in July 2000 in the UK, who wrote that 'if we confer in courts and governments the final decision of the percentage of nicotine that individuals are allowed to consume, by the same logic we want to authorise the courts and governments to determine the licitness or illicitness of the calories consumed in the family diet'. No public health professional should reduce their effort to control the harmful effects of tobacco as a result of this type of argument, but it is important to be aware of all the possible arguments against a public health programme and to focus on the morally unassailable high ground of ensuring that those who want to stop are helped to do so and that young people become adults without starting smoking as a rite of passage.

Further resources

Jha P and Chaloupka FJ (2000). The economics of global tobacco control. *BMJ*, **321(7257)**, 358–61. (In *BMJ Special Edition 1999*, **321**, 7257, 5 August 2000.)

Pollock D (1999). *Denial and delay: the political history of smoking and health 1951–1964, scientists, government and industry as seen in the papers of the UK Public Records Office*. Action on Smoking and Health (ASH), London.

UK Action on Smoking and Health. www.ash.org.uk/ (accessed 3 September 2000).

References

1. *UK Department of Health Statistical Bulletin*. Statistics on smoking: England 1976 to 1996. Bulletin 1998/25. Published July 1998. www.doh.gov.uk/public/smoking.htm (accessed 3 September 2000).

2. *UK Department of Health Statistical Bulletin*. Statistics on smoking: England, 1978 onwards Bulletin 2000/17. Published August 2000. www.doh.gov.uk/public/sb0017.htm (accessed 3 September 2000).

3. Pierce JP, Gilpin EA, Emery SL, *et al.* (1998). Has the California tobacco control program reduced smoking? *JAMA*, **280**, 893–9.
4. Personal communication. Cambridge Public Health Seminar, Institute of Public Health, 1999.
5. Cochrane Library: Cochrane Database of Systematic Reviews (CDSR) (2000). *Cochrane Collaboration. Cochrane Library*, **Issue 3**. Update Software, Oxford.
6. *The World Health Report, 1999. Making a difference.* Chapter 5: Combating the tobacco epidemic. World Health Organization, Geneva, 1999. www.who. int/whr/1999/en/report.htm (accessed 3 September 2000).

9.7 Diabetes: developing a local strategy

Margaret Guy

Introduction

All health authorities in England are now required to develop local strategies for improving the health of the population, reducing inequalities in health, and improving health services.[1] This case study describes how diabetes was selected as a priority by one London health district and the subsequent development of a strategy for improving the health of people with diabetes resident within the district. It illustrates some of the concepts described in earlier chapters.

Key features of the district

The diabetes strategy was developed in a diverse area of London which includes both areas of inner city deprivation and affluent suburbs. There are marked variations in the health status of the population–these closely mirror the marked variations in their socio-economic status. Nearly 40% of the population of approximately 500,000 residents are from black and minority ethnic groups–11% are of African or African Caribbean origin and 19% are of Asian origin.

How was diabetes chosen as a local priority?

Priorities were selected for initial action in the district's health improvement programme. The process for identifying these priorities involved a number of steps:

Production of an inventory of potential priorities

An inventory of potential priorities was produced which reflected the key health issues identified in Public Health Annual Reports, as well as discussions with local stakeholders.

For each potential priority, a brief description was given of:

- work already undertaken to assess the level of need
- strategies and initiatives already in progress
- reasons for inclusion in the health improvement programme
- expected health benefits.

Agreement of criteria for selecting initial priorities

Criteria were then agreed against which potential priorities were appraised. (Box 9.7.1.)

Box 9.7.1 **Criteria against which potential priorities were appraised**

- the proposed priority should be a national priority and/or a major issue within the district, e.g.:
  - a major determinant of health/ill-health
  - a major cause of premature death and/or poor health
  - a major cause of public concern
  - a major cost to society
  - a care group or population subgroup with particular needs
  - an issue where marked inequalities/variations exist
- there should be an existing strategy or initiative on which to build
- there should be effective interventions offering potential scope for health improvement
- it should be possible to set targets and to monitor progress
- the issue should ideally involve as many partners as possible.

Agreement of local priorities for initial action

Conferences were then organized to agree which of these potential priorities should be chosen. All those involved in improving the health of the local population within the district were invited to attend.

A consensus was reached as to which priorities should be included in the health improvement programme: six priority areas were chosen, one of which was diabetes. Strategies were then agreed with all relevant local players for each priority area.

The case for diabetes being a local priority

It was possible to make a very strong case for identifying diabetes as a local priority, particularly because of the ethnic diversity of the local population.[2]

Shortly after the decision was taken to make diabetes a local priority, it was announced that a national service framework for diabetes was to be developed in England, making it also a national priority.

The case for including diabetes as a local priority is summarized in Box 9.7.2.

Box 9.7.2 **The case for including diabetes as a local priority**

- diabetes is one of the most common chronic disorders in the UK, affecting at least 2% of the population[3]
- diabetes and its complications can cause severe problems for affected individuals:
  - it is a leading cause of blindness, kidney failure, and limb amputation, particularly in people of working age
  - it greatly increases the risk of coronary heart disease and stroke
  - it can also threaten the successful outcome of pregnancy
- diabetes is a particular challenge within the district because of the ethnic diversity of the population—diabetes is three to four times more common amongst people of Asian, African, and African Caribbean origin[4]
- the prevalence of diabetes is predicted to increase further as the population ages[5]—this will be a particular issue within the district if those of Asian descent remain (prevalence increases with age, particularly in those of Asian descent—more than 25% of people aged over 65 of Asian origin have diabetes)
- the prevalence of diabetes varies across the district—the impact of these variations is compounded by the difficulties accessing services experienced by older people and ethnic minority groups, especially those for whom English is not their first language
- there is real scope for health improvement:
  - increasing evidence that the onset of Type 2 diabetes can be prevented or delayed by promoting healthy weight management and physical activity, particularly in subgroups of the population at increased risk of developing diabetes[6]
  - robust evidence that meticulous metabolic control can prevent or delay the onset of the complications of diabetes—the UK Prospective Diabetes Study[7,8,9] has confirmed that tighter control of blood glucose and blood pressure can significantly improve health outcomes in people with Type 2 diabetes; this mirrors the results of the US Diabetes Control and Complications Trial[10,11] for the control of blood glucose in people with Type 1 diabetes
  - increasing evidence that surveillance for and careful management of cardiovascular risk factors, including smoking, hypertension, physical inactivity, and obesity, as well as the regular surveillance for and early treatment of the complications of diabetes, can improve outcome[12]

- the organization of diabetes services is complex and involves all sectors of the health service. Many other agencies also have an important role to play both in the prevention of diabetes and the provision of services to affected individuals, including social services and housing departments, providers of leisure facilities, schools and colleges, and voluntary and community groups

- a substantial body of guidance is already available on the recommended management of diabetes[13,14,15] and the monitoring of the quality and outcome of care provided[16]

- much work has already been undertaken within the district— a local diabetes advisory group had been in place for several years.

The development of the diabetes strategy

The development of the diabetes strategy was co-ordinated by the local diabetes advisory group, which includes representatives from all local partners with a role to play in reducing the impact of diabetes within the district.

Any strategy should address the following four questions:

(a) where are we now?

(b) where do we want to be?

(c) how are we going to get there?

(d) how will we know whether we have got there?

The following steps were therefore taken to develop the diabetes strategy:

(a) Where are we now?—establishing the baseline situation

A detailed assessment of the current situation was undertaken.

(b) Where do we want to be?—agreeing shared aims and objectives

The overall aim and specific objectives of the strategy were then agreed by all those with a role to play in reducing the impact of diabetes within the district. (Box 9.7.3.)

(c) How are we going to get there?—agreeing an action plan

The Local Diabetes Advisory Group agreed a rolling programme of action for achieving each of these objectives, which included specific milestones. It was agreed that progress would be reviewed annually.

Box 9.7.3 **Aims and objectives of the strategy**

Overall aim

To reduce the impact of diabetes on the local population by:

- preventing or delaying the onset of Type 2 diabetes
- maximizing the health of those with diabetes, so that they are enabled to achieve a quality of life and life expectancy similar to that of the general population
- reducing inequalities across the district in health outcomes for people with diabetes.

Specific outcome objectives

- to reduce premature mortality attributable to diabetes and its complications
- to decrease the incidence of the long-term complications of diabetes
- to decrease the incidence of the acute metabolic complications of diabetes
- to decrease the incidence of adverse pregnancy outcomes.

Specific process objectives

- ensure that local initiatives are in place to prevent or delay the onset of Type 2 diabetes
- promote the early diagnosis of those with diabetes
- ensure that all those with diagnosed diabetes have access to appropriate education
- maintain metabolic control at as near physiological levels as possible
- provide regular surveillance for and appropriate management of cardiovascular risk factors
- provide regular surveillance for long-term complications, thereby enabling their early identification and effective management
- promote strict blood glucose control before conception and throughout pregnancy in women with pre-existing diabetes and ensure the early diagnosis and effective management of gestational diabetes
- ensure that people with disabilities resulting from diabetes and its complications receive appropriate care and support.

It was also acknowledged that the implementation of this action plan would be supported by a number of other underpinning strategies including those for:

* organizational development
* workforce planning
* information and information technology
* deployment of resources
* clinical governance.

(d) How will we know whether we have got there?— monitoring progress

Although the ultimate aim of the strategy is to improve long-term health outcomes for people with diabetes, the relatively low prevalence rates for some of these outcomes mean that they can only be usefully interpreted at regional and national levels. Furthermore, many of these outcomes have long time-scales.

In order to assess progress in the shorter term, it was therefore agreed to monitor annually:

* indicators of the quality of the process of diabetes care
* indicators of the outcome of diabetes care.

Examples of indicators which can be used to monitor the process and outcome of care are set out in Table 9.7.1.

Table 9.7.1 Indicators of the process and outcome of care.

1. Process indicators of the quality of diabetes care	
Level of ascertainment	Age-standardized prevalence rates of diagnosed diabetes for whole population and specific subgroups
Annual review coverage	% patients in whom the following have been assessed within the last year: body mass index, dietary management, tobacco consumption, urinalysis for proteinuria, blood pressure, HbA_{1c}, serum lipids and creatinine, visual acuity and fundoscopy, feet
Patient satisfaction	Measures of patient satisfaction with the care received and the way in which this care is delivered
2. Indicators of the outcome of care	
Well-being and quality of life	Measures of psychological and physical well-being, knowledge of diabetes, and self-care performance
Glycaemic control	% patients in each treatment group with an HbA_{1c} within acceptable range

Table 9.7.1 (continued)

Glycaemic control (*continued*)	% patients requiring hospital admission for ketoacidosis within previous year
	% patients requiring professional attention for hypoglycaemia in last year
Prevalence of cardiovascular risk factors	% patients who smoke, are overweight
	% patients with hypertension, raised cholesterol, raised triglycerides
Markers of microvascular complications	% patients with proteinuria/microalbuminuria, raised creatinine
	% patients who have retinopathy
	% patients with absent food pulses, reduced sensation, foot ulceration
Intermediate outcomes	% patients with angina, claudication, symptomatic neuropathy, impotence
Pregnancy outcomes in women with pre-existing or gestational diabetes	Abortion rates: spontaneous and for congenital abnormality
	Stillbirth and perinatal/neonatal mortality rates in infants of diabetic mothers
	Incidence of congenital abnormalities: minor and major
Outcomes with long time-scales	% patients who have had a myocardial infarction
	% patients who have had a stroke
	% patients with visual impairment
	% patients with severe visual impairment
	% patients with end stage renal failure
	% patients who have had an amputation
	Age-specific mortality rates in people with diabetes

References

1. UK Department of Health (1998). *Health improvement programmes— planning for better health and better health care*, (Health Service Circular: HSC 1998/167). UK Department of Health, London.

2. *Health Improvement Programmes—an opportunity to improve the health of people with diabetes. Including diabetes as a local priority in Health Improvement Programmes.* Guidance prepared by Dr Margaret Guy on behalf of the British Diabetic Association. October 1998.

3. Williams DRR (1994). Diabetes mellitus. In *Health care needs assessment*, (ed. A Stephens and J Raftery). Radcliffe Medical Press, Oxford.

4. *Counting the cost: the real impact of NIDDM.* A King's Fund report commissioned by the British Diabetic Association. British Diabetic Association, London, 1996.

5. Amos A, McCarty DL, and Zimmet P (1997). The rising global burden of diabetes and its complications: estimates and projections to the year 2010. *Diabetic Medicine*, **14**, S1–S85.

6. Hamman RF (in press). Prevention of Type 2 diabetes mellitus. In *The evidence base for diabetes care*, (ed. WJ Herman, AL Kinmonth, NJ Wareham, and R Williams).

7. UK Prospective Diabetes Study Group (1998). United Kingdom Prospective Diabetes Study. Intensive blood-glucose control with sulphonylureas or insulin compared with conventional treatment and risk of complications in patients with Type 2 diabetes (UKPDS 33). *Lancet*, **352**, 837–53.

8. UK Prospective Diabetes Study Group (1998). United Kingdom Prospective Diabetes Study. Effect of intensive blood-glucose control with metformin on complications in overweight patients with Type 2 diabetes (UKPDS 34). *Lancet*, **352**, 854–65.

9. UK Prospective Diabetes Study Group (1998). United Kingdom Prospective Diabetes Study. Tight blood pressure control and risk of macrovascular and microvascular complications in Type 2 diabetes: UKPDS 38. *BMJ*, **317**, 703–12.

10. Diabetes Control of Complications Trial Research Group (1993). The effect of intensive treatment of diabetes on the development and progression of long-term complications in insulin-dependent diabetes mellitus. *New England Journal of Medicine*, **329**, 977–86.

11. Diabetes Control of Complications Trial Research Group (DCCT) (1996). Lifetime benefits and costs of tight control therapy as practised in the diabetes control and complications trial. *JAMA*, **276**, 1409–15.

12. Clark CM Jr and Lee DA (1995). Prevention and treatment of the complications of diabetes mellitus. *New England Journal of Medicine*, **332**, 1210–7.

13. European Diabetes Policy Group 1998 (1999). A desktop guide to Type 1 (insulin-dependent) diabetes mellitus. *Diabetic Medicine*, **16**, 253–66.

14. European Diabetes Policy Group 1999 (1999). A desktop guide to Type 2 diabetes mellitus. *Diabetic Medicine*, **16**, 716–30.

15. Guy M (ed.) (1997). *Recommendations for the management of diabetes in primary care*. British Diabetic Association, London.

16. Home P, Coles J, Goldacre M, Mason M, and Wilkinson E (ed.) (1999). *Health outcome indicators: diabetes mellitus*. Report of a working group to the Department of Health. National Centre for Health Outcomes Development, Oxford.

9.8 Depression: a public health issue

Rachel Jenkins

Introduction

According to the Global Burden of Disease model,[1] 10% of the world's disability is due to unipolar depression. The high prevalence,[2] severity, duration,[3] and accompanying disability[4] of depression means that it can never be remotely viable to tackle this public health challenge through the exclusive use of specialist care. In even the richest of nations, specialist care can usually only cater for around 10% of people with affective disorders.

On the other hand, ignoring depression as a public health problem would be foolish. The costs of depression are immense in terms of psychological distress, repeated GP consultation,[5] sickness absence,[6] labour turnover,[7] reduced productivity, and reduced physical health. Depression also has a major impact on families, through marital problems and damage to children. In addition, depression contributes to high-risk behaviours such as reckless driving, violent crimes, and substance abuse, as well as to suicide attempts and suicide.

Objectives

The development of strategies to reduce the burden of mental illness in the United Kingdom provides a good case study of public health practice in the control of chronic disease. This case study is designed to illustrate the principles of developing and implementing a national strategy, and develops many of the themes discussed in the handbook, from the measurement of health status and needs, through the setting of public health objectives and targets, the management of change, and the evaluation of public health programmes.

Developing public health objectives

An early step in the development of the programme in the UK involved developing a set of clear objectives, based on review of the epidemiology and effectiveness literature, and professional and other opinion (see chapter 3.2).

The process was stimulated by WHO's Health for All by the Year 2000 strategy.[8]

The objectives set were:

- to reduce the incidence and prevalence of depression
- to reduce the mortality associated with depression

- to reduce the extent and the severity of other problems associated with depression, including
  - poor physical health
  - impaired social functioning
  - poor social circumstances
  - family burden
- to ensure appropriate services and interventions are provided
- to tackle stigma and create a positive climate in which to seek and obtain help
- to research causes, consequences, and the care of depression.

Following earlier work, the current health strategy 'Our Healthier Nation' sets a target of reducing deaths due to suicide, and puts further emphasis on promotion and prevention as well as treatment and rehabilitation

Setting objectives however is only the first step, and an overall strategy was needed to achieve these objectives.

Developing an implementation strategy

The overall implementation strategy to tackle depression is multi-factorial. The strategy should include:

- gaining national and local commitment to action (see chapter 3.3)
- creating working partnerships
- addressing the role of both primary and specialist care, and their interfaces with each other
- addressing other agencies such as social care, the police and the prisons
- taking action in the community, including schools and workplaces
- training and education
- mental health information systems
- research and development.

Gaining national commitment and creating partnerships

Obtaining public ownership of the scale of the problem is a key step in implementing the strategy. Government sponsored surveys are useful for a variety of reasons, including helping to obtain national and public ownership of important factual information, which is often a necessary precondition for action. Large-scale epidemiological surveys are useful to assess the scope for public health interventions, to assess the requirements for primary care, and to assess the use of existing specialist services. By repeating community surveys it is possible to monitor the health of the population and trends in disorders, and changes in potential risk factors.

The national psychiatric morbidity survey[9] was the first national survey in any country to collect data on prevalence, risk factors, and associated disability simultaneously in household, institutional, and homeless samples by use of standardized assessment techniques. The survey covered depression as well as other neurotic disorders and psychosis and alcohol and drug misuse.

The household survey found that one in six adults aged 16 to 64 years who live in private households had suffered from some type of neurotic disorder in the week before the survey interview, half of which was mixed anxiety depression.

Primary care education

The high prevalence of depression means that it is imperative to ensure appropriate education and training of primary care teams, to develop good practice guidelines with locally agreed criteria for referral and shared care, and to develop opportunities for prevention and early detection. There have been a number of initiatives to support this process.

The Department of Health, in collaboration with the Mental Health Foundation and the Gatsby Trusts, funded a senior mental health fellow in general practice for four years to cascade knowledge and skills about depression through GP tutors and course organizers. This scheme has now evolved into a Royal College of General Practitioners Unit for Mental Health Education in primary care, largely focused on depression. The Unit has developed to 'train the trainers' course for trainers (usually a GP and nurse working together) who then offer flexible, multi-disciplinary, practice-based training in their localities.

During the last decade, ways have been explored to involve nurses more fully in the care of depression. Several studies have demonstrated the feasibility of practice and community nurses extending their role and associated training to cover:

- follow-up support to people with depression. Adherence to anti-depressant medication is similar in patients receiving nurse and GP follow-up[10,11]

- the assessment and management of patients with generalised anxiety, phobias, and panic attacks[12]

- screening of mothers post-natally and providing non-directive counselling, which leads to significant improvements in the mental health of mothers.[13]

The UK Department of Health therefore took the further step of funding a national primary care nurse facilitator to take a national lead in mental health education for primary care nurses and facilitators. This has now evolved into two ongoing initiatives: one a self-financing national education centre for primary care nurses that works in close partnership with the educational centre for general practice, the other a mental health facilitator who, working with the national primary care facilitation programme, continues to provide support and education to the network of facilitators.

Facilitation studies

The Department of Health funded a number of developmental studies in primary care. One used an external nurse (health visitor) facilitator working with six inner city general practices to help GPs and their staff improve the early detection and prompt treatment of depression. Another used a practice nurse, also previously without mental health training, to take a mental health lead within the practice and to support her colleagues, and a third developed a depression audit package for primary care.[14,15]

The experience gained in these pilots was made widely available through the primary mental health toolkit, which contains tools designed by the project teams for the assessment and management of common mental disorders.[16]

Another important approach has been to encourage grass roots primary care practitioners to share their ideas and projects with each other. The Department of Health funded conferences about innovations in primary care mental health, leading to the development of a continuing database and network of innovations which is now sited at the Sainsbury Centre for Mental Health.

Use of good practice guidelines

These have proved a useful way of improving practice. A wide variety are currently available, including the GP toolkit derived from the developmental projects described above, and the WHO ICD-10* guidelines, which are being adapted for the UK and have been piloted in several sites.

Workplace

The principal issues in the workplace are similar to those in primary care; there is a high prevalence of depression and anxiety, a substantial proportion of which is undetected hidden morbidity, and that which is recognized is not always managed optimally and is one of the top three causes of sickness absence and the second most common cause of absences longer than 21 days. For a number of years therefore the Department of Health stimulated a programme of action, including:

- the establishment and leadership of an inter-agency group to co-ordinate activities in the workplace

- co-sponsored national conferences on mental health in the workplace[17,18]

- conducting a survey with the Confederation for British Industry (CBI) on the prevalence of mental health policies in companies

- a guide to employers to encourage the development of workplace health policies which include mental health, encouraging employers to value the mental health of their workforce, promote understanding of mental health issues and problems, reduce stigma, reduce workplace stress, improve detection and management of illness, including suicidal risk, and improve rehabilitation back to work[19]

- funding a fellow in occupational health to take a lead in improving the knowledge and understanding of occupational health teams about depression and other mental health issues—mental health topics were included for the first time in the professional exams for occupational physicians

- the UK Health and Safety Executive (HSE) has greatly expanded its work on stress as an occupational hazard, and has produced materials for employers giving advice on reducing workplace stress and improving support to employees—the first prosecution under the health and safety act for stress-related illness provided added impetus to the campaign

- action in the National Health Service included Department of Health funding of a stress fellowship in general practice, production by the Health Education Authority (now Health Development Agency) of an organizational stress audit package for NHS employers/employees, and an NHS research and development strategy which commissioned a number of studies on mental health in the NHS workforce.

Prisons

The recent prison survey[20] has demonstrated the high rates of depression in prisoners. Neurotic disorders (mostly depression and mixed anxiety depression) were found in 58% and 75% of male and female remand prisoners respectively and in 39% and 62% of male and female sentenced prisoners.

The policy of the government is to link more closely together the prison service health care providers and the NHS. Local health authorities will now be responsible for helping prison governors to commission and carry out a health care needs assessment of their prison. The Department of Health has provided funding to adapt the WHO ICD-10 guidelines for prisons.

Suicide prevention

Following publication of the Health of the Nation Strategy in 1992,[21] the overall suicide rate has fallen by 11.7% in five years when it was only expected to fall by 7% in ten years if previous trends had continued. The overall suicide prevention strategy has included:

- education of health and social care professionals about suicidal risk
- supporting high-risk groups (people with severe mental illness especially depression and co-morbid depression, those committing deliberate self harm, certain occupational groups such as doctors, vets, farmers, pharmacists, and nurses)
- consideration of methods of reducing access to the means of suicide
- development of primary and secondary care services
- research and audit of all suicides to feedback the lessons for prevention into future practice
- working with the media to encourage responsible reporting which does not glamorize nor report the method
- the National Confidential Enquiry into suicides and homicides by people with a mental illness[22] began collecting information on suicide in 1993. It has provided valuable insights into suicide, including the need for clarity of responsibilities, multi-disciplinary co-operation, communication, treatment compliance, risk-assessment skills, adequate staff numbers, audit programmes to maintain clinical skills, quality of patients' living environment, integration between the voluntary and statutory services, and risk associated with change in care regimens.

Conclusions

As the burden of infectious and acute disease has receded, the relative public health importance of chronic conditions is increasing. Mental conditions, and especially depression, impose an enormous burden of avoidable ill-health. Developing a control programme begins by recognizing that specialist health care alone cannot hope to deal with the problems faced. A comprehensive public health programme is needed, based on evidence, setting realistic objectives and targets. Action is needed in many sectors, including workplaces and prisons, as well as in health services. As ever, winning public and political support for such a strategy is important, and epidemiological data can help to achieve a shared set of 'facts' about the public health challenge. Repeating such surveys can also allow progression to be monitored and the programme to be evaluated, and such a repeat of the psychiatric surveys in England and Wales is currently under way.

References

1. Murray C and Lopez AD (1996). *The global burden of disease.* Harvard University/WHO, Boston, MA.

2. Üstün TB and Sartorius N (1995). The background and rationale of the WHO collaborative study on psychological problems in general health care. In *Mental illness in general health care*, (ed. TB Üstün and N Sartorius). Wiley, Chichester.

3. Mann AH, Jenkins R, and Belsey E (1981). The twelve month outcome of patients with neurotic illness in general practice. *Psychological Medicine*, **11**, 535–50.

4. Jenkins R, Bebbington P, Brugha TS, Farrell M, Lewis G, and Meltzer H (1998). British psychiatric morbidity survey. *Brit J Psychiatry*, **173**, 4–7.

5. Lloyd K, Jenkins R, and Mann AH (1996). The long-term outcome of patients with neurotic illness in general practice. *BMJ*, **313**, 26–8.

6. Jenkins R (1985). Minor psychiatric morbidity in civil servants and its contribution to sickness absence. *Brit J Ind Med*, **42**, 147–54.

7. Jenkins R (1985). Minor psychiatric morbidity and labour turnover. *Brit J Ind Med*, **42**, 534–9.

8. World Health Organization (1981). *Development indicators for monitoring progress towards health for all by the year 2000*. WHO, Geneva.

9. OPCS (ONS) (1985). *OPCS Surveys of psychiatric morbidity in Great Britain*, Reports nos. 1–8. The Stationery Office, London.

10. Wilkinson G, Allen P, Marshall E, Walker J, Browne W, and Mann AH (1993). The role of the practice nurse in the management of depression in general practice: treatment adherence to antidepressant medication. *Psychological Medicine*, **23**(1), 229–37.

11. Mann AH, Blizard R, Murray J, Smith JA, Botega N, Macdonald E, and Wilkinson G (1998). An evaluation of practice nurses working with general practitioners to treat people with depression. *Brit J Gen Pract*, **48**, 875–9.

12. Marks I (1985). Controlled trial of psychiatric nurse therapists in primary care. *BMJ*, **290**, 1181–4.

13. Holden JM, Sagovsky R, and Cox J (1989). Counselling in a general practice setting: controlled study of health visitor intervention in treatment of post natal depression. *BMJ*, **298**, 223–6.

14. Jenkins R (1992). Developments in the primary care of mental illness: a forward look. *Int Rev Psychiatry*, **4**, 237–42.

15. Reynolds K (1998). The role of the practice nurse in identifying and managing depression and liaising with voluntary groups. In *Preventing mental illness: mental health promotion in primary care*, (ed. R Jenkins and TB Üstün). Wiley, Chichester.

16. Armstrong E (1997). *The primary mental health care toolkit*. Royal College of General Practitioners, London.

17. Jenkins R and Coney N (1992). *Promoting mental health at work*. HMSO, London.

18. Jenkins R and Warman D (1993). *Developing mental health policies in the workplace*. HMSO, London.

19. UK Department of Health (1996). *ABC of mental health in the workplace*. HMSO, London.

20. Singleton N, Meltzer H, Gatward R, Coid J, Deasy D/Office for National Statistics (1998). *Psychiatric morbidity among prisoners in England and Wales*. The Stationery Office, London.

21. UK Department of Health (1992). *The Health of the Nation: a strategy for health in England*. Cm. 1986. HMSO, London.

22. UK Department of Health (1999). *Safer services: the national confidential inquiry into suicide and homicide by people with mental illness*. Department of Health, London.

9.9 **Injury prevention**

Joan Ozanne-Smith

Introduction

'Injuries are a large, and neglected, health problem in all regions'.[1]

Injury is a leading cause of premature mortality and substantial morbidity and disability world-wide. Globally, it is increasingly the major cause of death in children, adolescents, and young adults, in developing countries as well as developed countries.

Injury provides an ideal example to encapsulate the public health process from problem definition through to translating evidence into practice and the achievement of population health gains.

Objectives

By reading this chapter you will gain knowledge of the nature and dimensions of injury as a public health problem. In particular you will grasp its preventability by inter-sectoral action. Through knowledge of the principles and practice of injury prevention and proven counter measures and implementation strategies, you will be able to systematically implement, or advise on, interventions. You will also have the basis to measure whether or not the interventions have been successful.

Definition

Injury is damage to the body caused by (acute) exchanges with environmental energy that are beyond the body's resilience. The energy may be mechanical, thermal, electrical, ionizing radiation, or chemical (poisoning, asphyxiation). This definition applies to both unintentional and intentional injuries.

The word '*injury*' should be distinguished from the word '*accident*'. The use of the word 'accident' implies inevitability; this risks obscuring the preventable element of most accidents. For this reason many people prefer the use of the word 'injury'.

Injuries as an important public health issue

Injury is a threat to health in every country in the world and is currently responsible for 7% of world mortality. According to WHO predictions, this proportion is expected to rise by the year 2020.[1] In developed countries, injury is the leading cause of premature death before 75 years. The health care costs for injury are among the highest of all diseases, as is the loss of productivity, due to the youth of the age-group primarily affected.

The major causes of injury vary between countries, level of industrialization, age-group and by severity. In all countries, common causes of injury death are transportation, suicide, drowning (among young children), falls (among the elderly), and work-related, particularly in developing countries (see Table 9.9.1). More than 50% of injuries involve a consumer product.

Table 9.9.1 An example of classification of injuries by major cause.

Fatal
Suicide
Motor vehicle accidents
Falls
Homicide
Drowning
Hospitalized
Falls – same level
Falls – different level
Motor vehicle accidents
Self-inflicted
Interpersonal violence

Injury patterns are strongly influenced by exposure and other risk factors such as gender, age, developmental stage (children, older persons), socio-economic status, indigenous populations, and alcohol. Males are at higher risk of injury from most causes, largely due to greater exposure, which may be associated with risk-taking behaviours. Females are over-represented in older persons' falls, pharmaceutical overdose, and some sports and recreational injuries e.g. horse-riding.

Because of the high rates and lifetime costs of moderate to severe injuries, the cost is greatest for hospitalized injuries. This is exemplified by data from the state of Victoria, Australia shown in Figure 9.9.1.[2]

Understanding the issue

Injury typically results from a chain of events. Systematic review of pre-event, event, and post-event factors relating to the host, products, or activities and the environment potentially identifies both risk factors and intervention points. Intervention anywhere along this chain of events may prevent the injury.

This concept was developed as a simple matrix by Haddon in the 1960s[3] to describe motor vehicle crashes and has been modified for broader application (Figure 9.9.2). Application of the matrix to any injury problem provides categorisation of potentially modifiable risk factors and an overview of solutions.

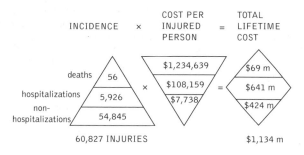

Figure 9.9.1 Cost of injury.
(Reprinted with permission from Monash University Accident Research Centre.[2])

	Factors		
Phases	Host	Products or activities	Environment
Pre-event			
Event			
Post-event			

Figure 9.9.2 Haddon's matrix.

Unlike many other health problems, preventive action is required in sectors other than the health sector. It is, therefore, necessary to describe the problem in terms appropriate to the responsible sector, such as settings (home, workplace, transport), activities (sport, leisure, work), injuries by body region (head injuries, eye injuries, hip fractures), products (motor vehicles, bicycles, stairs, lawnmowers, tractors, dogs, firearms, baby-walkers, pharmaceuticals).

Criteria to apply to the selection of interventions

Good evidence exists for many countermeasures and implementation strategies. The mix of strategies will depend on the particular issue, the scale and scope of the intervention, the possibility for collaboration with other key stakeholders, and other criteria listed below. A schema derived from the work of a WHO *ad hoc* working party conceptualizes injury within a 'burden box' (Figure 9.9.3).[4] Clearly, there are important considerations about where effort should be allocated. New knowledge continues to evolve and recent

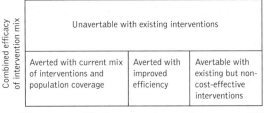

Figure 9.9.3 The burden box.
(Adapted from WHO Ad Hoc Committee on health research to future options.[4])

literature reviews and strategic plans should be accessed on particular issues.

Some of the challenges in injury prevention relate to influencing the factors affecting implementation such as:

- regulation
- enforcement
- industry codes to support voluntary standards
- organizational change
- market demand
- community awareness.

Intervention should be sustainable e.g. by institutionalization or regulation, and generalizable. Safety has been shown to be a selling point for motor vehicles and for sports participation. The application of incentives/disincentives (subsidies, penalties) may stimulate or enforce compliance.

Examples of successes and failures

Substantial success in injury prevention has occurred in road safety and much is transferable to other sectors. Successful interventions can be classified as:

- design/environmental (seat belts, airbags, dual highways, child-resistant packaging, pool fences, automatic cut-off switches on machinery, hip protectors, protective helmets, tractor roll-over protection, smoke alarms, protective eyewear)
- organizational (modified rules in junior sports, work practices to avoid fatigue, random breath testing for alcohol)
- behavioural (road-crossing skills, swimming competence, use of protective equipment).

Box 9.9.1 **Case study: carbon monoxide suicide from car exhausts**

Car exhaust gassing is a major method of suicide in many highly motorized countries, accounting for almost 20% of suicides in Australia in 1998. The epidemiology of car exhaust gas suicide has been published in a limited way for several countries since the 1980s.[5–9]

This method of suicide usually involves the application of a hose to the exhaust pipe of an idling vehicle, leading into the sealed-off vehicle cabin. This problem has continued in Australia, despite the implementation of catalytic converters to convert highly toxic carbon monoxide (CO) gas emissions to carbon dioxide and increasingly stringent regulation of the allowable parts per million of CO in exhaust gases.

Design changes to motor vehicles have been developed based on two concepts. A tailpipe design, which prevents the fitting of a hose to the exhaust system, has been published to make the design principles freely available to vehicle and after market parts manufacturers. Estimates of the benefits versus costs reveal that if such a device were fitted, which prevented 25–50% of these suicides, the cost could be recovered in two to four years.[10]

A second design intervention is based on the monitoring of vehicle cabin gasses by a sensor device linked to the engine management system of the vehicle. Levels of CO and CO_2 above, or O_2 below, acceptable safe levels trigger an alarm followed by automatic cut-off of the engine. Since recent literature suggests a link between levels of cabin gases and fatigue, this mechanism may have added benefits.

Neither of these designs has yet been implemented. It would take an estimated eight years in Australia for 100% of vehicles to be fitted with new design exhaust pipes and 11 years for cabin gas sensors to be fitted in 50% of vehicles.[11]

Steps for implementation:

- documenting the problem
- clarifying the evidence-based solutions
- setting clear goals, objectives, and performance indicators
- undertaking detailed benefits/cost estimates
- establishing a co-ordinating group of allies among key stakeholders (although motives for achieving the desired outcome may differ e.g. sales of an anti-fatigue or unhealthy air product)

- providing data and intervention information, including costs and benefits, to decision makers, partners, advocates
- ensuring ownership of the problem and solutions by stakeholders
- directly targeting design solutions to the motor vehicle industry
- opportunistic letters to key politicians
- identifying incentives and barriers to implementation
- government regulation of new motor vehicle design to prevent the possibility of unsafe cabin gas levels (performance standards)
- regulation of the fitting of the suicide-resistant tailpipe design on tailpipe replacement in existing motor vehicles—regulation is necessary, since such a development is unlikely to be driven by voluntary standards or the market place
- persistence; provision of public evidence of progress or lack of progress
- publication of results in the peer-reviewed literature.

Future strategies

Attention to alternative solutions, such as:

- further reductions in acceptable parts per million of CO, and regulating for the warming-up and idle mode of the motor
- influencing fleet owners to purchase protected vehicles
- further investigation of potential anti-fatigue and unhealthy air effects of cabin gas monitoring and alerting systems
- coroner's recommendations to industry and government following deaths by this means
- litigation by relatives of suicide victims
- further engagement of decision makers by processes such as a letter campaign following each death by this means.

Evaluation

Impact (intermediate effect) and outcome evaluation are achievable in injury prevention, since substantial health and economic gains are possible in the relatively short term. Injury data is available in most countries to measure outcomes at least for moderate and severe injuries. Impact measures are often available from secondary data sources; otherwise, observational studies or surveys should be conducted.

1. Process evaluation—quantified description of how impacts and outcomes are achieved.
2. Impact measures:
   - changes to motor vehicle design rules
   - uptake of the new, safe designs by manufacturers

- sales figures of the new, safe designs
- observational studies of these safer design features in motor vehicles.

3. Outcome measures:
   - changes to suicide and hospital admission rates from this method
   - any proportional shift to other methods of suicide or suicide attempt.

4. Cost–benefit analysis for deaths prevented (see chapter 2.6).

Barriers to implementation

Plenty of barriers exist in all public health implementation. With an injury strategy, the most common are:

- lack of jurisdictional ownership (not a transport problem)
- cost to manufacturers to tool-up to new designs although there may be no direct gains for this sector
- additional minor cost to purchase or repair price of vehicle
- ethical barriers to publicizing this issue, since publicity may inadvertently advertise this method of suicide.

Lessons learned

Clear problem definition, together with the identification of practical and cost-effective solutions, does not necessarily translate to practice. Implementation requires long-term strategies, typically over many years. Other injury prevention examples of lengthy implementation processes include seat belts, air bags, pool fences, smoke alarms, bicycle helmets, hot-tap water temperature controls, and many others.

This case study demonstrates the public health principles of problem definition, targeted intervention strategies, and evaluation.

Conclusion

Injuries cause a significant amount of preventable morbidity and mortality in every society in the world. With the application of public health principles and the co-operation of the relevant sectors, injury prevention presents great opportunities for success in the coming century.

Further resources

Barss P, Smith GS, Baker SP, and Mohan D (1998). *Injury prevention—an international perspective: epidemiology, surveillance, and policy.* Oxford University Press, Oxford.

Chapman S and Lupton D (1994). *The fight for public health: principles and practice of media advocacy.* BMJ Publishing Group, London.

Haddon W (1995). Energy damage and the 10 countermeasure strategies. *Injury Prevention*, **1**, 40–4.

Ozanne-Smith J and Williams F (ed.) (1995). *Injury research and prevention: a text*. Monash University Accident Research Centre, Clayton, Australia.

Robertson LS (1998). *Injury epidemiology—research and control strategies*. Oxford University Press, Oxford.

References

1. Murray C and Lopez A (1996). *The global burden of disease*, (Summary). Harvard School of Public Health, Boston MA.

2. Watson W and Ozanne-Smith J (1997). *The cost of injury to Victoria*. Monash University Accident Research Centre Report No. 124. Monash University, Clayton, Australia.

3. Robertson L (1983). *Injuries causes, control strategies and public policy*. Lexington, Massachusetts.

4. World Health Organization (1996). *Investing in health research and development*. Report of the Ad Hoc Committee on health research relating to future intervention options. WHO, Geneva.

5. Clarke R and Lester D (1987). Toxicity of car exhausts and opportunity for suicide: comparison between Britain and the USA. *JECH*, **41**, 114–20.

6. Lester D and Abe K (1989). Car availability, exhaust toxicity and suicide. *Annals of Clinical Psychiatry*, **1**, 247–50.

7. Ostrom M, Thorsen J, and Eriksson A (1996). Carbon monoxide—suicide from car exhausts. *Soc Sci Med*, **42(3)**, 447–51.

8. Routley V (1998). *Motor vehicle exhaust gassing suicides in Australia: epidemiology and prevention*. Monash University Accident Research Centre Report No. 139. Monash University, Clayton, Australia.

9. Thielade P, Steenberg J, Kofoed P, Schrann J, and Morgen C (May 1998). *Automobile exhaust as a suicide means: experience in a Danish population*. Fourth World Conference on Injury Prevention and Control, Amsterdam.

10. Routley V (1994). Non-traffic motor vehicle related injuries. *Hazard* edition 20, Victorian Injury Surveillance System, Monash University Accident Research Centre, Monash University, Clayton, Australia.

11. Routley VH and Ozanne-Smith J (1998). The impact of catalytic converters on motor vehicle exhaust gas suicides. *Med J Australia*, **168(2)**, 65–7.

Classics in public health practice

We offer a list of about 100 classic references in public health. It is an unsystematic collection from the editors' and authors' collections of references over the last 25 years. Some of these 'classics' were drawn from a project entitled 'Classics in Public Health: a database of seminal articles and books in public health selected by public health professionals in the Anglia and Oxford region', run in 1995 by the Healthcare Libraries Unit of Oxford University, UK. Send us your favourites for inclusion in the next edition on the evaluation card.

RM, DP, CSG

Acheson D (1988). *Public health in England*. HMSO, London.

Beaglehole R, Bonita R (1997). *Public health at the crossroads*. Cambridge University Press, Cambridge.

Berwick DM (1991). Controlling variation in health care: a consultation from Walter Shewhart. *Medical Care*, 29(12), 1212–25.

Berwick DM, Leape LL (1999). Reducing errors in medicine. *BMJ*, **319**, 136–7.

Beveridge W (1942). *Social insurance and allied services*. HMSO, London.

Black N (1992). Research, audit, and education. *BMJ*, **304**, 698–700.

Brook RH, Ware JE Jr, Rogers WH, et al. (1983). Does free care improve adults' health? Results from a randomized controlled trial. *N Engl J Med*, **309**, 1426–34.

Caldwell J (1986). Routes to low mortality in poor countries. In: *Population and development review 12*. Center for Population Studies of the Population Council, New York.

Davis DA, Thomson MA, Oxman AD, Haynes RB (1982). Evidence for the effectiveness of CME. A review of 50 randomized controlled trials. *JAMA*, 268(9), 1111–7.

Defoe D (1991). A journal of the plague year. (First published 1722). Penguin, Harmondsworth.

Doll R, Peto R (1976). Mortality in relation to smoking: 20 years' observations on male British doctors. *BMJ*, 2(6051), 1525–36.

Doyal L (1995). Rights and equity: moral quality in healthcare rationing. *Quality in Health Care*, **4**, 273–83.

Dubois RW, Brook RH (1998). Preventable deaths: who, how often, and why?. RAND Corporation, Los Angeles, California. *Annals of Internal Medicine*, 109(7), 582–9.

Eddy DM (1990). Clinical decision making: from theory to practice. Designing a practice policy. Standards, guidelines, and options. *JAMA*, **263**, 3077–84.

Eddy DM (1990). Clinical decision making: from theory to practice. Resolving conflicts in practice policies. *JAMA*, **264**, 389–91.

Eddy DM (1991). What care is 'essential'? What services are 'basic'? *JAMA*, **265**, 782, 786–8.

Eddy DM (1994). Principles for making difficult decisions in difficult times. *JAMA*, **271**, 1792–8.

Editorial (1994). Population health looking upstream. *Lancet*, **343**, 429–30.

Egolf B, Lasker J, Wolf S, Potvin L. (1992). The Roseto effect: a 50-year comparison of mortality rates. *Am J Pub Health*, **82**, 1089–92.

Enkin M, Keirse MJN, Chalmers I (1989). A guide to effective care in pregnancy and childbirth. Oxford University Press, Oxford.

Florey CD (1993). Sample size for beginners. *BMJ*, 306(6886), 1181–4.

Freiman JA, Chalmers TC, Smith H Jr, Kuebler RR (1978). The importance of beta, the type II error and sample size in the design and interpretation of the randomized control trial. Survey of 71 'negative' trials. *N Engl J Med*, 299(13), 690–4.

Gray JAM (1997) *Evidence-based healthcare - how to make health policy and management decisions*. Churchill Livingstone, London.

Greco PJ, Eisenberg JM (1993). Changing physicians' practices. University of Pennsylvania School of Medicine, Philadelphia 19104. *N Engl J Med*, 329(17), 1271–3.

Greenhalgh T (1997). *How to read a paper - the basics of evidence based medicine*. BMJ Books, London.

Ham C, Hunter DJ, Robinson R (1995). Evidence based policy making. *BMJ*, **310**, 71–2.

Hurwitz B (1999). Legal and political considerations of clinical practice guidelines. *BMJ*, **318**, 661–4.

Khaw K (1994). Genetics and environment: Geoffrey Rose revisited. *Lancet*, **343**, 838–9.

King M (1990). Health is a sustainable state. *Lancet*, **336**, 664–7.

Le Grand J (1993). Can we afford the welfare state? *BMJ*, **307**, 1018–9.

Logie D (1992). The great exterminator of children. *BMJ*, **304**, 1423–6.

Lomas J (1993). Making clinical policy explicit. Legislative policy making and lessons for developing practice guidelines. *International Journal of Technology Assessment in Health Care*, 9(1), 11–25.

Lomas J, Sisk JE, Stocking B (1993). From evidence to practice in the United States, the United Kingdom, and Canada. *Milbank Quarterly*, **71**, 405–10.

Mant D, Fowler G (1990). Mass screening: theory and ethics. *BMJ*, 300(6729), 916–8.

Mathers N, Hodgkin P (1989). The gatekeeper and the wizard: a fairy tale. *BMJ*, **298**, 172–4.

Metz CE (1978). Basic principles of ROC analysis. *Seminars in Nuclear Medicine*, 8(4), 283–98.

Mulley AG, Eagle KA (1988). What is inappropriate care?. *JAMA*, **260**, 540–1.

Mulley AG, Mendoza G, Rockefeller R, Staker L (1996). Involving patients in medical decision making. *Quality Connection*, **5**, 5–7.

Murray C, Lopez AD (1997). Mortality by cause for eight regions of the world: Global Burden of Disease Study. *Lancet*, **349**, 1269–76.

Neuhauser D, Lweicki AM (1975). What do we gain from the sixth stool guaiac?. *N Engl J Med*, 293(5), 226–8.

Oxman AD, Thomson MA, Davis DA, Haynes RB (1995). No magic bullets: a systematic review of 102 trials of interventions to improve professional practice. *Can Med Assoc J*, **153**, 1423–31.

Palmer CR (1993). Probability of recurrence of extreme data: an aid to decision-making. *Lancet*, 342(8875), 845–7.

Phelps CE (1993). The methodologic foundations of studies of the appropriateness of medical care. *N Engl J Med*, 329(17), 1241–5.

Rennie D Flanagin A (1992). Publication bias the triumph of hope over experience. *JAMA*, 267(3), 411–2.

Rose G (1985). Sick individuals and sick populations. *International Journal of Epidemiology*, 14(1), 32–8.

Rose G (1986). Epidemiology and health care planning: their place in medical education. *J R Soc Med*, **79**, 631–3.

Rose G (1990). The population mean predicts the number of deviant individuals. *BMJ*, **301**, 1031–4.

Rosen R (1993). *A history of public health*. Johns Hopkins, Baltimore MA.

Rothman KJ, Greenland S (1998). *Modern epidemiology* (2nd edn). Lippincott-Raven, Philadelphia.

Schön DA (1983). *The reflective practitioner: how professionals think in action*. Temple Smith, London.

Sackett DL, Haynes RB, Guyatt G, Tugwell P (1991). *Clinical epidemiology; a basic science for clinical medicine*. (2nd edn). Little and Brown, Boston, MA.

Smith AFM (1996). Mad cows and ecstasy: chance and choice in an evidence-based society. *J R Statist Soc*, **159**, 367–83.

Smith R (1991). Where is the wisdom? (editorial). *BMJ*, **303**, 798–9.

Smith R (1994). Towards a knowledge based health service. *BMJ*, **309**, 217–8.

Sox H, Blatt MA, Higgins MC, Marton KI (1998). *Medical decision making*. Butterworths, London.

Stevens A, Gabbay J (1991). Needs assessment needs assessment. *Health Trends*, 23(1), 20–3.

Tarlov AR, Ware JE Jr, Greenfield S, Nelson EC, Perrin E, Zubkoff M (1989). The medical outcomes study. An application of methods for monitoring the results of medical care. *JAMA*, 262(7), 925–30.

Timmins N (1996). *The five giants - a biography of the welfare state*. Fontana Press, London.

Tufte E (1983). *Visual display of quantitative information*. Graphics Press, Connecticut.

Tufte E (1990). *Envisioning information*. Graphics Press, Connecticut.

Tufte E (1997). *Visual explanations*. Graphics Press, Connecticut.

West R (1987). High death rates: more deaths or earlier deaths? *J R Coll Physicians Lond*, **21**, 73–6.

White K, Connolly J (1992). *The medical school's mission and the population's health: medical education in Canada, the United Kingdom, the United States, and Australia*. Springer-Verlag, New York.

White K (1994). *Healing the schism: epidemiology, medicine, and the public's health*. Springer-Verlag, New York.

Sources of reference

This list is highly selective, and, due to the highly volatile nature of the internet (in sections 1–10), highly susceptible to change. Send us your favourites for inclusion in the next edition on the evaluation card.

DP, CSG, CS-J, RM, AB

1. Research and evidence

Bandolier www.jr2.ox.ac.uk/Bandolier
Centre for Evidence Based Medicine www.cebm.jr2.ox.ac.uk
Clinical Prevention cait.cpmc.columbia.edu/texts/gcps
Cochrane hiru.mcmaster.ca/cochrane/default.htm
Effective Care Bulletins www.york.ac.uk/inst/crd
Netting the Evidence www.shef.ac.uk/~scharr/ir/netting.html
PubMed www.ncbi.nlm.nih.gov/Pubmed/
UK National Research Reg www.doh.gov.uk/research/nrr.htm
Consumers in Research www.hfht.org/ConsumersinNHSResearch
The UK National Electronic Library for Health www.NELH.nhs.uk

2. Clinical guidelines

AHCPR www.guideline.gov
Canadian www.cma.ca/cpgs
e-guidelines www.eguidelines.co.uk
Scottish www.sign.ac.uk
New Zealand www.nzgg.org.nz/index.htm
North of England Guidelines www.ncl.ac.uk/~ncenthsr/publicn/publicn. htm

3. Inequalities

UK Department of Health www.doh.gov.uk/inequalities
Acheson on Inequalities www.official-documents.co.uk/document/doh/ih/ih.htm
UK Health Action Zones www.haznet.org.uk

4. Professional development in public health practice

www.public-health.com
www.ukph.org

5. Determinants of health

www.who.dk/document/e59555.pdf

6. Health development

UK Health Development Agency www.hda-online.org.uk

7. Leadership in public health

www.RIPHH.org.uk
www.APHA.org
www.cphl.org
www.pha2000.org

8. Priority setting

www.bham.ac.uk/HSMC/publicns/priority.doc

9. Public health in the media

BBC www.bbc.co.uk news health site news.bbc.co.uk/hi/english/health/default.stm
Quackwatch www.quackwatch.com/index.html

10. Other agencies and organizations

UK National Institute for Clinical Excellence (NICE) www.nice.org.uk
Commission for Health Improvement www.chi.nhs.uk
UK Public Health Observatories www.pho.org.uk
Australasian Faculty of Public Health Medicine www.racp.edu
UK Faculty of Public Health Medicine www.fphm.org.uk
Public Health Association of Australia www.phaa.net.edu
UKPHA www.ukpha.org.uk

A gateway to many of the institutions, agencies and organizations in the Australian health field www.prometheus.com

11. Public health agencies in the UK

11.1. National Poisons Information Service

The National Poisons Information Service (NPIS) comprises six Poisons Centres (Belfast, Birmingham, Cardiff, Edinburgh, London and Newcastle). They provide a year-round, 24-hour a day service for health care staff on the clinical aspects of patients who may have been poisoned.

The NPIS can be contacted on 0870 600 6266. Enquiries are routed to the nearest regional unit.

11.2. The National Focus for Work on Response to Chemical Incidents

The National Focus (www.natfocus.uwic.ac.uk) runs a surveillance service of chemical incidents throughout England and Wales. It also provides a link between the RSPUs and government, and liaises between RSPUs in incidents involving more than one region.

The National Focus can be contacted on 029 2041 6388 or by e-mail at nfocus@uwic.ac.uk

Regional Service Provider Units for Chemical Incidents (RSPUs) are organizations which provide support to subscribing Health Authorities in responding to and managing chemical incidents. They provide a 24-hour a day, 365 days a year toxicological, environmental, epidemiological and chemical emergency management service. There are five RSPUs covering the UK. For example, the RSPU for the West Midlands region is The Chemical Hazards Management and Research Centre (CHMRC) based at the University of Birmingham (www.ad.bham.ac.uk/chmrc). The CHMRC can be contacted via its hotline on 020 7394 5112.

11.3. UK Environment Agency

The Environment Agency (www.environment-agency.gov.uk/) is responsible for all environmental issues in the UK. They are responsible for the implementation of Integrated Pollution Prevention Control (IPPC) which involves protecting public health from the effects of industrial pollution. They are also responsible, in conjunction with the Health and Safety Executive (HSE), for implementing the emergency planning legislation for major industrial processes.

The Environment Agency runs Regional Control Centres to deal with environmental pollution incidents. These can be contacted via the Environment Agency's hotline (0800 80 70 60). They also operate 'Floodline' (0845 988 1188) to handle enquiries about problems caused by flooding. General enquiries can be made by calling 0845 133111.

11.4. UK Health and Safety Executive

Responsible for implementation of health and safety legislation in most major activities and businesses. HSE is involved in emergency planning for industrial complexes and has access to considerable expertise in the fields of toxicology and emergency planning

11.5. Drinking Water Inspectorate

The Drinking Water Inspectorate (www.dwi.detr.gov.uk) ensures that the water companies in England and Wales supply water that is safe to drink and meets the standards set in the Water Quality Regulations.

They also investigate complaints from consumers, and incidents that affect or could affect drinking water quality.

They can be contacted on 020 7944 5956 or by e-mail at: dwi_enquiries@detr.gov.uk

11.6. UK Food Standards Agency (FSA)

The Food Standards Agency (www.foodstandards.gov.uk) provides advice and information to the public and to the government on food safety, in addition to enforcement and monitoring of food standards.

They can be contacted on 020 7270 8960 (out of hours emergencies) or by e-mail at helpline@foodstandards.gsi.gov.uk.

11.7. Environmental Health Departments (EHDs)

EHDs have responsibility for a range of issues that impact upon public health including air, water, food, and housing quality. They also have an important role in emergency situations. Each EHD will have its own emergency contact arrangements with which the Health Authority should be familiar.

11.8. National Chemical Emergency Centre (NCEC)

The National Chemical Emergency Centre (www.the-ncec.com) operates a national 24-hour chemical incident response centre, supported by the UK Department of The Environment Transport and the Regions (DETR) (now Department of Transport, Local Government and the Regions (DTLR)) and the Chemical Industries Association (CIA). The service is by subscription only.

The NCEC can be contacted on 01235 463060 or by e-mail at ncec@aeat.co.uk

11.9. The Water Research Centre

The Water Research Centre (www.wrcplc.co.uk) provides consultancy on water and waste management issues.

They can be contacted on 01793 865000 or 01491 571531 and by e-mail at solutions@wrcplc.co.uk

11.10. The UK Public Health Laboratory Service (PHLS)

The Public Health Laboratory Service (www.phls.co.uk) provides advice and support for the effective management of outbreaks of communicable diseases. They also provide advice on policy development, and the application of new technologies and methods.

Contact details are available from the PHLS website at www.phls.co.uk/whoweare/directory/index.htm

The PHLS also runs the **Communicable Disease Surveillance Centre (CDSC)**. This was established in 1977 to undertake national surveillance of communicable disease and to provide epidemiological assistance and co-ordination in the investigation and control of infection in England and Wales.

12. Agencies outside the United Kingdom

12.1. United States Environmental Protection Agency (USEPA) (USA)

The USEPA (www.epa.gov) is responsible for all environmental issues in the USA. Its website provides databases, newsletters, and other information concerning environmental protection.

12.2. Centers for Disease Control and Prevention (CDC) (USA)

The Centers for Disease Control and Prevention (www.cdc.gov) provides information on a number of areas in public health, such as infectious disease, environmental health, and health promotion, and serves as the national focus for public health issues in the United States.

12.3. Agency for Toxic Substances and Disease Registry (ATSDR) (USA)

The ATSDR (www.atsdr.cdc.gov) is concerned with the public health implications of hazardous substances. The website provides a number of services including databases of hazardous chemicals and toxicity standards.

12.4. The Chemical Safety and Hazard Investigation Board (USA)

The Chemical Safety and Hazard Investigation Board (chemsafety.gov) is an independent federal agency that investigates chemical incidents and provides information on the prevention of such incidents. This agency is also mandated to provide assistance to agencies outside the USA.

The Board can be contacted at info@csb.gov.

12.5. The National Institute for Occupational Safety and Health (NIOSH) (USA)

NIOSH (www.cdc.gov/niosh) is responsible for conducting research and making recommendations for the prevention of work-related disease and injury. A number of databases related to occupational health and safety, including occupational standards for chemicals, are available from their website.

12.6. The Food and Drug Administration (FDA) (USA)

The FDA (www.fda.gov) provides information on a number of subjects ranging from food and drug safety and disease, to devices that emit radiation (cellular phones, etc.).

13. Other sites relating to food and environmental health

13.1. UK Sites

BSE Inquiry www.bse.org.uk
Eurosurveillance Weekly www.eurosurv.org
Institute of Food Science and Technology (IFST) www.easynet.co.uk/ifst
Ministry of Agriculture, Fisheries and Food www.maff.gov.uk
Food Standards Agency www.foodstandards.gov.uk/index.htm

13.2. Other European Sites

What's New at DG XXIV Consumer Policy, Consumer Health Protection inc. Food Safety europa.eu.int/comm/dg24
Scientific Committee on Food, DG XXIV European Commission europa.eu.int/comm/dg24/health/sc/scf/index_en.html
DG XII Biotechnology, European Commission europa.eu.int/comm/dg12/biotech/biotnew.html
EC Evaluation of Food Control Systems in Member States europa.eu.int/comm/dg24/health/afh/afh08_en.html
European Food Information Council www.eufic.org
European Union www.europa.eu.int
WHO Regional Office for Europe www.who.it/programmes/food_safety.htm

13.3. International Sites

Centre for Nutrition Policy and Promotion www.usda.gov/cnpp
Environmental Protection Agency (EPA) www.epa.gov
Food and Drug Administration (FDA) www.fda.gov/default.htm
United States Department of Health and Human Services www.os.dhhs.gov
United States Department of Agriculture (USDA) www.usda.gov
Australian New Zealand Food Authority (ANZFA) www.health. gov.au/anzfa
Consumers International www.consumersinternational.org
Food and Agriculture Organisation of the United Nations (FAO) www.fao.org
International Food Information Council (IFIC) ificinfo.health.org
Joint FAO/WHO Food Standards Programme (Codex Alimentarius Commission) www.fao.org/waicent/faoinfo/economic/esn/codex/Default.htm
World Health Organization (WHO) www.who.int

14. and finally...

if all else fails, try:
... the Boy Scouts' Public Health Badge Handbook ... (unfortunately, now out of print, but it's very good, if you can find it!)

Abbreviations and glossary

This list aims to standardize some of the more frequently used terms in this book, marked by an asterisk * in the text on their first appearance in a chapter. The glossary is restricted to words or phrases with a technical meaning in the broad field of public health practice. Selected resources follow the list below, including a recommended general dictionary, a guide to usage, and of primary importance, Last's *Dictionary of Epidemiology*. Many terms below are defined at greater length in the latter. While we have intended to provide a sufficient list here, the annotation '(see Last)' indicates either that we have closely followed the *Dictionary of Epidemiology* or that it contains a more elaborate description that may be particularly helpful.

After abbreviations or acronyms, terms that are capitalized also have a glossary entry, appearing in alphabetical order.

AHCPR	Agency for Healthcare Policy and Research, now AHRQ (www.ahrq.gov, accessed 14 May 2001)
AHRQ	Agency for Healthcare Research and Quality (www.ahrq.gov, accessed 14 May 2001)
AIDS	Acquired Immune Deficiency Syndrome
BSE	Bovine Spongiform Encephalopathy
Case-mix	An index of the type of illnesses managed in a health care facility
CDSR	Cochrane Database of Systematic Reviews – part of the Cochrane Library co-ordinated by the International Cochrane Collaboration (see chapter 2.3 and www.cochrane.org, accessed 28 March 2001)
CHD	Coronary heart disease
CHI	see COMMISSION FOR HEALTH IMPROVEMENT
Cinahl	An electronic database (see chapter 2.3)
Clinical Governance	A framework for continuous quality improvement
Clinical Indicators	Measurements of aspects of clinical care related to quality

CME	Continuing medical education
Cochrane Collaboration	The international organization that prepares and disseminates systematic reviews of the effects of health care interventions (www.cochrane.org, accessed 28 March 2001)
Commission for Health Improvement (UK)	A UK body that assures, monitors and helps improve the quality of patient care by undertaking reviews of clinical governance (www.chi.nhs.uk, accessed 2 April 2001)
Co-morbidity	The simultaneous presence of two or more health disorders
Cost-benefit analysis	An analysis in which the economic and social costs of medical care and the benefits of reduced loss of net earnings due to preventing premature death or disability are considered (see Last)
CPD	Continuing Professional Development
CRD	Centre for Reviews and Dissemination, York, UK (www.york.ac.uk/inst/crd, accessed 11 May 2001)
DALY	see DISABILITY-ADJUSTED LIFE YEAR
DARE	Database of Abstracts of Reviews of Effectiveness (see chapter 2.3)
Diagnosis-related group (DRG)	Classification of hospital patients according to diagnosis and intensity of care required, used by insurance carriers to set reimbursement scales (see Last)
Disability	Temporary or long-term reduction of a person's capacity to function (see Last)
Disability-adjusted life year	Measure adopted by the World Bank to estimate the burden of disease by combining premature mortality and disability (see Last)
Dose	The stated quantity of a substance to which an organism is exposed
DRG	see DIAGNOSIS-RELATED GROUP
ECG	Electrocardiogram
EIA	Environmental Impact Assessment
EMBASE	A European electronic database of health related scientific references (see chapter 2.3).

	This database has a significant (~40%) overlap with MEDLINE, but has a more European and pharmacological emphasis
ESD	Ecologically sustainable development
EU	European Union
Evaluation	A process that attempts to determine as systematically and objectively as possible the relevance, effectiveness, and impact of activities in the light of their objectives (see Last)
Evidence-based health care/ medicine/public health	Systematic use of evidence derived from published research and other sources for management and practice
Exposure	A measure of the actual contact with an agent (usually chemical, physical or biological)
Expressed needs	Needs expressed by action e.g. visiting a doctor
FAO	Food and Agriculture Organization (of the United Nations)
Felt needs	What people consider and/or say they need
Focus group	Small, convenient sample of people brought together to discuss a topic or issue with the aim of ascertaining the range and intensity of their views, rather than arriving at a consensus (see Last)
GATT	General Agreement on Tariffs and Trade
GDP	Gross Domestic Product
Goal	A general statement of direction and intent (usually measurable) (see chapter 3.2)
GP	General Practitioner
Handicap	Reduction in a person's capacity to fulfil a social role as a consequence of an impairment or disability, or other circumstances (see Last)
Hazard	The intrinsic capacity of an agent, a condition or a situation to produce an adverse health or environmental effect
Health	The extent to which an individual or a group is able to realize aspirations and satisfy needs, and to change or cope with the environment. Health is a resource for everyday life, not the objective of living; it is a positive concept, emphasizing social and personal resources

	as well as physical capabilities. Your health is related to how much you feel your potential to be a meaningful part of the society in which you find yourself, is adequately realized (see Last)
Healthcare Resource Groups	Classification of patients according to severity and intensity of care required, used by insurance carriers (or equivalent) to compare resource use throughout a health system
Health Impact Assessment	An assessment process to look at the impact on health of Government policies or other actions, completed or projected. (see chapter 1.6)
Health Improvement Programme	(HImP) (UK) an action programme to improve health and health care locally, led by the local Health Authority, and designed to help partnership working
Health outcome	Health status, sometimes related to the effects of health care or other interventions
HeaLY	Healthy life years. A composite indicator that incorporates morbidity and mortality into a single number (see Last)
HIA	see HEALTH IMPACT ASSESSMENT
HImP	see HEALTH IMPROVEMENT PROGRAMME
HRG	see HEALTHCARE RESOURCE GROUPS
IARC	International Agency for Research on Cancer
ICD-9 (CM)	International Classification of Disease, edition 9 (Clinical Modification)
ICD-10	International Classification of Disease, edition 10
IDT	International Development Target
Impairment	A physical or mental defect at the level of a body system or organ. Contrast with Disability and Handicap (see Last)
MEDLINE	An electronic database that provides citations, sometimes including abstracts, from the biomedical literature (beginning 1966)
National Institute for Clinical Excellence (NICE)	Part of the UK National Health Service (NHS) - its role is to provide patients, health professionals and the public with authoritative, robust and reliable guidance on current 'best practice' (www.nice.org.uk, accessed 11 May 2001)

National Service Framework	(UK) National Service Frameworks set national standards and define service models for a specific service or care group, put in place programmes to support implementation and establish performance measures against which progress within an agreed timescale will be measured (www.doh.gov.uk/nsf/, accessed 2 April 2001)
NeLH	(UK) National Electronic Library for Health (www.nelh.nhs.uk, accessed 2 April 2001)
NGO	Non-governmental organization
NHS	National Health Service
NICE	see NATIONAL INSTITUTE FOR CLINICAL EXCELLENCE
Normative needs	Needs as defined by a health professional
OECD	Organization for Economic Cooperation and Development
PCG	Primary Care Group
PCT	Primary Care Trust
PDP	Personal Development Plan
Public health	The science and art of improving the population's health through the organised efforts of society (see introduction). Public health practice is the emphasis in this handbook, while public health may also be considered as a discipline or a social institution (see Last)
Public health practitioner	In this handbook, includes anyone working in the broad field of public health, neither defined by formal qualifications nor restricted to a professional group. (*The term 'public health professional' could be contradictory, as the traditional definition of professional implies unique control over an important core of knowledge*)
PubMed	A service of the National Library of Medicine, provides access to over 11 million citations from MEDLINE and additional life science journals. PubMed includes links to many sites providing full text articles and other related resources (www.ncbi.nlm.nih.gov/PubMed/, accessed 11 May 2001)
QALY	Quality-adjusted life year

RCT	Randomized controlled trial
Risk	The probability that a particular adverse event occurs during a stated period of time, or results from a particular challenge. It can never be reduced to zero
Screening	The systematic application of a test or inquiry, to identify individuals at sufficient risk of a specific disorder to benefit from further investigation or direct preventive action among persons who have not sought medical attention on account of symptoms of that disorder
SIDS	Sudden Infant Death Syndrome
SMR	Standardised mortality ratio (see Last)
Stakeholders	Persons or organizations with an interest that may affect the outcome of an activity. Responses to stakeholders may include collaboration, involvement, monitoring or defence
STD	Sexually transmitted disease
Surveillance	The ongoing, systematic collection, collation and analysis of data and the prompt dissemination of the resulting information to those who need to know so that an action can result
SWOT	(Analysis of) strengths, weaknesses, opportunities and threats
Target	A specific change, intended within a given time period (see chapter 3.2)
UNESCO	United Nations Economic, Social and Cultural Organization
UNICEF	United Nations Children's Fund
URL	Uniform resource locator (technical name for a Web address)
WHO	World Health Organization

Further resources

Burchfield RW (ed.) (1999). *Fowler's modern English usage*, (revised 3rd edn). Clarendon Press, Oxford.

Last JM (ed.) (2001). *A dictionary of epidemiology*, (4th edn). Oxford University Press, Oxford.

New Oxford dictionary of English (1998). Oxford University Press, Oxford.

World Health Organization. Health Promotion Glossary www.who.int/hpr/docs/glossary.pdf (accessed 12 September 2000).

When a word causes more confusion than clarity, it is time to stop using it.

Wittgenstein 1889–1951

Index